DREAMS, SLEEP, AND CONSCIOUSNESS

Dreams, Sleep, and Consciousness presents the first scientifically based explanation of how dreams, sleep, and consciousness interconnect since the beginning of the neuroimaging era. This groundbreaking book introduces a fully developed neurocognitive theory of dreaming that encompasses the development of dreaming in children and provides detailed quantitative findings demonstrating how dreams reveal personal concerns.

The book features two innovative theoretical frameworks. The new "adaptive inactivity theory of sleep" explains why the sleeping brain shows varying activation levels and how this enables dreaming. The "multistate hierarchical model of consciousness" explains both why consciousness occurs and how dreaming fits within this three-level theory. Key features include comprehensive coverage of dreaming during the sleep-onset process and detailed analysis of the waking/arousal process, revealing how rapidly consciousness returns despite morning grogginess—the optimal time for dream recall.

This essential resource targets undergraduate and postgraduate students in psychology, neuroscience, sleep medicine, and consciousness studies. It provides invaluable new ideas for researchers in sleep laboratories, clinicians specializing in sleep disorders, and neuroscientists investigating consciousness. The book also provides crucial insights for anyone interested in dream research, cognitive neuroscience, or sleep medicine.

G. William Domhoff is Distinguished Professor Emeritus and Research Professor at the University of California, Santa Cruz. Professor Domhoff has written five books on dreams: *The Mystique of Dreams* (1985), *Finding Meaning in Dreams* (1996), *The Scientific Study of Dreams* (2003), *The Emergence of Dreaming* (2018), and *The Neurocognitive Theory of Dreaming* (2022).

DREAMS, SLEEP, AND CONSCIOUSNESS

Interweaving the Neurocognitive Theory of Dreaming with New Theories of Sleep and Consciousness

G. William Domhoff

Routledge
Taylor & Francis Group
NEW YORK AND LONDON

Designed cover image: Getty Images

First published 2026
by Routledge
605 Third Avenue, New York, NY 10158

and by Routledge
4 Park Square, Milton Park, Abingdon, Oxon, OX14 4RN

Routledge is an imprint of the Taylor & Francis Group, an informa business

ISBN: 9781041225690 (hbk)
ISBN: 9781041225621 (pbk)
ISBN: 9781003732969 (ebk)

DOI: 10.4324/9781003732969

Typeset in Sabon
by Newgen Publishing UK

CONTENTS

ABOUT THE AUTHOR

G. William Domhoff is Distinguished Professor Emeritus and Research Professor at the University of California, Santa Cruz. He received his B.A. in psychology from Duke University in 1958, his M.A. in psychology from Kent State University in 1959, and his Ph.D. in psychology from the University of Miami in 1962. He then became an assistant professor of psychology at California State University in Los Angeles in 1962. He next joined the faculty at the University of California, Santa Cruz, when the campus opened in July, 1965, where he is affiliated with both the Department of Psychology and the Department of Sociology. He was promoted to distinguished professor in 1993 and retired from teaching at the end of the Spring Quarter in 2019. He was at various times a visiting professor at the University of California, Santa Barbara, the University of Paris 8 Vincennes Saint-Denis, and Colgate University.

Professor Domhoff has written five books on dreams: *The Mystique of Dreams* (1985), *Finding Meaning in Dreams* (1996), *The Scientific Study of Dreams* (2003), *The Emergence of Dreaming* (2018), and *The Neurocognitive Theory of Dreaming* (2022).

He is also the author or co-author of 17 books in the field of political sociology, including *Who Rules America?* (1967–2023); *The Higher Circles* (1970); *The Bohemian Grove and Other Retreats* (1974); *The Powers That Be* (1979); *The Power Elite and the State* (1990); *State Autonomy or Class Dominance?* (1996); *Class and Power in the New Deal* (2011, with Michael J. Webber); *Diversity in the Power Elite* (2018, with Richard L. Zweigenhaft); and *The Corporate Rich and the Power Elite in the Twentieth Century* (2020).

ACKNOWLEDGMENTS

As with my other books over the past 30 years, I am indebted to my research assistant, Adam Schneider, who created the many tables and graphics that appear in the book and also carried out new research for one of the chapters on dream content. I also relied on his editing suggestions.

I am very grateful to Darren M. Lipnicki, a cognitive neuroscientist at the Centre for Healthy Brain Ageing at the University of New South Wales, who does work on dementia and Alzheimer's, as well as dream research. He was kind enough to read the whole manuscript in detail, and to make innumerable valuable suggestions on issues large and small, and thereby greatly improved the accuracy and readability of the manuscript.

I heartily thank dream researcher Tony Zadra at the University of Montréal for his careful reading of the chapter on dream recall, and for taking the time for a long telephone conversation in which he provided me with new ideas and angles on several vexing issues related to dream recall. I also extend my thanks to psychologist Benjamin Storm, an expert on memory and forgetting at the University of California, Santa Cruz, for his many insights and comments on the issue of forgetting. I also thank memory researcher Bjorn Rasch of the University of Fribourg for comments on memory consolidation during NREM sleep that caused me to think further on some issues.

In addition, I am grateful to dream researcher Tore Nielsen at the University of Montréal for reading the chapter on sleep, and for expressing his doubts on several key issues. Dream researcher Patrick McNamara of Boston University read several relevant paragraphs on one of his areas of expertise (dreams during N2 sleep) and provided valuable advice on how to approach this difficult and unresolved topic.

I deeply thank researcher and lecturer Rob Cooper in the Medical Physics and Biomedical Engineering Department at the University of London for reading passages in three different chapters about a new neuroimaging technology that he led the way in developing. His corrections and reassurances concerning the likely usefulness of this technology for studying neurocognitive networks during mind-wandering and dreaming gave me the confidence to make the suggestions that are put forth in these three chapters.

I am also grateful to neuroimaging researcher Matt Dixon, currently a postdoctoral researcher at Stanford University, for his useful additions and clarifications related to issues raised in several fine articles that he wrote with his dissertation mentor, Kalina Christoff, and others, at the University of British Columbia. In addition, I thank Kalina Christoff for the reassuring feedback she gave me on my presentation of her views at various places in the book.

The most important influence on my views on sleep, Jerry Siegel, of the Semel Institute at the University of California, Los Angeles, has been a creative and indefatigable sleep researcher for over 50 years. I thank him for his colleagueship in patiently answering my endless questions about sleep over the past two decades, along with his more recent efforts to help me understand key aspects of his new adaptive inactivity theory of sleep. Similarly, I thank emotions and consciousness researcher Joseph LeDoux of New York University for responding to my questions in numerous emails over the past four years concerning his Multistate Hierarchical Model of Consciousness.

Finally, I am pleased to thank my longtime—now retired—sociology editor, Dean Birkenkamp, and my current sociology editor at Routledge, Mike Gibson, for sending the manuscript to Ceri McLardy, who is now the psychology publisher at Routledge, after many years as a cognitive and neurocognitive psychology editor.

I wrote this book without a contract so I would not feel any guilt if I did not finish it, or if it took a very different direction than I originally intended. I therefore feel relieved, elated, and lucky that Dean and Mike steered me to Ceri, who could not be a more ideal person for publishing a book such as this one, and I am grateful for her support.

1

AN INTRODUCTION TO THE THREE THEORIES UTILIZED IN THIS BOOK

The purpose of this book is to place an updated version of a recent theory of dreaming within the context of a new theory of sleep on the one side and a new theory of consciousness on the other. The three theories—the neurocognitive theory of dreaming, the adaptive inactivity theory of sleep, and the multistate hierarchical model of consciousness—were developed separately and independently by three psychologically trained empirical researchers on the basis of three very different research literatures. All three theories reached their current formulations between 2019 and 2023 (Domhoff, 2022, 2023; LeDoux, 2019, 2020a; Siegel, 2022b, 2022d).

The discussion of the three theories in this introductory chapter, along with an indication of how they can be interwoven, attempts to provide readers with a sense of the issues and questions that animate the following nine chapters. In addition, the chapter provides a first look at the methods and systematic findings that will be used in the effort to answer the questions that will arise for readers as they examine the various aspects of each of the three theories. Put another way, the many issues that are left unanswered in this chapter will be addressed in succeeding chapters.

Before turning to the overviews of the three theories and how they can be related to each other, it should be added that the book makes every attempt to use replicated findings that derive from studies with large sample sizes and clearly defined and established means of analyzing the data. There is also a preference for concepts and conclusions that are based on the use of two or more different methods. Finally, it should be emphasized that this book provides a synthesis of the three separate theories, so it is of necessity selective in dealing with the wide range of theories and the growing bodies of literature that exist in all three fields of studies that it draws upon.

DOI: 10.4324/9781003732969-1

The Neurocognitive Theory of Dreaming

The neurocognitive theory of dreaming was developed on the basis of neuroimaging studies of the sleeping brain in the late 1990s, as well as new research on the impact of brain lesions on dreaming (Domhoff, 2000b, 2003, Chapter 1). In particular, it focused on the periods of "Rapid Eye Movement" (REM) sleep that occur four to six times in the course of a night's sleep, along with "the conceptual system of schemata and scripts" that "generates the process of dreaming" (Domhoff, 2003, p. 9). It also had a developmental dimension from the outset and a focus on quantitative studies of dream reports that were collected in both laboratory and non-laboratory settings (e.g., Foulkes, 1982; Hall, 1966b; Hall et al., 1982; Hall & Van de Castle, 1966).

The theory was later updated on the basis of a growing wave of waking neuroimaging studies, a meta-analysis of neuroimaging studies of REM sleep, and further quantitative studies of dream content (Domhoff, 2022). The neurocognitive theory of dreaming now suggests that dreaming is based on the cognitive process of "simulation," defined as "a particular kind or subset of thinking, which involves imaginatively placing oneself in a hypothetical scenario and exploring possible outcomes" (Schacter et al., 2008, p. 42). Simulations also can be defined as "imaginative constructions of hypothetical events or scenarios" (Buckner et al., 2008, p. 20). In fact, these definitions sound like they were created with dreaming in mind.

The defining feature of dreaming is therefore the sense of being a participant in, or an observer of, an unfolding series of events. These simulated events often take place in vivid sensory environments and almost always include other humans and/or animals (Domhoff, 2022, p. 8, for this definition of dreaming.). Then, too, dreaming is sometimes thought of as an actual experience for a few seconds after awakening, even while at least partially realizing that it didn't "really" happen.

Given this unique sense of what a dream is like, it is therefore not a dream if a participant in a sleep-dream laboratory study reports seeing an image of her mother after an awakening by the experimenter. This image most likely occurred during "Non-REM 3" (N3) sleep, which is also called "slow-wave sleep." It is also a different kind of mental experience if a participant reports thinking about a conversation with his sister or brother during the previous one or two days. This type of report is sometimes made after an awakening from "Non-REM 2" (N2) sleep, which is a more activated stage of sleep than N3 sleep.

And it is still another experience—a dream—for a participant to report after an awakening from REM sleep, when the brain is sometimes even more activated than it is during waking, that she was standing in her family's backyard, discussing a sporting event with her father, while he was building a small shed. To further complicate matters, that hypothetical dream might have been experienced during N2 sleep in the 1.5–2.5 hours before the morning awakening, when brain activation levels are gradually increasing to wake-like levels.

Dream researchers therefore have been aware since the early 1960s that it is important to phrase their questions to the participants in their studies in ways that make clear that they "want to know about the extent and quality" of the participants' "mental experience during the period of sleep preceding the awakening" (Rechtschaffen et al., 1963, p. 409). They therefore use phrases such as "what were you experiencing just before I called you" and "was there anything going through your mind just before I called you?" (Foulkes & Vogel, 1965, p. 232; Rechtschaffen & Foulkes, 1965, p. 1151). It is through this type of open-ended approach that dream researchers learned that the participants sometimes are seeing a static image of a person or object, or thinking about a discussion that occurred during the previous day or two. They also learned that most participants in effect define what they had been experiencing as a "dream" if the experience included visual, auditory, or kinesthetic imagery, or if they felt as if they were in a different physical setting than they were actually in at the time they reported the dream (Foulkes, 1962, p. 17).

As the examples in the preceding paragraphs make clear, the neurocognitive theory of dreaming leads to the conclusion that it is not useful to define dreaming as simply any form of mental activity that occurs during sleep. This is because several different forms of cognitive activity occur during sleep (Kamiya, 1961, for a detailed account of the various forms of cognitive activities during sleep, and especially for a summary on pp. 168–170; Pagel et al., 2001, for the several different definitions of dreaming). In addition, there are still other forms of cognitive activity that can occur during brief arousals from sleep and in various atypical events during sleep. They include such frightening events as "night terrors" and "sleep paralysis," both of which can become confused with dreams (e.g. Avidan, 2017; Domhoff, 2022, pp. 6–8, for a brief summary of the various non-dream types of experiences during the night; Iranzo, 2022; Yale Medicine, 2024).

Then, too, people suffering from severe insomnia have atypical activation patterns during sleep (Kay et al., 2016). In some cases, people insist they are awake, even though EEG (electroencephalogram) studies suggest they are asleep (e.g., Aquino et al., 2024; Bressera et al., 2025; Kay et al., 2016, for overviews of different types of insomnia). Still other studies make clear that post-traumatic stress disorder (PTSD) patients, who suffer from frequent nightmares, have expanded activation networks during sleep (Domhoff, 2022, pp. 47, 237 for a summary of past findings; Ebdlahad et al., 2013; Germain et al., 2013; Mysliwiec et al., 2014; Simor et al., 2013). The nighttime events mentioned in this and the previous paragraph are discussed in Chapter 9.

All of these different cognitive activities and events during a person's nighttime in bed—some of which occur while they are asleep, some while they are awake for a few seconds to several minutes—have to be set to one side for the time being to develop a plausible theory of dreaming. That is, it is first of all necessary to develop a "foundational" theory of dreaming, which involves a full focus on "understanding core processes" in everyday non-patient populations (Ochsner & Kosslyn, 2014b, p. 482). Only then is it possible to develop "translational" models that can be applied to one or another atypical kind of dreaming.

The interweaving of the neurocognitive theory of dreaming with the adaptive inactivity theory of sleep and the multistate hierarchical model of consciousness in this book provides an opportunity to strengthen the theory by demonstrating its compatibility with what is known about both sleep and waking consciousness. This interweaving makes it possible to show how the neurocognitive network that gives rise to dreaming comes to be ascendant over the waking multistate consciousness network as the sleep-onset process unfolds. The neurocognitive network that supports dreaming is also ascendant during the periodic REM periods, and often during the N2 sleep that occurs most frequently during the 1.5–2.5 hours before the spontaneous morning awakening. (During slow-wave N3 sleep, which occurs most frequently in the middle of the night, no neurocognitive network is connected enough to generate more than static imagery or an isolated thought, according to the neurocognitive theory of dreaming.)

In addition, the neurocognitive theory of dreaming is strengthened by research on the "arousal networks" that make it possible for a rapid return to self-aware consciousness during the spontaneous morning awakening. These studies also show that there is a slower return to full alertness, which helps to explain why this groggy period of drifting waking thought often leads to dream recall. These very useful findings, along with studies of brain lesions that lead to the loss of consciousness, are discussed in Chapter 8.

The interweaving of the neurocognitive theory of dreaming with the new theory of sleep and the new theory of consciousness also makes it possible for the neurocognitive theory of dreaming to explain how dreaming relates to waking consciousness. Looked at from the perspective of waking consciousness, dreaming can be understood as an intensified form of mind-wandering, imagining, and daydreaming that does not include the component of self-awareness. This conclusion brings dreaming closer to what is known about waking human thought than was possible in the past. This comparison of dreaming with waking consciousness is presented in Chapter 9.

The Adaptive Inactivity Theory of Sleep

The adaptive inactivity theory of sleep provides an excellent nighttime context for the neurocognitive theory of dreaming. First and foremost, this theory can explain the varying causes of brain activation during sleep, which provide the necessary support for the neurocognitive network that produces dreaming. To begin with, it can explain the activation levels and functional connectivity among neural substrates that make the neurocognitive process of dreaming possible in the 4–6 REM periods that occur each night. Second, it can also explain the activation levels and functional connectivity that make dreaming possible at various times during the sleep-onset process, and in N2 sleep in the approximately 1.5–2.5 hours before spontaneous morning awakenings.

In addition, it is consistent with the discovery that the sleep cycle in humans living in indigenous societies without electricity is linked to the ambient temperature cycle, not to the light–dark cycle, as it is in other known diurnal primates. Similarly, it can explain why humans in indigenous societies without electricity sleep for nearly an hour longer in the cold winter months than they do in the warm summer months.

According to the adaptive inactivity theory, sleep first of all can be understood as one instance of a more general strategy of energy conservation that is pervasive in the long evolutionary histories of both plants and the earliest animals, well before mammals and birds first appeared (Siegel, 2022b, 2022d). By characterizing adaptive inactivity in terms of reduced metabolism and decreased energy consumption, the theory places the phenomenon of sleep in the context of issues that are essential to all life forms—the acquisition, use, and conservation of energy.

Also, the theory can explain why there is a periodic occurrence during sleep of the highly activated form of sleep called REM sleep, for which there is as yet no generally accepted adaptive function. The evolutionary explanation for REM sleep suggested by the adaptive inactivity theory of sleep—the restoration of a waking-level brain temperature that keeps the brain at adequate activation levels for waking functioning—is based on comparative, lesion, and experimental studies that are discussed in Chapter 6. It is parsimonious and plausible within the context of currently available evidence.

At the same time, the adaptive inactivity theory is fully compatible with the various cellular-level adaptive processes that occur during sleep in many, but not all, mammals. According to the adaptive inactivity theory, these other adaptive processes were added to sleep later in the evolutionary history of mammals. Moreover, there is no evidence that any of these other adaptive theories of sleep can explain the activation patterns that support dreaming during the sleep-onset process and NREM 2 sleep late in the sleep period, as well as during REM sleep.

Further, the adaptive inactivity theory of sleep is the only adaptive theory of sleep that systematically addresses the large variations in sleep duration among mammals, which range from about 20 hours a day in one species of bats to as little as 2.1 hours per day in African bush elephants, and to little or no sleep at all in at least some species of dolphins and porpoises. It can also explain the relatively short sleep periods (5.7–7.1 hours) and the aforementioned seasonal variations in the amount of sleep that are experienced by humans living in two indigenous hunting-gathering societies in the southern half of Africa, and one indigenous hunting-horticultural society in the southern half of South America. The theory presents evidence and analysis to suggest that sleep duration is shaped by the energy-acquisition, predator-avoidance, and temperature-maintenance strategies that are necessary for survival within a specific ecological niche.

Drawing upon the adaptive inactivity theory of sleep, dreaming during the sleep-onset process can be explained by the brain temperatures that remain at or near waking levels during these few transitional minutes. Thanks to the theory's emphasis on REM sleep as a brain-heating mechanism, it can explain dreaming during REM periods on the basis of the elevated temperatures and high activation levels in specific brain areas, which occur about every 90 minutes during the course of the sleep period and together account for about 20%–25% of total human sleep time. Finally, the theory can explain the dreaming that occurs during N2 sleep in the 1.5–2.5 hours before a spontaneous morning awakening. It does so on the basis of the built-in, 24-hour pattern of circadian rhythms, which gradually raise brain temperatures in preparation for spontaneous morning awakenings.

The adaptive inactivity theory of sleep also makes it possible to explain why there is little or no dreaming during N3 sleep. This low-activation, slow-wave stage of sleep cannot sustain the functional connectivity among the relevant neural substrates that is necessary for the neurocognitive process of dreaming to occur. This emphasis on lower brain temperatures in N3 sleep, which occupies about 35%–40% of total sleep time in humans, also makes it possible to explain the reports of static imagery or isolated thoughts after N3 awakenings in the middle of the night.

The adaptive inactivity theory is discussed in detail in Chapter 6 and used to understand several unique features of human sleep at the outset of Chapter 7.

The Multistate Hierarchical Model of Consciousness

Just as the adaptive inactivity theory of sleep provides an excellent nighttime basis for the neurocognitive theory of dreaming, the multistate hierarchical model of consciousness provides an ideal theoretical framework for explaining how dreaming relates to self-reflective, self-knowing *waking* consciousness (LeDoux, 2019, 2020a).This theory is based on a further extension of a "higher-order" theory of consciousness that was developed by several colleagues (Brown et al., 2019, Lau & Rosenthal, 2011, LeDoux, 2017, #3331; LeDoux & Lau, 2020; LeDoux et al., 2020, for empirical evidence developed by psychologists and neuroscientists that supports a "higher -order" approach).

The higher-order network has the capacity to carry out the self-reflective thought that makes self-knowing consciousness possible. In making these claims, the theory draws specifically upon the emphasis on "one kind of consciousness (autonoetic) that characterizes the workings of one kind of memory (episodic)," as stated by memory theorist Endel Tulving (2005, p. 5). The theory thereby focuses on exactly the kind of self-aware, self-reflective consciousness that is of relevance in distinguishing between consciousness and dreaming. More specifically, the theory explains how it is possible for individual participants to reflect upon the fact that they are thinking specific thoughts about themselves. In addition, they can make verbal reports to researchers about these self-related thoughts, with "verbal self-report" serving as the most crucial evidence for "measuring conscious experiences" (LeDoux & Brown, 2017, p. E2017).

The multistate hierarchical model of consciousness consists, first, of lower-order sensory networks, which receive and then send forward new sensory information from both the external world and the body. This sensory information is then processed by the episodic, semantic, and schematic cognitive networks at the intermediate level. These intermediate-level networks then "re-represent" the newly updated and revised schemas and concepts to the higher-order network, which makes decisions based on the new information. Taken together, it is this multistate hierarchical model that explains self-reflective, self-knowing consciousness. An overview of the multistate hierarchical model is presented in Figure 1.1.

The multistate hierarchical model of consciousness encompasses the neurocognitive theory of dreaming within its intermediate level (Domhoff, 2023, for the initial statement of the relationship between the two theories). The intermediate level not only includes the memory networks and cognitive schemas mentioned in the previous paragraph. It also includes much of the self-system and the neural substrates that support simulation, imagination, mind-wandering, and daydreaming.

Within the context of the multistate hierarchical theory, the relative deactivation of the higher-order network throughout the sleep period immediately suggests that dreaming is not a form of autonoetic (self-knowing) consciousness. Instead, it is a form of fact-knowing ("noetic") consciousness, which relies on semantic memory, as discussed more fully in Chapter 9 as part of a comparison of dreaming and consciousness (Domhoff, 2023; see LeDoux & Lau, 2020, for a discussion of noetic and autonoetic memory; and Tulving, 2005, for an original statement of these ideas). The truncated nature of the neurocognitive network that supports dreaming, limited as it is to several of the neural substrates that support the intermediate networks, explains the relative absence of both external sensory in-puts in dreams and

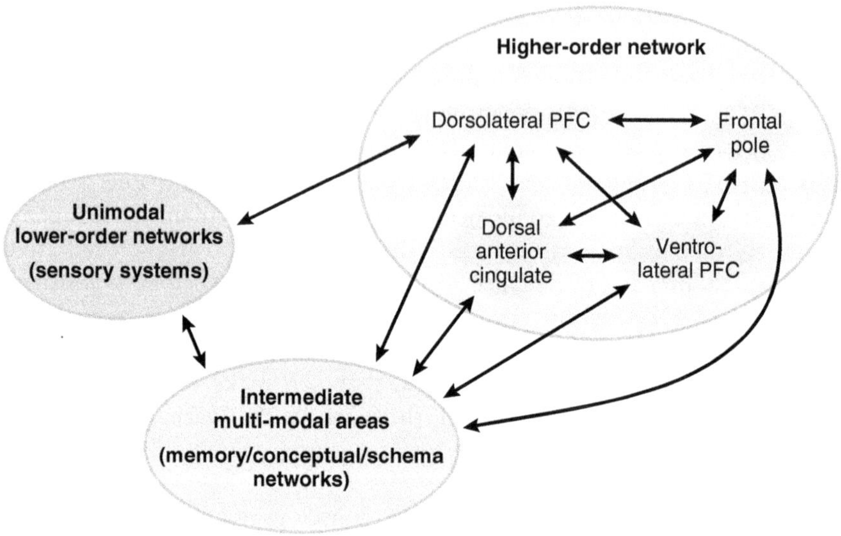

FIGURE 1.1 A schematic graphic of the relationships among the levels in the multistate hierarchical model of consciousness: The unimodal lower-order networks, the multi-modal intermediate areas, and the higher-order network.

Source: Adapted with permission from LeDoux (2020a).

the absence of reflective self-awareness concerning the dreamer's current state. It also explains several other cognitive deficiencies in dreaming, such as the absence or near absence of episodic memories and figurative thinking. These conclusions are supported on the basis of empirical studies that are discussed in Chapter 9.

This new context for the neurocognitive theory of dreaming is very useful because it makes possible more fine-grained comparisons of dreaming and consciousness. In particular, the strong emphasis on memory systems in the multistate hierarchical model contrasts with the perceptual emphasis that is found in several theories of consciousness (LeDoux & Lau, 2020, for a critique of perception-oriented theories of consciousness; Seth & Bayne, 2022, for a general comparison of theories of consciousness, in which several theorists concern themselves with visual perception).

Although the higher-order network is the final level that is necessary for consciousness to occur, it is also important to repeat that the neural substrates in the intermediate level are essential. This is because consciousness is the property of the overall network, which consists of many brain areas and subnetworks working together. Consciousness therefore is not possible unless the areas at the intermediate level are mature and intact. This point will become readily apparent in Chapter 8, in which the loss of consciousness due to specific lesions in areas at the intermediate level is discussed as part of the general emphasis on arousal networks in that chapter.

The Default Network as Building Block and Red Thread

With the neurocognitive theory of dreaming now situated between the adaptive inactivity theory of sleep on the one side and the multistate hierarchical model of consciousness on the other, the remainder of this introductory chapter provides further basic background information that relates to all three of the theories discussed above. It does so by focusing on the only waking neurocognitive network—the *default network*—that is in part activated at specific times during sleep. The default network is unique in that it is an essential part of the intermediate level in the multistate hierarchical model of consciousness and is also the primary basis for dreaming.

The default network was first discovered in the early 2000s and has been a source of increasing attention ever since (Gusnard et al., 2001; Gusnard & Raichle, 2001; Raichle et al., 2001). It consists of "multiple interacting subsystems," and the main neural substrates that support it are well established, but the full scope of the neural substrates that support the default network is a work in progress (Andrews-Hanna et al., 2014, pp. 33–35 for the quoted phrase and the updates between 2003 and 2014; Girn et al., 2024, for an analysis that expands the default network). Twenty years after its discovery, one of the pioneers in mapping the default network reported evidence that its discovery "has revolutionized our understanding of the workings of the human brain" (Menon, 2023, p. 2469).

The existence of the default network first came to the attention of dream researchers around 2005–2007 (e.g., Maquet et al., 2005; Pace-Schott, 2007, pp. 137–140). Its likely importance to dreaming was clear to an increasing number of dream researchers just a few years later (e.g., Domhoff, 2011; Eichenlaub et al., 2014; Fox et al., 2013; Hartmann, 2011). Still, the high probability that portions of the default network are essential in the understanding of dreaming and dream content has been only gradually and partially acknowledged by many dream researchers. In this book, though, the default network is a central building block in developing a better understanding of both dreaming and waking consciousness. It provides the red thread that runs throughout the rest of the book.

As noted earlier in the chapter, the neurocognitive theory of dreaming first of all builds upon neuroimaging studies of both the waking and sleeping brain. This combination of waking and sleeping neuroimaging studies makes it possible to delineate the neurocognitive network that engenders dreaming in considerable detail. Due to the discovery of the default network in the early 2000s, it is now possible to say that the neurocognitive network that supports dreaming is based on relatively activated neural substrates located in *portions* of the frontal medial and parietal regions of the brain that are part of the default network, along with *portions* of the sensory network and the sensorimotor network. (The somewhat cumbersome and awkward-sounding term—"relatively activated," along with its counterpart, "relatively deactivated"—is used in cognitive neuroscience to make clear that brain areas and neurocognitive networks do not turn "on" or "off" but instead are only more or less activated in terms of their relationships to each other.)

More specifically, the neurocognitive network that produces dreaming includes (1) several of the areas in two subsystems within the default network, which are called the *dorsomedial prefrontal cortex subsystem* and the *medial temporal cortex subsystem*; (2) the secondary visual cortex, which lies within the larger sensory network; and (3) a movement-supporting region within the sensorimotor network, called the caudate nucleus, which is involved in motor control, learning, and other functions in waking life. Figure 1.2 presents an

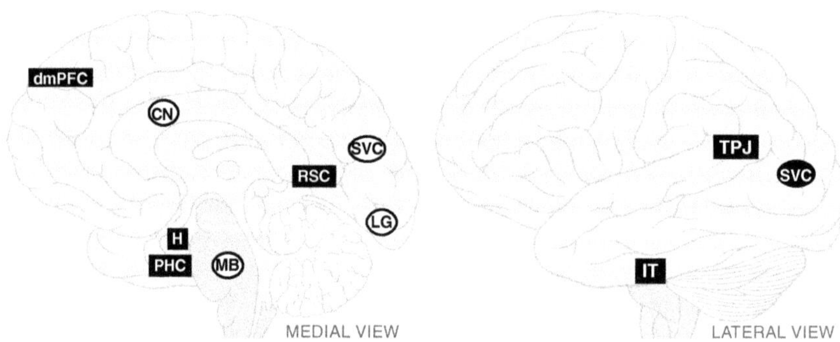

Substrates within the default mode network	Dorsomedial prefrontal cortex subsystem	• Dorsomedial prefrontal cortex	dmPFC
		• Inferior temporal cortex	IT
		• Temporoparietal junction	TPJ
	Medial temporal cortex subsystem	• Hippocampus	H
		• Parahippocampal cortex	PHC
		• Retrosplenial cortex	RSC
Substrates not in the default mode network	Occipital cortex	• Secondary visual cortex (V2-V5)	SVC
		• Lingual gyrus (visual processing)	LG
	Subcortical regions	• Caudate nucleus (movement)	CN
		• Pons/midbrain (arousal, activation)	MB

FIGURE 1.2 Several of the main neural substrates that subserve the neurocognitive process of dreaming.

Notes: For a more detailed account of the neural substrates that underlie dreaming, see Fox et al. (2013), Uitermarkt et al. (2020), and Domhoff (2022).

overview of several of the main neural substrates that give rise to dreaming whenever they are sufficiently activated to be functionally connected to each other and thereby constitute a neurocognitive network for dreaming. But it also has to be cautioned that the exact contours of the neurocognitive network that supports dreaming are not as yet fully established.

Further, it is important to add, as will be discussed in detail in Chapter 2, that this network only becomes fully ascendant if the higher-order network that directs waking thought—which is considered to be part of the *frontoparietal control network (FPCN)* in this book, for reasons that will be discussed below—has become relatively deactivated. This relative deactivation of the FPCN is accompanied by the relative deactivation of portions of the default network that link with the FPCN. These relative deactivations within the border regions of the default network are the final step in creating the isolation of the portions of the default network that make dreaming possible.

During directed waking thought, the various areas in the default network that support dreaming are entirely at the service of the several brain networks involved in perception and cognition. For example, areas in the default network have a major role in semantic memory schemas and conceptualizing, and still others support language and mental imagery (Bar, 2011; Moulton & Kosslyn, 2011). Neural regions within the default network also provide support for the "social brain," which is the cognitive system that makes possible the complex social relations that characterize human groups (Amft et al., 2015, p. 1031; Lieberman, 2013). Importantly, the neural substrates underlying the default network are also essential in supporting the self-system (Abraham, 2013; Levorson et al., 2025; Meyer & Lieberman, 2018; Tan et al., 2022). The default network's involvement in semantic memory, mental imagery, the social brain, and the self-system is highly relevant to the neurocognitive theory of dreaming because the cognitive capacities it supports are the basis for the quantitative findings on dream content that are discussed in Chapters 3 and 4.

However, when the FPCN is not fully focused on the many types of external and internal stimuli that arrive continuously every second of the day, the two subsystems in the default network mentioned above, the dorsomedial prefrontal cortex subsystem and the medial temporal cortex subsystem become relatively more activated in comparison to the externally oriented networks in the brain. It is at this point that mind-wandering and/or daydreaming may occur. The increased activation of the two subsystems of the default network at this time also has been shown to be relevant to dreaming by a waking neuroimaging study in which the participants were asked to think, first, about the person's present situation (called the "present self" condition), and then about personal situations that would arise in the future (the "future self" condition) (Andrews-Hanna, Reidler, Sepulcre, et al., 2010).

This experimental study found that the dorsomedial prefrontal cortex subsystem is preferentially activated when the participants were asked to think about their "present self"; on the other hand, the medial temporal cortex subsystem is preferentially activated when the participants are thinking about their "future self" (Andrews-Hanna, Reidler, Sepulcre, et al., 2010, pp. 554, 559). According to the neurocognitive theory of dreaming, portions of these two subsystems work together to produce dreaming when the FPCN is relatively deactivated (Domhoff, 2022, Chapter 2; Domhoff & Fox, 2015; Fox et al., 2013).

As discussed in the next subsection, the FPCN and the default network are not the only neurocognitive networks that are active during waking. Important though they are, they are only two of seven networks that are essential in providing a more complete description of perception and cognition.

The Seven-Network Framework for Analyzing Perception and Cognition

The neurocognitive theory of dreaming and the multistate hierarchical model of consciousness can be augmented and refined when they are encompassed within an empirically derived seven-network parcellation for analyzing perception and cognition. Framing the understanding of both dreaming and consciousness within the seven-network framework makes it possible to draw upon a wider literature in neurocognitive psychology. It also makes the neurocognitive theory of dreaming and the multistate hierarchical model of consciousness more accessible and familiar to a wider range of neurocognitive researchers. This framework was derived from neuroimaging data collected from 1000 participants, which is now available as part of the large Harvard Dataverse collection of brain scans (Buckner et al., 2014, on the Dataverse; Yeo et al., 2011, for the first full presentation of the seven-network parcellation).

The analysis further showed that many studies of perception and cognition can be organized and understood on the basis of the complex and constantly changing interactions among these seven basic networks. A number of studies using varying methods have reported a similar network structure (L. Fan et al., 2021; Gordon et al., 2016; Paquola et al., 2025; Power et al., 2011; Schaefer et al., 2018; Uddin et al., 2019; Yan et al., 2023; Yuan et al., 2024).

Five of the seven networks are nonlinear, nonhierarchical, and complexly intertwined "association" networks. They are based on neural substrates that are located in several different parts of the brain. These association networks are often identified as central points ("nodes") in the overall brain network because they are frequently part of the shortest pathways that link various brain regions (Bertolero et al., 2018; Bullmore & Sporns, 2009; Watts & Strogatz, 1998). The two sensory networks, on the other hand, are localized in specific brain regions and function in a linear and hierarchical fashion (Domhoff, 2022, pp. 16–22, for a detailed discussion of the network organization of the human brain in the context of the neurocognitive theory of dreaming). The names of these seven networks, and a brief characterization of each of them in terms of their roles in waking thought and perception, are provided in Table 1.1.

The primary function of the FPCN, which is briefly characterized in the first row of Table 1.1, is to synthesize the information that it receives from other brain networks and to make decisions and issue top-down commands on the basis of this information. It is also the basis for the sense of self-knowing (the sense that a person is having a certain thought)—which is, at the very least, a key element of consciousness, a topic that is discussed more fully in Chapter 9. More generally, the FPCN serves executive functions in relation to the other six networks and is often called the "executive network." In this book, it is shown to be the main basis for the higher-order network in the multistate hierarchical model of consciousness.

The conclusion that the FPCN is the main basis for the higher-order network first of all draws upon a large-scale synthesis of a wide range of studies, which suggests that areas within the FPCN are responsible for both

TABLE 1.1 The seven networks involved in perception and cognition

Network	*Organizational form*	*Main functions supported*
Frontoparietal control network (FPCN)	Associational, interweaved	Top-down control, hierarchical reasoning, executive regulation
Default network	Associational, interweaved	Internally focused, semantic memory, self-system, imagination
Salience/ventral network	Associational, interweaved	Attention-shifting, alerting
Dorsal attention network	Associational, interweaved	Focused thought, task-oriented
Limbic network	Associational, interweaved	Memory, reward, empathy
Visual network	Hierarchical, linear	Processes information on static and moving objects, spatial information
Sensorimotor network	Hierarchical, linear	Processes external physical stimuli and internal sensations

Notes: The associational networks are "small-world" networks, which are characterized by clustering, short paths between neurons, and a large general component (Bertolero et al., 2018; Bullmore & Sporns, 2009; Domhoff, 2022, p. 16 for a summary; Watts & Strogatz, 1998). The importance of small-world networks in understanding dream content in individual dream series is discussed in Chapter 4.

consciousness and directed thought (Levy, 2024). This synthesis leads to the conclusion that all of the "most recent theories underlying the concept of consciousness/awareness" rely on "a largely distributed network of brain regions in which the lateral prefrontal cortex plays an important role" (Levy, 2024, p. 797). Second, it concludes that "The way the involvement of the lateral prefrontal cortex in consciousness/awareness is usually described fully overlaps with what is required to achieve a goal-directed behavior" (Levy, 2024, p. 797).

In other words, the FPCN supports consciousness as well as directed thought and hierarchical reasoning, which are the building blocks for top-down commands. This synthesis then places the anterior regions of the prefrontal cortex, which are the final necessary regions that make human consciousness possible, squarely within the FPCN (Levy, 2024, pp. 797, 799, 806). Still other work discussed in Chapter 9 of this book is consistent with this conclusion and more fully explains why it is useful to place the higher-order network within the FPCN (e.g., Burgess et al., 2007; Christoff, 2014; Christoff & Gabrieli, 2000; Christoff et al., 2003; Dixon et al., 2014b, 2018; Henseler et al., 2011; LeDoux, 2019, pp. 256–257).

As will be detailed in Chapter 2, the FPCN has a very close working relationship with the second network characterized in Table 1.1, the default network, which is in turn an important part of the intermediate level in the multistate hierarchical model of consciousness (Andrews-Hanna et al., 2014, p. 31, Box 2, and pp. 34–35, for the ways in which the seven-network analysis augmented and reshaped prior understandings of the contours of the default network). And, as already noted above, and is reemphasized here, portions of the default network are central to the neurocognitive theory of dreaming because they provide the main basis for dreaming when the FPCN is relatively deactivated. In addition, and as also noted earlier, portions of the default network are essential to consciousness. Finally, the default network also has a role in the arousal process that underlies spontaneous awakenings from sleep, as will be discussed in Chapter 8.

The FPCN is importantly aided by two "attention networks," which help it maintain focus and attention on external tasks. The *dorsal attention network* and the *salience/ventral network*—which are listed in Table 1.1—also work closely with the FPCN in modulating the default network, as discussed in Chapter 2. The *limbic network*, which is the fifth and final of the association networks, contributes to many different processes, such as reward and memory, and also has a role in the creation of emotions, which are discussed in Chapter 9.

The Activation and Arousal Networks in the Brain

As the use of the word "activation" in several places in the first few pages of this chapter makes clear, the seven brain networks could not function without sufficient cortical activation. This activation derives from several interacting neurophysiological networks in subcortical areas of the brain. These networks have their starting point in the brainstem, an area at the base of the brain that is about the size of an adult human thumb. More exactly, the origins of the activation networks are located in the upper levels of the brainstem in two adjacent areas, the *pons* and the *midbrain.*

The neurochemical activation signals originating in the pons/midbrain, which are called "neurotransmitters," are sent ("propagated") to the basal forebrain and the hypothalamus. After receiving further input from the basal forebrain, the hypothalamus propagates its neurochemical information to the thalamus, which has many connections with cortical brain regions. Figure 1.3 provides an overview of the brain areas that constitute the "engine room" of the brain.

The brain areas depicted in Figure 1.3 are not only involved in brain activation during waking. They also are involved in the sleep-onset process and in the generation of REM periods during sleep. Further, these same small areas are essential to arousal from sleep, which leads to the almost instantaneous return to waking consciousness. (The sleep-onset process is discussed in Chapter 5, the REM-generation network is discussed in Chapter 6, and arousal from sleep, as mentioned above, is discussed in Chapter 8.)

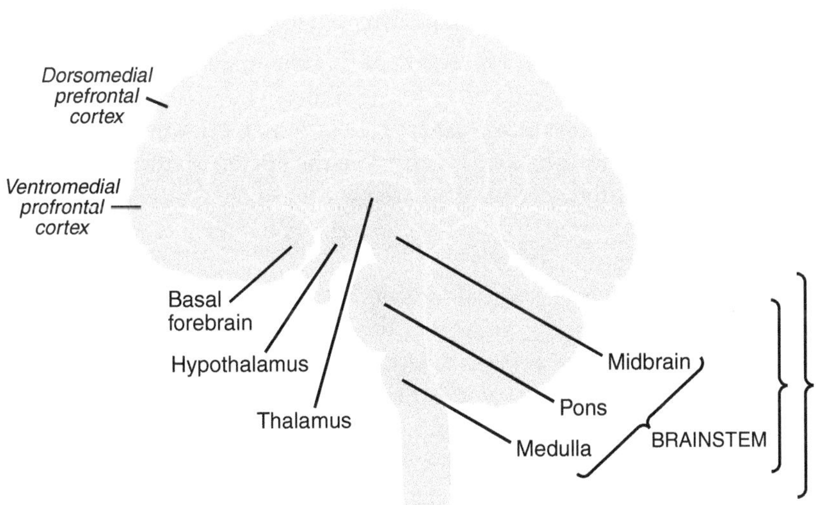

FIGURE 1.3 Six subcortical areas of the brain that are essential in brain activation and deactivation.

Note: Two cortical areas in the default network (in italics) are shown for perspective.

The Importance of Lesion Studies in Demonstrating Causality

Although the neurocognitive theory of dreaming relies heavily on neuroimaging research, it also makes use of studies of brain lesions, which can be caused by brain injuries, brain diseases, or surgical procedures. In effect, lesion studies based on accidents or brain diseases are similar to a series of accidental "experiments," in which the impacts of "focal" (small, circumscribed, narrowly focused) brain lesions in all parts of the brain are assessed. By asking patients if their lesions have led to any changes in their dreaming, these studies provide crucial first-person testimony with regard to the areas in the brain that are and are not necessary for normal adult dreaming. In the case of lesions created by surgical procedures, they are often meant to treat brain conditions such as seizures, which are usually caused by epilepsy. In the case of surgical lesions that are made for scientific purposes, they are carried out on non-human mammals after being approved by institutional review boards at universities or governmental agencies.

Not coincidentally, studies of both sleep and consciousness also make use of both experimental and accidental lesions. For example, experimental lesions in the lateral pons and lower midbrain in animal models lead to the complete loss of REM sleep. These studies thereby established that the small network in the upper brainstem, which was discussed above, is both necessary and sufficient for REM sleep to occur (Siegel, 2022c, pp. 68, 73). Accidental brain lesions in the brainstem and the default network, which can lead to "disorders of consciousness"—the clinical category for the various types of loss of consciousness, based on lesions in different brain regions—also have been important in studying foundational parts of the consciousness network. As noted in the previous section of this chapter, the impact of some of these lesions is discussed in Chapter 8 (e.g., Edlow et al., 2024; Fernández-Espejo et al., 2012; Laureys et al., 2005; J. Li et al., 2021; Vanhaudenhuyse et al., 2011; Vogt & Laureys, 2005). Lesions in the FPCN, on the other hand, usually lead to more subtle defects in consciousness, such as attention deficits and deficiencies in planning, for reasons stated in Chapter 9 (LeDoux et al., 2020, p. 255; Odegaard et al., 2017).

In the case of dreaming, lesion studies first of all provide independent support for the neuroimaging findings concerning the neural substrates that support the neurocognitive process of dreaming. These studies also provide causal evidence that portions of the default network are both necessary and sufficient to produce dreaming in adolescents and adults when there is (1) a relative deactivation of the other six brain networks; (2) an occlusion of external stimuli; and (3) a sufficient level of brain activation. Similarly, lesion studies can provide causal evidence that lesions in specific areas in the secondary visual cortex are necessary for visual imagery to occur during dreaming. Lesions in these areas also can have specific causal effects

TABLE 1.2 A few of the regions of the brain needed and not needed for dreaming

Region of brain	*Neurocognitive network*	*Effect on dreaming of lesions in this area*
Ventromedial prefrontal cortex	Default network	Loss of dreaming
Temporoparietal junction	Default network	Loss of dreaming
Medial occipitotemporal cortex	Sensory network	Distortion or loss of visual imagery
Primary visual cortex	Sensory network	No impact
Dorsolateral prefrontal cortex	Frontoparietal control network	No impact

on particular aspects of visual imagery, such as the loss of the ability to recognize faces.

Stated very generally, accidental, medical, and experimental studies show that lesions in areas that provide support for the neurocognitive network that generates dreaming lead to the loss of dreaming, or to the alteration of dreaming. This is direct causal evidence for the importance of these regions for dreaming. On the other hand, focal lesions in any brain area outside of this neurocognitive network do not have any impact on the continuance of dreaming. These findings are of major significance. They provide direct causal evidence that "experimental" lesions outside the neurocognitive network that supports dreaming, whether due to accidents or diseases, do not alter this network. Table 1.2 provides an overview of the location of a few of the lesions that do and do not impact dreaming.

More generally, the neurocognitive theory of dreaming, by drawing upon both neuroimaging studies and lesion studies, claims that dreaming, like consciousness, is a property of a specific neurocognitive network. If that network is not intact, dreaming is defective in some way or does not occur at all. The use of both neuroimaging and lesion studies can also be understood in methodological terms as providing "convergent validity," in which two very different methodologies lead to the same result (Cronbach & Meehl, 1955, for one early statement of this important methodological approach in psychology).

Studies of the Development of Dreaming in Children and Adolescents

In addition to neuroimaging and lesion studies, the neurocognitive theory of dreaming also draws upon maturational studies of the default network, laboratory studies of the development of dreaming, and studies of the development of waking cognition in children from preschool through middle school. These studies separately and unexpectedly discovered that (1) the

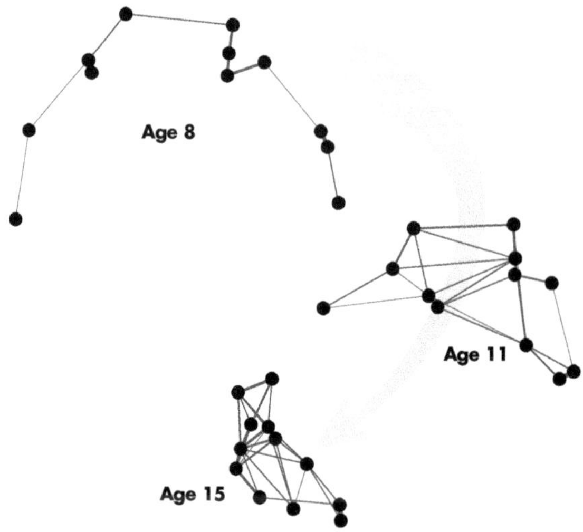

age	dream content
3–5	Dreaming is very rare if not non-existent; static imagery; very short
5–7	Social interactions occur, but dreamer is often not in the action
7–9	Dreamer more often has a central role in the dream; longer reports
9–11	Dreams adult-like in frequency and complexity
13–15	Dreaming becomes more adult-like in content as well as complexity

FIGURE 1.4 Maturation of connectivity in the default network from ages 8 to 15.

Note: The networks become "smaller" at each age in this fictive configuration in order to depict the increasing functional connectivity within the default network.

Source: Adapted from Fair et al. (2009), under CC BY license.

default network does not reach an adult-like maturational level until ages 9–11 and (2) that dreaming is a gradual cognitive achievement that is not adult-like in frequency and complexity until that same age period (Domhoff, 2022, Chapters 6 and 7). Figure 1.4 provides a graphic overview of the changes in the default network from ages 8 through 15, and the table below the illustration presents an overview of the gradual development of dreaming.

Moreover, waking developmental studies by cognitively oriented psychological scientists show that children do not fully demonstrate "abstract, psychological self-knowledge" until ages 9–11 (Ross et al., 2024, p. 12). More generally, the cognitive capacities that support mental imagery, imagination, and simulation are not adult-like until late childhood. The importance of the maturation of the default network and the development of various cognitive capacities to the development of both dreaming and waking consciousness are discussed in Chapter 9.

Taken together with the neuroimaging and lesion studies discussed above, these studies of children provide further evidence of convergent validity for the neurocognitive theory of dreaming by adding a third independent method that leads to the same results. This triangulation of three separate methodologies—each with different strengths and weaknesses—further strengthens the overall analysis because they all lead to the same results (e.g., Webb et al., 1966/1981/2000, for one of the classic formulations of this "triangulation approach" to hypothesis testing).

Using Expectations about Dream Content to Test the Neurocognitive Theory of Dreaming

To test expectations about the likely nature of dream content that derive from the neurocognitive theory of dreaming, this book makes use of systematic findings on dream content that are based on quantitative content analyses of many thousands of dream reports collected in both laboratory and non-laboratory settings (e.g., Domhoff, 1996, 2022, Chapters 3 and 4; Hall & Van de Castle, 1966). These replicated findings on dream content make it possible to examine, for example, the extent to which the dreamer's current and ongoing personal concerns appear in dreams, and the degree to which the dreamer's waking social networks are reproduced in dreams. These results are discussed in Chapters 3 and 4.

In addition, the findings on dream content can be combined with more recent neuroimaging, lesion, and developmental discoveries to explain why dreaming has no adaptive evolutionary function, which has been the consensus view among cognitively oriented dream researchers since the early 1990s (e.g., Antrobus, 1993; Blagrove, 1992, 1996; Foulkes, 1993). Instead, it seems more likely that dreaming is an evolutionary by-product of the rapid selection for increasingly complex social cognition, imagination, and an enhanced self-system over the past 70,000–250,000 years. All of these recent cognitive adaptations provided enormous adaptive advantages for a bipedal, tool-making hominid that lived in increasingly larger social networks in extensive wooded grasslands and later in even more challenging ecological contexts (e.g., Hallett et al., 2025; Hare, 2017, p. 166; Henn et al., 2011). These adaptations add up to an enlarged, rewired, and more densely connected set of brain regions that could, for the first time in mammalian history, bring together the past and the present to imagine alternative ways to think and behave in the future.

In this view, waking simulations are a cognitive process that allows people "to mentally 'try out' different ways that upcoming events might play out without engaging in actual behaviors," a process that is sometimes called "episodic simulations" or "episodic prospecting" (Spreng et al., 2018, p. 23). In addition, the various regions of the brain that are in good part responsible for these new waking capabilities, which are largely located in the default network, also facilitated far greater cooperation, collaboration, and collective innovative advances in material culture than were possible for earlier hominids (e.g., Hare, 2017; Hare & Woods, 2020; Wrangham, 2019). When placed within this larger context, dreaming has an honorable lineage as a result of being a by-product of these important evolutionary adaptations.

In drawing these conclusions, however, it is also essential to note that the adaptive functions supported by the default network also involve interactions between the default network and the FPCN, as explained in Chapter 9. Thus, the waking adaptive evolutionary value of the default network does not necessarily carry over to the portions of the default network that are active during dreaming, as shown by discussions of the inadequacies of all adaptive theories of dreaming at various points in Chapters 2 and 10. That said, the dreaming brain often dramatizes waking personal concerns, as demonstrated in Chapters 3 and 4, such as ongoing grievances with family members and acquaintances. Dreams therefore have psychological meaning even though the process of dreaming is an evolutionary by-product.

Although dreaming does not appear to have any evolutionarily adaptive value, an impressive array of anthropological and historical studies carried out in several different parts of the world over the past 165–170 years nonetheless reveal that the puzzling and sometimes frightening nature of dreams has led humans to create both collective and personal uses for dreams. People in an extensive range of indigenous societies concluded that dreams are part of another world, a world in which a person's wandering soul meets other wandering souls. Dreaming thereby becomes one basis for believing in an afterlife, and also a basis for religion, for healing ceremonies, and for foretelling the future (e.g., Benjamin, 2014; Bulkeley, 2008; D'Andrade, 1961; Gregor, 1981b; LaBarre, 1972; Tylor, 1871/1958). Dreams are also used by some artists, poets, novelists, and many others as a basis for creative work or for a greater understanding of themselves (e.g., Barrett, 2001; Blagrove et al., 2019; Edwards et al., 2013; Epel & Nichols, 1993; Townley, 1998).

Conclusion

In addition to supporting the neurocognitive theory of dreaming, the robustness of the similar findings that result from these three very different methodologies—neuroimaging studies, lesion studies, and developmental studies—creates doubts about several theories of dreaming that were developed in the pre-neuroimaging era. To begin with, these three sets of findings, when joined with quantitative studies of dream content, refute clinical theories of dreaming, which blossomed in the first half of the 20th century (e.g., Freudian and Jungian theory). This point is discussed in more detail, with regard to Freudian theory as the prototype, in Chapter 10.

The new findings also create doubts about the post-1960s, neurophysiologically oriented theories that rely on the neural substrates that support REM sleep as their sole or primary basis. These REM-oriented neurophysiological theories tend to downplay or ignore neurocognitive networks and to doubt or ignore the psychological meaning that can be found in dream reports. The implications of systematic findings on dreaming and dream content for REM-oriented theories are discussed in Chapter 10.

Finally, the findings on dreaming and dream content that support a neurocognitive theory of dreaming also lead to grave doubts about theories claiming that waking activities and the events of the day are the stuff of dream content. Their emphasis on the incorporation of waking activities as the basis for dream content rests on the implicit assumption that the cognitive processes that are available during dreaming are by and large similar to those that operate during waking. This wake-state bias thereby downplays the imaginative nature of dreaming and ignores or minimizes the limitations on cognitive functioning during dreaming (Windt, 2015, pp. 9, 200, 309–310, 500, for the concept of a wake-state bias). The incorporation theory is discussed briefly in a later section of Chapter 4 and then analyzed more fully in Chapter 10.

Having presented overviews of the three theories, the methodologies used in studying them, and a glimpse of the empirical evidence that supports them now completed, it is possible to turn to more detailed discussions of the many claims that have been made in this chapter. This journey begins with an empirically based discussion of the contours of the unique neurocognitive network that supports dreaming. The claim of uniqueness for this network has important implications.

2

THE UNIQUE NEUROCOGNITIVE NETWORK THAT MAKES DREAMING POSSIBLE

This chapter demonstrates that a unique functional brain network gives rise to dreaming. The discovery of this functional neurocognitive network unfolded over a period of several years. Strikingly, the research that led to this discovery was initiated and largely carried out by neuroscientists who had not previously been involved in the study of dreams. With regard to the importance assigned to the default network in this book, it is also noteworthy that one of the researchers who was involved in this work from the outset calls the discovery of the default network "serendipitous" (Buckner, 2012).

In addition to delineating and explaining the neurocognitive network that generates dreaming, the chapter emphasizes that this network can become relatively ascendant only if the frontoparietal control network (FPCN) has reduced its tight control of the default network. Put another way, the FPCN and the default network work in tandem, but the FPCN is always "in charge," except during the sleep-onset process and sleep itself. Their relationship is discussed in a later section of the chapter.

The conclusion to this chapter draws two important implications from the nature of this unique neurocognitive network, both of which provide further support for the neurocognitive theory of dreaming. First, the uniqueness of the network outlined in this chapter means that dreaming cannot be usefully compared to seemingly similar states, such as hallucinations, neurosis, psychosis, drug states, meditation, or hypnosis. Each of those states is now known to be supported by its own unique neurocognitive network, and all of those different neurocognitive networks are more similar to each other than they are to the neurocognitive network that supports dreaming. Second, several of the findings presented in this chapter raise difficult questions for several hypotheses concerning the possible adaptive function of dreaming.

DOI: 10.4324/9781003732969-2

Visual Imagery and Dreaming

The dorsomedial and medial temporal subsystems of the default network are the essential components of the neurocognitive network that produces dreaming, as stressed in Chapter 1 and demonstrated fully in later sections of this chapter. However, the chapter nonetheless begins with a three-part analysis of the network of secondary visual cortices that is responsible for the visual imagery in dreams. This starting point is due to the fact that visual imagery has been studied for many more decades than other parts of the neurocognitive network that produces dreaming. It therefore provides an indication of what might be possible in the future in terms of understanding the neurocognitive network for dreaming as a whole.

Scientific studies of the visual system began over 400 years ago, and visual imagery more specifically has been studied since 1879 (Yellout, 2007). And, as might be expected, based on the importance of vision and visual imagery in waking life, the mental imagery during dreaming is overwhelmingly visual (Kerr, 1993; Zadra et al., 1998). By way of contrast, auditory imagery appears in only half of all dream reports, and olfactory, gustatory, and tactual imagery appear in less than 2%–3% of the dream reports from sighted people in large-scale studies of both lab and non-lab dream reports (Snyder, 1970; Zadra et al., 1998).)

Moreover, the relative absence, or complete absence, of visual imagery during dreaming in some people provides further useful information, as discussed below. Taken together, these two sources of information first of all show that visual perception and visual imagery are based on different networks. As a result, there are people with good eyesight who lack the cognitive ability to create visual imagery, including preschool children. There are also people who have visual imagery but cannot see.

To start with, a waking neuroimaging study of six male participants, ages 19–27, who were asked to carry out both perceptual and visual imagery tasks while their brains were being scanned, demonstrated that the primary visual cortex is not part of the neural network that supports visual imagery (Kosslyn et al., 1997, pp. 327, 331–332). Consistent with these waking-state findings, neuroimaging studies have determined that the primary visual cortex is relatively deactivated throughout sleep, including rapid eye movement (REM) sleep, whereas the visual imagery network is active during REM sleep, a stage of sleep from which dreams are reported after 80%–85% of laboratory awakenings (Braun et al., 1998; Maquet, 2000; Maquet et al., 1996).

Thus, both waking and sleeping neuroimaging studies reveal that there are essential differences between the neural networks that support visual perception on the one hand and visual imagery on the other. The two networks share some neural substrates, but they are not one and the same network.

It therefore follows that the visual imagery that appears during dreaming cannot be considered to be "visual perception." As demonstrated below, this conclusion is further supported by lesion studies, developmental studies of visual imagery, developmental studies of dreaming in young children, studies of blind dreamers, and studies of the eye movements that occur during REM sleep. These different types of studies provide evidence of convergent validity for this conclusion and enhance confidence in neuroimaging studies relevant to dreaming.

Lesion Studies Provide Replications and a Form of Convergent Validity on Visual Imagery

Although the results from neuroimaging studies of the differences between perception and visual imagery are impressive in and of themselves, it is essential to add that these findings have been supported by a very different methodology with a long and honored role in the development of neurology and the neurosciences.

The first and most important study of a sighted person, who by definition had an intact visual perceptual system, but who lacked visual imagery during waking as well as during dreaming, was carried out in a sleep-dream laboratory in the late 1970s (Kerr et al., 1978). The study concerned a 21-year-old woman who suffered from Turner syndrome, which arises from a chromosomal defect that occurs in some women. This chromosomal defect sometimes damages regions in the neurocognitive network that generates visual imagery.

In addition to taking several waking tests that assess the ability to create visual imagery, the participant was also awakened 14 times during REM and twice during the sleep-onset process over the space of four nights in a sleep-dream laboratory and asked to report her dreams. The participant recalled dreams after most of these awakenings and reported the complex interactions that went on in them—including with a man unknown to her, who surprisingly said he loved her—but in no instance was there any visual imagery (Kerr et al., 1978, pp. 250, 255).

A few years later, the same research team also studied a patient with brain lesions that limited him to static visual imagery. He, too, was given a series of waking tests of visual imagery and then studied in the sleep-dream lab by means of REM awakenings, which confirmed his lack of normal visual imagery in dreaming (Kerr & Foulkes, 1981). These two well-controlled laboratory studies augment the neuroimaging studies that revealed the different networks that support visual perception and visual imagery.

The findings from these two studies were later confirmed in a large-scale, systematic study of the retention, alteration, or loss of dreaming in 361 people who were not mental patients. Nor had they been subjected to any neurological procedure before they arrived at a neurology clinic in Cape Town between 1985 and 1989. Instead, they came to the clinic because they had been in accidents that caused neurological injuries, or else had developed neurological symptoms that led them to seek treatment.

Before being fully examined and having CAT scans of their brains—this study was carried out in the pre-neuroimaging era—the patients were asked if their dreaming had been affected in any way by their new medical problems. Most did not report any changes in their dreaming, which is very useful information that will be discussed in a more relevant context later in the chapter. Further, most of those who did report changes in their dreaming did not mention any changes in visual imagery, which is equally useful information that will be discussed later in the chapter. However, two of the patients reported changes in the visual aspects of their dreaming. Their visual defects were consistent with the sleep-dream laboratory studies discussed above.

In particular, one of these patients had static visual imagery based on neurological lesions that was "strikingly reminiscent" of the static imagery of the participant in the earlier-mentioned laboratory study, who had static visual imagery during both waking and dreaming (Kerr & Foulkes, 1981; Solms, 1997, p. 105). The neuropsychologist who studied the 361 walk-in patients also found further support for the findings concerning defects in visual imagery in dreaming in 13 cases in the neurology literature that went back to the 1880s. Some of these patients experienced the complete loss of visual imagery during dreaming. Others had specific lesions that led to unusual impairments in visual imagery during both waking and dreaming, including static visual imagery and the loss of facial imagery (Solms, 1997, Chapters 2 and 3).

This large-scale lesion study also supported the fact that the visual perception network is separate from the visual imagery network by identifying 38 patients who had suffered lesions in primary visual areas and lost their ability to perceive movement in waking life. Despite this waking visual perceptual disability, these 38 patients nonetheless continued to experience visual imagery of movement in dreams, as determined by questioning the patients about this specific issue (Solms, 1997, p. 125).

The Gradual Development of Visual Imagery in Children

The findings from adult neuroimaging studies and adult lesion studies are further supported in a canonical developmental study that included 24 participants (half were female, half were male) in each of four groups (preschool children, ages 4 years, 5 months to 6 years, 3 months); elementary school children, 7 years, 8 months to 9 years, 3 months; teenagers, ages 13–15; and adults, ages 18–57). Since it is the youngest group that is the most important in relation to studies of the development of visual imagery in dreaming, it is relevant to point out that this preschool group, ages 4–6, was recruited from private schools in Cambridge, MA, the home of Harvard and MIT. It therefore seems very likely that these children were from families that wanted to provide their children with every possible opportunity to develop their cognitive abilities (Kosslyn et al., 1990, p. 997).

Nevertheless, the children ages 4 years, 5 months to 6 years, 3 months are described as "relatively poor" at generating, scanning, and rotating objects using visual imagery, although they were found to be "relatively good at maintaining images" once they generated these images (Kosslyn et al., 1990, p. 995). To provide one useful example, this youngest group took twice as long as the 8-year-olds in generating a simple visual image (9.4 vs. 4.5 seconds). Moreover, even though the children in the second age group (ages 7 years, 8 months to 9 years, 3 months) could generate a visual image twice as fast as the preschool children, they took twice as much time as the 14-year-olds, and even the 14-year-olds did a little less well than the adults (Kosslyn et al., 1990, p. 1000, Figure 1, from which the comparison percentages were estimated). One of these large differences, which concerned the time to develop a visual image of simple letters of the alphabet, such as the letter "C," is shown in Figure 2.1. The younger and older groups also differed widely on the visual imagery tasks of mental rotation and scanning, which are not included in Figure 2.1 (Kosslyn et al., 1990, pp. 1000, 1005, 1007, 1009).

Two other studies support these cross-sectional developmental findings. In the first study, 20 4-year-olds (mean age 4.8), 20 6-year-olds (mean age

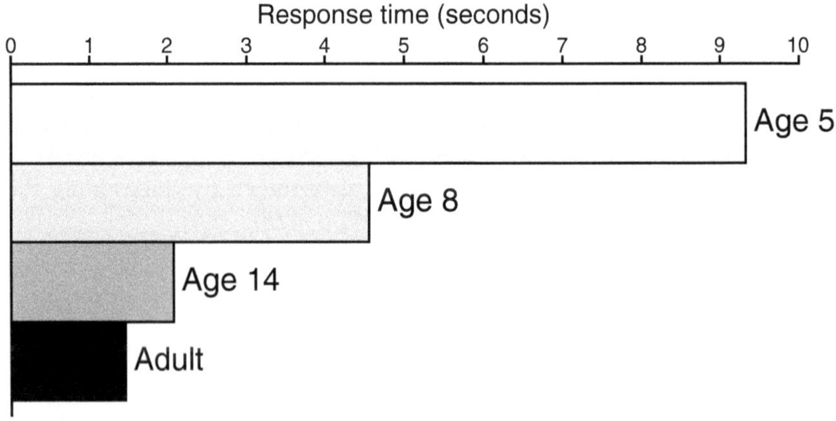

FIGURE 2.1 Preschool children take much longer to generate a simple visual image than do school-age children, teenagers, or adults.

Source: Based on information from Kosslyn et al. (1990, Figure 1).

6.6), and 20 young adults were compared on their ability to do a mental rotation task. The task involved comparing drawings of monkeys shown on a computer screen—one always upright, the other rotated to varying degrees—to determine if they were holding up the same or different arms in the various frames. Only 25% of the 4-year-olds and 33% of the 5-year-olds in the study were successful, compared to 75% of the 6-year-olds and 90% of the young adults (Estes, 1998, pp. 1349, 1353; Frick et al., 2013, p. 386). Smaller studies using slightly different methods came to similar conclusions (Childs & Polich, 1979; Dean et al., 1983; Kail et al., 1980). The few studies that claim otherwise (e.g., Marmor, 1975; Möhring & Frick, 2013; Quinn & Liben, 2014) could not be replicated using the same method the three dissenting studies used (Dean & Harvey, 1979), or else had methodological flaws (Frick et al., 2013; Frick et al., 2014, for critiques).

The conclusion that perception and visual imagery are based on slightly different networks is further supported by several studies of young children's proficiency in generating and rotating objects using visual imagery. For example, as part of a study of 80 children who were involved in a cross-sectional sleep-dream laboratory study, which is discussed below, only 10% of the 20 5-year-olds were able to carry out a mental rotation task. On the other hand, 75% of the 20 8-year-olds could do the task. The investigators concluded that "the possibility of kinematic [i.e., motion] imaging emerges somewhere between 5 and 8 years of age, rather than being generally well-developed in 5-year-olds" (Foulkes et al., 1989, p. 450).

Studies of Blind Dreamers Provide Further Evidence for the Importance of the Visual Imagery Network

The systematic waking-state findings on the development of visual imagery in children receive dramatic support from numerous studies concerning the presence or absence of visual imagery in the dreams of people who were born blind or became blind at differing ages in their childhoods (e.g., Hurovitz et al., 1999; Kerr, 1993; Kerr & Domhoff, 2004; Kerr et al., 1978, 1982; Kirtley, 1975; Meaidi et al., 2014). These studies can be considered analogous to clinical lesion cases in that they are based on accidents of nature or accidents that occur during life activities. They first of all show that there is an absence of visual imagery in the otherwise normal dreams of people who are born blind, or who lose their sight before age 4. On the other hand, people who become blind at age 7 or thereafter retain visual imagery in their dreams, although the percentage of their mental imagery that is visual gradually declines over the decades (Hurovitz et al., 1999, for the study with the largest database and a summary of past studies; Kirtley, 1975, for a full history of blindness studies).

Moreover, people who become blind after age 7 "continue to be able while awake to conjure up mental images of persons, objects, and events, and they continue to dream in imagery" (Foulkes, 1999, p. 15). This point includes waking and dreaming visual imagery of people they met *after* they became blind, which further supports the earlier claim in this chapter, based on both neuroimaging and lesion studies, that the human visual imagery network is not the same as the human visual perceptual system (Kerr, 1993, pp. 30–35). Put another way, if people who become blind after age 7 can imagine a person, they sometimes can create a visual image of that person during dreaming.

The importance of visual imagery in dreaming, and the absence of any visual perception during sleep, was further demonstrated from a highly original angle in a rigorous all-night electroencephalogram (EEG) study of 11 adult blind participants, using scalp electrodes pasted near their eyes (Christensen et al., 2019). Five of the participants were congenitally blind, and six were "late blind"; that is, they became blind between the ages of 8 and 40. These two types of blind participants were matched with a control group of 11 normally sighted participants.

The eye movements of the participants during REM sleep were recorded through the use of automatic detectors. The recordings were analyzed in terms of "eye-movement coverage," which was "computed as the percentage of eye movement time in each sleep stage" (Christensen et al., 2019, p. 1). The researchers first of all found that the congenitally blind and late-blind participants did not differ in their eye movement activity. The finding that the late blind also had the same amount and type of eye movements as the congenitally blind strongly suggests that these eye movements have a random stereotypic quality that does not relate to visual imagery during dreaming.

In addition, those participants who became blind after age 8 reported far more visual imagery in their morning reports than did the congenitally blind participants, according to an analysis of a morning questionnaire that all participants had filled out for a month before their two nights in the sleep-dream laboratory (Christensen et al., 2019, pp. 4–5). More specifically, the congenitally blind participants reported "very few or no visual dream elements," which is consistent with findings on imagery in past studies (Christensen et al., 2019, p. 5; Hurovitz et al., 1999). The authors conclude that their results do "not support the visual scanning of dreams hypothesis" (Christensen et al., 2019, p. 1). Instead, their results "suggest a 'dissociation' between eye movements and visual dream content in blind individuals" (Christensen et al., 2019, p. 1).

Systematic Lab Studies of REM Eye Movements Also Support Dissociation

Systematic lab studies focused on the nature of eye movements during waking and dreaming, along with a sleep-dream lab study that compared atypical eye movement patterns to dream content, support the idea that there is a dissociation between eye movements and visual dream content in sighted individuals as well as in blind dreamers. The physiologist who first discovered REM in 1953 (Aserinsky, 1996; Aserinsky & Kleitman, 1953) demonstrated the lack of any relationship between sleeping and waking eye movements in a further study in which he and his co-workers analyzed 192 rapid eye movements and 288 waking "saccades" (Aserinsky et al., 1985, p. 4). ("Saccades" is the technical term for the eye movements that occur during waking when the eyes move quickly to focus on a new "fixation" point in the environment.)

A comparison of saccades with the rapid eye movements during REM sleep is essential in terms of assessing the scanning hypothesis of dreams. Simply put, the scanning hypothesis states that the darting, seemingly random, eye movements during REM sleep are saccades, or very much like saccades. However, the detailed study under discussion here demonstrated that rapid eye movements are significantly slower than their waking counterparts and differ in their amplitude as well. The slowdown was not due to either eye closure or to the surrounding darkness (Aserinsky et al., 1985, p. 1). This conclusion was further supported by the measurement and analysis of 700 additional eye movements during various waking situations. The authors conclude their detailed study, and their exhaustive review of the highly technical literature on saccades, by wondering why rapid eye movements "behave so differently if they are simply the unmodified motor concomitant of visual imagery in dreaming" (Aserinsky et al., 1985, p. 9). An earlier trio of experts who specialize in eye function came to the same conclusion (Jacobs et al., 1970, 1972).

The fact that rapid eye movements are not related to visual imagery during dreaming also has been demonstrated in a sleep-dream laboratory experiment based on four participants, three women and one man. They were awakened by the first of the two experimenters 75 times over the space of 15 nights each to report "what they were experiencing" just before the awakening occurred immediately after a series of highly unusual eye movements. The four highly atypical eye movement patterns were (1) "predominantly horizontal"; (2) "predominantly vertical"; (3) "alternately horizontal and vertical"; and (4) "predominantly oblique" (Moskowitz & Berger, 1969, p. 613).

Then the second experimenter, who had been involved in ten published laboratory studies of eye movements during REM sleep in humans and rhesus monkeys between 1961 and 1969, attempted blind matching among various subsets of the data. However, he could not do better than chance using the binomial theorem as the test of statistical significance. Then he examined "each of nine reports" that contained "very clear descriptions of visual events," which "should have been associated with distinctive patterns of eye movement according to the 'scanning hypothesis'." Only three of the nine appeared to match correctly with the EOG (electrooculogram) records, and the others were "totally inappropriate to the dream events" (Moskowitz & Berger, 1969, p. 614).

For example, one of the "totally inappropriate" cases was the opposite of what would be expected if rapid eye movements are consistent with the content of the dream. The EOG record showed horizontal eye movements, but the participant reported that she was looking up and down at "vertical rows of buttons at a distance of about two feet" (Moskowitz & Berger, 1969, p. 614). This example provides a strong demonstration of why the occasional matches or near matches that inevitably occur by chance cannot be taken seriously within the context of statistically insignificant results. It shows in a dream-related way that the aforementioned study of 192 instances of rapid eye movements and 288 waking saccades is right in saying that waking eye movements are not at all like random bursts of eye movements during REM sleep (Aserinsky et al., 1985).

There is one final piece of evidence that refutes the idea that the eye movements during REM sleep relate to visual imagery during dreaming. As briefly noted in a subsection in Chapter 1, it was discovered in a five-year longitudinal laboratory study that the young participants had few or no dreams during their preschool years. But they did have adult-like rapid eye movements at this age, which led the researcher to make awakenings during "REM-bursts" in an unsuccessful attempt to maximize the chances of obtaining a dream (Foulkes, 1999, pp. 92–93).

At ages 5–7, however, these same 14 children did report dreams with visual imagery in them. This is because, recalling an earlier subsection of this chapter, children ages 5–7 are more proficient at generating visual imagery than they are before age 5 (e.g., Foulkes et al., 1989; Frick et al., 2013; Kosslyn et al., 1990). The fact that adult-like rapid eye movements are present in preschool children who seldom or never dream shows once again, this time from a developmental angle, that the random bursts of eye movements that occur during REM sleep have nothing to do with either visual imagery or dreaming.

The several different types of studies of visual imagery discussed in this section also reveal that the visual imagery that occurs during waking and dreaming is as similar as it could possibly be hoped for by neurocognitively oriented sleep-dream researchers. Thanks to the excellent and very detailed data on visual imagery that has accumulated over many decades, this conclusion demonstrates just how fully delineated the neurocognitive network that produces dreaming actually is. For a variety of reasons, the information on other parts of the neurocognitive network that generates dreaming is not yet as exact and detailed. But in principle there is every reason to believe that the full neurocognitive network that produces dreaming will be as well understood at some point in the future as the visual imagery portions of that network are understood right now.

The research on visual imagery also may point the way for future studies of the functioning of a subcortical area, the caudate nucleus, which is part of the neurocognitive network that creates dreaming. Little is known about the caudate nucleus in terms of its involvement in dreaming, except for the fact that it is very likely involved in creating kinetic (movement) imagery during dreaming, just as areas in the caudate nucleus are involved in the initiation of movement during waking. (The caudate nucleus has other functions as well during waking.)

Most of all, perhaps, the differentiation of visual imagery from visual perception during waking, and also from the random bursts of rapid eye movements during REM sleep, brings the neurocognitive network that produces dreaming into the realm of imagery and imagination. The neurocognitive theory of dreaming is thereby differentiated from the theory that claims dreaming is a direct reaction to REM sleep, which is discussed in Chapter 9.

The Frontoparietal Control Network and the Default Network during Waking

As stressed at the outset of this chapter, the relationship between the FPCN and the default network is critically important in understanding the nature of dreaming, as well as when dreaming occurs. This section therefore uses detailed waking-state studies of this relationship to provide the initial evidence for the essential point that the FPCN is relatively deactivated *and* the relevant portions of the default network are relatively activated during dreaming. More specifically, there is a negative correlation (an "anti-correlated relationship") between the FPCN and the neurocognitive network that gives rise to dreaming.

In making this assertion, it should be stressed that such negatively correlated relationships between neurocognitive networks are frequent and meaningful during waking life, too. Moreover, regions within the default network exhibit "the highest degree of cortex-wide negative connectivity" during waking (M. Li et al., 2021, p. 1). Thus, there is nothing atypical about finding an anti-correlated relationship between the FPCN and the neurocognitive network that produces dreaming.

During waking, the FPCN uses the lack of incoming sensory stimulation as the occasion to lighten its control on the default network's inclination to mind-wandering and daydreaming. On the other hand, the FPCN tightens its control of the default work whenever the two attention networks signal that it should focus its attention on incoming sensory information or directed waking thought. The close relationship between the FPCN and the default network during relaxed waking—"the resting state"—is evidenced first of all by a connectivity correlation of .70 between the two networks in a study of 38 participants. Among several clustering analyses carried out by these researchers, the study included an algorithm that produced seven networks that are similar to those found in the seven-network framework presented in Table 1.1 (Lee et al., 2012, p. 7; Yeo et al., 2011). Based on the seven-network analysis, the connectivity correlation between the FPCN and the default network was higher than any other connectivity correlation that was used (Lee et al., 2012, p. 2). On the other hand, the default network was negatively correlated with the dorsal attention network (–.74), the ventral/salience network (–.20), the sensory (visual) network (–.60), and the somatosensory network (–.82) during the resting state (Lee et al., 2012, p. 2).

The causal relationship between the FPCN and the default network is demonstrated in an experimental study that used transcranial magnetic stimulation to alter their relationship in two different ways. First, excitatory transcranial magnetic stimulation of the FPCN decreased its connectivity to the default network, as measured by changes in brain activity revealed by fMRI scans (Chen et al., 2013, p. 19944). This change is exactly what would be expected when the FPCN becomes more activated and ascendant. On the other hand, inhibitory stimulation of the FPCN increased the activation level of the default network. This latter change is highly relevant in terms of developing a neurocognitive theory of dreaming because the increase occurred "primarily within the medial prefrontal portion" of the default network, which is an area that is known to be important in supporting both mind-wandering and dreaming (Chen et al., 2013, p. 19944).

In keeping with these findings, still another study used a combination of fMRI and EEG technologies to study the relationship between the FPCN and the default network during relaxed waking thought and drowsiness. This combination of measurement methods makes it possible to detect rapid changes in neurocognitive networks because the EEG has excellent temporal resolution (in milliseconds), which complements the excellent spatial resolution of fMRI (Warbrick, 2022, for the advantages and disadvantages of simultaneous EEG and fMRI, and the many methodological complexities in combining them). Based on findings from the scans of ten young adults (six women, four men), the study first of all found that parts of the posterior cingulate cortex, an area within that default network that interfaces with attention networks, decouple from the dorsal attention network during mind-wandering (Chang et al., 2013).

This decoupling leads to a stronger negative correlation between the anterior portions of the default network and the dorsal attention network than any two of the several network combinations that the researchers compared (Chang et al., 2013, p. 230). In addition, the anterior regions of the default network become more connected with each other and more activated at the same time as the posterior cingulate cortex is decoupling from the dorsal attention network. This change is important because the dorsal attention network is involved in constraining the default network during focused waking thought.

To complete the picture, the decoupling of the posterior cingulate cortex from the dorsal attention network is accompanied by a simultaneous disconnection from regions in the posterior thalamus and a nearby area involved in attention shifts, the precuneus. (The precuneus, an area underlying the default network that is involved in supporting episodic memory and self-reflection during waking, does not figure prominently in this book because it is relatively deactivated throughout sleep.) These findings were conceptually replicated shortly thereafter in a waking neuroimaging study that used a different methodology to "confirm that the previously reported negative correlations between the dorsal attention and default networks are intrinsic to the brain and not the result of statistical manipulations" (Carbonell et al., 2014, p. 343).

The conclusions concerning the relative deactivation of the portions of the posterior cingulate cortex during REM sleep that interact with the dorsal attention network are supported in separate neuroimaging and high-density EEG studies. They, too, found a negative correlation between the relevant area in the posterior cingulate cortex and the medial prefrontal cortex (Chow et al., 2013, p. 10301, for the fMRI findings; Perogamvros et al., 2017, pp. 1769, 1772, for the high-density EEG findings).

These results are relevant to the neurocognitive theory of dreaming because they support earlier neuroimaging findings showing that both the FPCN and portions of the posterior cingulate cortex are also less active during REM sleep (Braun et al., 1997; Maquet et al., 1996). Put another way, these results provide part of the neurocognitive explanation for why the portions of the default network that give rise to imagination and dreaming are able to wander freely through the semantic memory network whenever they are activated during sleep. The rest of the explanation is based on the fact that the source of spontaneous cognition is located in a key area underlying the default network, the temporal lobe, as determined by electrical stimulation studies that made use of implanted electrodes in numerous epileptic patients (Curot et al., 2018, pp. 9–10; Domhoff, 2022, p. 32, for a summary; Fox, 2018, pp. 170, 173, for the most comprehensive findings).

In addition, the simultaneous disconnection from regions in the posterior thalamus mentioned above is also relevant from the perspective of the neurocognitive theory of dreaming. Areas in the posterior thalamus are part of the other waking attention network, the salience/ventral network, which interacts with the dorsal attention network in helping the FPCN to restrain the default network (e.g., Crawford, 2022). The salience/ventral network also has an extremely important alerting function—think Red Alert!—that is essential in preparing every organ in the body for immediate action in response to both internal and external danger signals (Chang et al., 2013; Di

& Biswal, 2015; Menon & Uddin, 2010; Seeley et al., 2007; Uddin, 2015). On the other hand, when the two attention networks are relatively deactivated, and the anterior regions of the default network have greater connectivity, the stage is set for either spontaneously generated mind-wandering during waking or dreaming during the activated portions of the sleep period.

More generally, the relationships among the dorsal attention network, the salience/ventral network, the thalamus, the posterior cingulate cortex, and anterior areas in the default network are at the nexus of several basic processes that will be discussed in this and later chapters. As discussed at the outset of Chapter 5, they are part of the transition process that begins when people gradually fall asleep. Then, too, as discussed at the outset of Chapter 8, they are integral to the arousal process when sleep ends. Finally, they are also relevant to understanding the nature of REM sleep, a topic that will be discussed a little later in this chapter and in Chapter 6. These brain areas thereby play a role in making both dreaming and consciousness possible.

EEG Correlates Provide Useful Electrophysiological Indicators of Dreaming

The increased functional connectivity and relative activation in the anterior areas of the default network, along with the relative deactivation of the dorsal attention network and the salience/ventral network, are most readily revealed by the changing frequencies of two EEG rhythms, the alpha rhythm and the theta rhythm. This finding is important because these two rhythms (which are also called "waveforms" and "brain waves") provide electrophysiological signals that can be used to infer the activation level of the default network (Chang et al., 2013, p. 227). That is, they serve as "indicators," which are also known as "biomarkers."

EEG waves can be faster or slower, as measured by an international standard for the frequency of periodic oscillations of sound and electrical waves per second ("hertz"). (This measure for frequency is also sometimes expressed as "cycles per second" ("cps").) Brain waves also differ in terms of their size or "amplitude" (i.e., the "height" of the wave), which is measured in microvolts. Table 2.1 includes a graphic of the two brain waves—the alpha wave and the theta wave—that often appear during relaxed waking thought, drowsiness, and/or dreaming. Several other brain waves that occur during sleep or waking will be discussed at the appropriate, more contextualized, moments when they appear in later chapters.

Alpha waves are mentioned frequently in this book because they often appear during relaxed waking thought and the sleep-onset process, or even on some occasions during sleep. As the alpha wave slows to its lower boundaries (7–9 Hz), it is usually replaced by theta waves (4–7 Hz), which

TABLE 2.1 Two EEG waveforms that relate to mind-wandering, drowsiness, and REM sleep

Name of pattern	*Frequency*	*Description*	*Illustration*
Alpha	8–13 Hz	Alpha waves are often present in drifting waking thought. They are also found in the sleep-onset process and sometimes in REM.	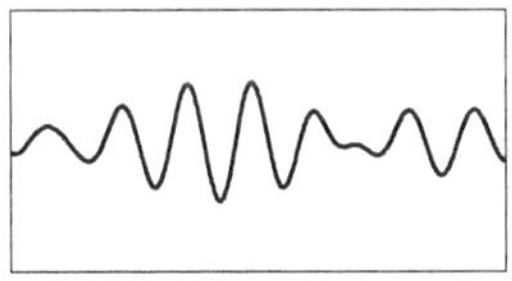
Theta	4–8 Hz	Theta waves are sometimes present in drifting waking thought, are present in the later half of the sleep-onset process, and are prominent in REM sleep.	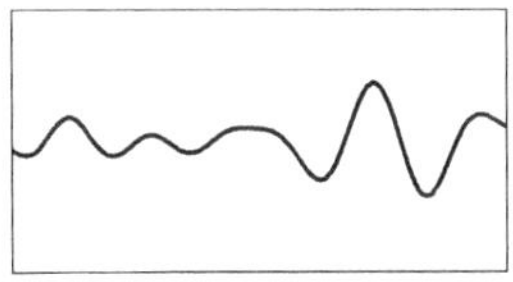

first appear during drowsiness. This finding is highly useful with regard to the neurocognitive theory of dreaming because "increased theta power was associated with increased functional connectivity between nodes of the default network, particularly within anterior regions," according to the analysis of drowsiness that was discussed previously (Chang et al., 2013, p. 230).

This finding supports the earlier conclusion that "frontal theta activity can be seen as an EEG index of default network activity" during the resting state (Scheeringa et al., 2008, p. 242). Theta waves also appear during REM sleep, a topic that is discussed in the next section of this chapter (Armitage, 1995). They also appear at later points in the sleep-onset process, when participants are most likely to report dreaming, as discussed in Chapter 5 (e.g., Badia et al., 1994; De Gennaro et al., 2004; Hori et al., 1994; Marzano et al., 2011; Vecchio et al., 2017). Theta waves may be the closest thing there is to an EEG indicator of dreaming, but they are far from perfect, especially when compared to the more detailed findings that neuroimaging studies provide.

Neuroimaging Studies of Dreaming During REM Sleep

The possibility that dreaming might have a more specific basis than "the brain" was first discovered in neuroimaging studies carried out in the late 1990s (Braun et al., 1997, 1998; Maquet, 2000; Maquet et al., 1996; Nofzinger et al., 1997). Although the results did not always agree exactly, they usually included the dorsomedial prefrontal cortex, the ventromedial prefrontal cortex, parts of the posterior cingulate cortex, and the hippocampus, the latter of which is the source of continuous theta waves during REM sleep.

Moreover, the general findings were confirmed in a meta-analysis that compared regions in the waking-state default network, which were determined by an examination of 18 resting-state neuroimaging studies of the default network, with six PET-scan studies of REM sleep (Fox et al., 2013, pp. 7–8). The study concluded that dreaming during REM sleep very likely "amplifies the same features that distinguish mind-wandering from goal-directed thought" (Fox et al., 2013, p. 1). As might be expected, the most activated areas during REM sleep were even more activated than they are in restful waking. They include areas in the medial prefrontal cortex, the inferior parietal cortex, and the medial temporal lobe (Fox et al., 2013, p. 6, Table 2).

The meta-analysis also confirmed that regions in the posterior cingulate cortex were relatively deactivated during REM sleep, which is consistent with the drowsiness findings reported in the previous section (Chang et al., 2013). At the same time, the region in the posterior cingulate cortex that lies next to the lingual gyrus, an important area in the generation of visual imagery, is relatively activated. Although other parts of the secondary visual cortices discussed in the previous section were not included in this meta-analysis, it did find that many areas involved in the high-level processing of visual imagery, such as the lingual gyrus and the parahippocampal region, are active during REM sleep (Fox et al., 2013, p. 9). In addition, two small areas in the upper brainstem, the pons and the midbrain, which were briefly mentioned in Chapter 1 as the source of the activation that makes REM sleep possible, were also shown to be more active in REM than N3 sleep.

The results of the meta-analysis were confirmed by an analysis that compared a resting-state neuroimaging study in which the participants were not sleep deprived with the findings from several neuroimaging studies of REM sleep (Uitermarkt et al., 2020). Its results are important because they show once again that sleep deprivation, which is necessary in helping participants in REM sleep studies to fall asleep within noisy neuroimaging scanners, did not alter the relevant aspects of REM sleep in the early PET-scan studies.

The use of the REM neuroimaging studies to examine the functional neurocognitive network that gives rise to dreaming does not imply that dreaming only occurs during REM sleep. Instead, the neuroimaging studies of REM sleep provide the best starting point because dreaming has been linked to REM sleep again and again in EEG-based sleep-dream laboratory studies since the 1950s (Dement, 1965, for an early summary; Nielsen, 2000, for a large-scale analysis of numerous studies since the early 1960s that led to similar findings on REM sleep).

As two later chapters demonstrate, the neurocognitive network that produces dreaming is also activated during the sleep-onset process and N2 sleep, although not as frequently or as evenly as it is during REM sleep. This point is relevant because it shows that the two key issues from a neurocognitive point of view are (1) brain activation levels and (2) the functional connectivity of the neurocognitive network that produces dreaming. In other words, dreaming cannot be reduced to or limited to REM sleep.

Lesion Studies Relating to Areas in the Default Network

As already shown in the section on visual imagery, lesion studies can provide strong convergent evidence for findings based on neuroimaging studies. This section further demonstrates this point by drawing upon several lesion studies, which show that the dorsomedial prefrontal subsystem of the default network is necessary for dreaming to occur. That is, if the neural substrates that support this subsystem are damaged, whether in its anterior or posterior regions, then people report that they no longer experience dreaming. And, as stressed in the Introductory chapter, these studies provide causal evidence that portions of the default network are necessary for dreaming to occur.

The first of these studies was a "natural experiment" in that the experimental group was created by someone other than the experimenter, which in this case means neurosurgeons, as explained shortly (APA, 2023, for this definition of a natural experiment). The researchers were also able to create a control group of participants who were very similar to the experimental group, except that they did not have any brain lesions (Jus, Jus, Villeneuve, et al., 1973). In addition, this section also discusses the loss of dreaming in two subsets of patients with lesions in two different regions within the default network, who were part of the same group of 361 neurological patients from which cases were drawn in the earlier section on visual imagery (Solms, 1997, Chapter 16). The section also includes two additional confirmatory case studies of the loss of dreaming from early in the 21st century (Bischof & Basset, 2004; Poza & Marti-Masso, 2006).

The natural experiment that provides the starting point for this section is the first and perhaps most systematic lesion evidence demonstrating that the dorsomedial prefrontal cortex subsystem is essential for dreaming. This well-controlled study was carried out 50 years ago in order to evaluate the frequent clinical observation that psychiatric patients on whom prefrontal lobotomies had been performed often reported the loss of dreaming for varying periods of time after the operation (Jus, Jus, Villeneuve, et al., 1973, p. 277; Solms, 1997, Chapter 5). At that time, of course, the researchers did not know that the patients they were studying had received an operation that directly impacted the dorsomedial prefrontal cortex subsystem.

The experimental group (n = 13, 12 of whom were men) consisted of hospitalized schizophrenics who had received a refined and more limited form of a prefrontal lobotomy, called bimedial leucotomy, 10–22 years previous to the sleep-dream study (Jus, Jus, Villeneuve, et al., 1973, p. 279;

Poppen, 1948, for the full details concerning the nature of the operation by the originator of this procedure). The control group also consisted of hospitalized schizophrenics, 12 men and one woman, who had not been treated with any surgical procedures. This control group was carefully matched with the experimental group for "age, sex, duration of illness, clinical symptomatology, and type of psychopharmacological treatment," and for scores on memory tests and intelligence tests (Jus, Jus, Villeneuve, et al., 1973, p. 279).

The surgical lesions were carried out as last-alternative options for consenting patients who felt constantly besieged by their symptoms, mostly recurrent thoughts, in the era before psychiatric medications provided a better treatment option. However, there were many negative outcomes using the first-generation methods of carrying out prefrontal lobotomies. It is therefore important to note in terms of assessing the value of the results in this study that the bimedial method used with these particular patients was found to be "superior in treatment of chronic mental illness to either conventional bilateral lobotomy or unilateral lobotomy," according to a study of the outcomes of all types of lobotomies over a nine-year period (Greenblatt & Solomon, 1952, p. 262).

This study further noted that bimedial leucotomy patients showed "dramatic" reductions in symptoms such as anxiety and impulsivity and were "more interested in interaction, more alive to group needs, more productive and organized in their activities than patients receiving the other operations" (Greenblatt & Solomon, 1952, p. 262). Still another study of 35 bimedial cases showed that 65% of them had shown "significant" improvement in a five-year follow-up study, with most of them living outside of a hospital setting (Paul et al., 1956, pp. 51–52). Similarly, a team of Canadian neurosurgeons concluded that this procedure was predominantly successful in relieving an ongoing state of "tortured self-concern" for 44 patients who were studied one to seven years after their bimedial procedures (Baker et al., 1970, p. 41).

Three dependent variables were examined—EEG records of the night's sleep, post-awakening verbal reports of sleep quality, and nighttime verbal reports of the presence or absence of dreaming after awakenings from each REM period over the course of two non-consecutive nights. The participants in both the experimental and the control group had normal, uninterrupted non-REM/REM EEG records, and the members of both groups reported after the morning awakening that they slept well. It therefore can be concluded with confidence that the participants in both the experimental and control groups had normal sleep, as evidenced by both the EEG records and the self-reports provided by the participants.

However, only one of the 13 participants in the experimental group reported a dream from 97 REM awakenings overall, and another three reported four instances in which they thought they might have been dreaming. (The fact that some participants in the experimental group might report dreams was anticipated on the basis of earlier clinical reports stating that some lobotomized patients later reported the recovery of dreaming.) In sharp contrast, 10 of the 13 participants in the control group reported at least one dream. In addition, one participant in the control group reported that he thought he had been dreaming after six of nine awakenings over the two-day period.

The study was then replicated with ten of the participants in the experimental group and ten of the participants in the control group. This time they were given reserpine, a medication that was thought at the time to enhance memory. The same large differences between the two groups were found (Jus, Jus, Gautier, et al., 1973).

Other Lesion Studies Support the Role of the Dorsomedial Prefrontal Cortex Subsystem in Dreaming

The results of the natural experiment and the follow-up replication study using a subset of the original participants are supported by several of the findings in the earlier-mentioned systematic study of 361 people who came to the neurology clinic in Cape Town. When asked if their dreaming had been affected in any way by their new medical problems, eight of the patients who said they had experienced the complete loss of dreaming had narrowly circumscribed (focal) lesions that impacted the same prefrontal brain regions that were severed by bimedial prefrontal leucotomies. In addition, two other patients with lesions in the same brain regions reported a large diminution in the frequency of dreaming (Solms, 1997, pp. 138, 145–146). These findings support the conclusion that lesions in anterior areas of the dorsomedial prefrontal cortex subsystem lead to the loss of dreaming.

Based on 45 other patients who reported the loss of dreaming, the study in Cape Town further discovered that focal lesions in and around the temporoparietal junction, which is also part of the dorsomedial prefrontal cortex subsystem, can lead to the loss of dreaming. The loss of dreaming in some of these cases proved to be for relatively short time periods, which lasted until the swelling caused by the lesion had dissipated. Overall, the researcher who did the study hypothesized that injuries to the temporoparietal junction might be sufficient to cause the loss of dreaming (Solms, 1997, pp. 141–145).

Two later case studies of individuals who had lost dreaming supported the hypothesis that lesions confined to the temporoparietal junction are sufficient to cause the long-term loss of dreaming (Bischof & Basset, 2004; Poza & Marti-Masso, 2006). This finding is of additional interest because this is the area that one group of high-density EEG researchers view as a "hot spot" in the brain that is central to both dreaming and consciousness (e.g., Boly et al., 2017; Perogamvros et al., 2017).

As already noted above, it is also necessary to examine the many areas of the brain in which lesions do *not* have any impact on dreaming, according to verbal reports by the patients. These patients in effect provide a control group that is essential in demonstrating the causality of the lesions inside the default network. Put another way, the first-person verbal reports by these patients eliminate these regions as potential candidates for inclusion in the dream-creation network.

First and foremost, the Cape Town study showed that a key underpinning of the FPCN, the dorsolateral prefrontal cortex, is not needed for dreaming. This conclusion is consistent with the neuroimaging findings revealing that the FPCN is negatively correlated during drowsiness and sleep with the portions of the default network that give rise to dreaming (e.g., Chang et al., 2013; Uitermarkt et al., 2020). Still another region, one that is sometimes claimed to be important to dreaming, the amygdala, which is involved in emotion, was found to be unnecessary for dreaming by the Cape Town researcher and his co-workers in a later study. Their findings are based on eight patients with Urbach–Wiethe disease, a genetic disorder that attacks the basolateral amygdala, an area that is involved in the creation of emotions during waking (Blake et al., 2019). All of the patients continued to dream.

The several independent lesion studies discussed in this subsection can be summarized with two generalizations. First, lesions within the dorsomedial prefrontal cortex subsystem lead to the loss of dreaming, sometimes permanently, sometimes temporarily, depending on the site of the lesion. The several studies that support this conclusion are consistent with the idea that the dorsomedial prefrontal cortex subsystem is necessary for dreaming. Second, based on studies of lesions *outside* the neural substrates that support dreaming, which have no impact on dreaming according to the patients' verbal reports, it can be concluded that these areas are not necessary for dreaming. These lesion findings—summarized in Figure 2.2—thereby provide direct causal evidence as to the relevance or irrelevance for any given neural substrate in supporting the neurocognitive network that gives rise to dreaming.

Although few or no focal lesion studies related to dreaming have been reported in the past several years, a study of 52 adults (16 women and 36 men), who had suffered traumatic brain injuries of varying severity, supports these findings. Using the Glasgow Coma Scale and the length of the patients' post-trauma amnesia as a starting point, and a follow-up questionnaire filled out by these patients about 4.2 years after their brain injury, the researchers found that patients who suffered severe brain traumas were much more likely to state that they "never dreamed" than were those who suffered milder brain traumas (Fisher-Hicks et al., 2025).

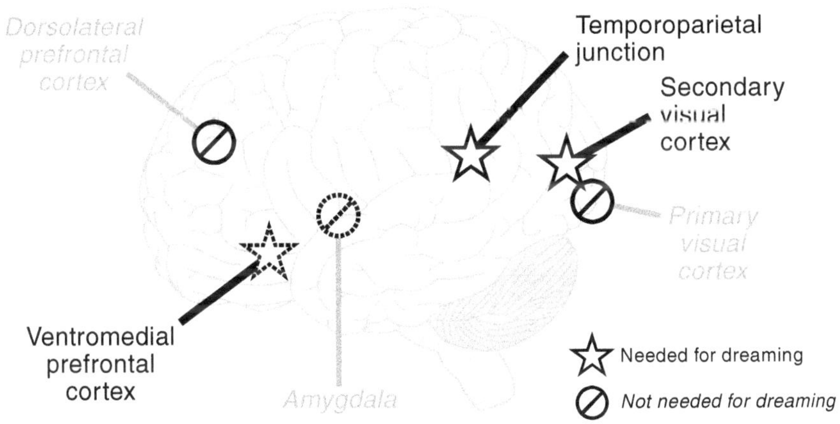

FIGURE 2.2 Brain regions needed and not needed for dreaming.

Notes: The dotted lines indicate that the ventromedial PFC and amygdala are located in the medial region of the brain, not on the lateral surface that is shown in this graphic. Five of the six brain areas included in this graphic are also the basis for Table 1.2.

Brain Maturation and Cognitive Development Are Necessary for Dreaming

The combination of neuroimaging and lesion studies of adults provides strong convergent evidence for the existence of a specific neurocognitive network that gives rise to dreaming. In this section the neuroimaging and lesion evidence is further supported by (1) studies of the gradual maturation of the default network, which demonstrate that it is not adult-like in its functional connectivity until ages 9–11, and not fully adult-like until ages 13–15; (2) waking studies showing that the development of complex cognitive skills, such as the ability to form concepts, make use of narrative thinking, and think imaginatively, occurs only gradually; and (3) studies demonstrating that children do not dream with adult-like frequency, length, and complexity until they are ages 9–11.

The Gradual Maturation of the Default Network

Although the basic outlines of the default network can be detected in infants and preschool children, most of its maturation occurs after the ages 4–7 (Bulgarelli et al., 2020; Gao et al., 2009; He et al., 2019). The importance of the elementary school years in the development of the default network was first discovered in a seminal cross-sectional study of the default network that spanned the ages from 7–9 to 19–31, with 66 participants at age 7–9, 54 participants ages 10–15, and 91 participants who ranged in age from 19 to 31 (Fair et al., 2008; Fair et al., 2009). The medial prefrontal cortex,

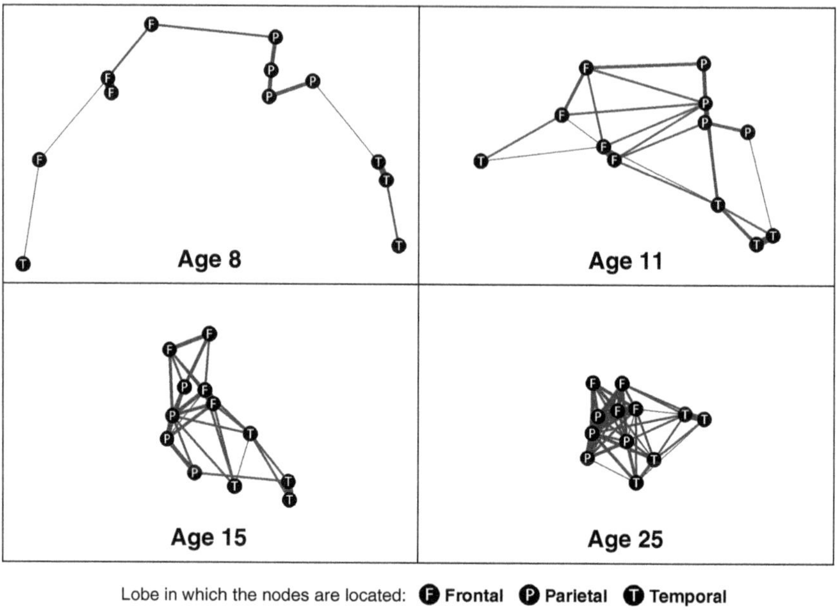

FIGURE 2.3 Maturation of connectivity in the default network from ages 8 to 25.

Source: Adapted from Fair et al. (2009), under CC BY license.

Notes: The networks become "smaller" at each age in this fictive configuration in order to depict the increasing functional connectivity within the default network. Also note that the neural substrates in the frontal and parietal lobes are only weakly connected at age 8 and that the neural substrates in the temporal lobe do not become well-connected with each other until age 15.

one of the default network's most central areas in adults, and an area that is involved in dreaming, was on the periphery of the network at ages 7–9 and only indirectly connected to the networks' parietal areas (Fair et al., 2009). Similarly, a study of social cognition between ages 6 and 12 concluded that the default network matures slowly during this age period (Moraczewski et al., 2020). Figure 2.3 provides a closer look of the maturation of the default network at ages 8, 11, 15, and 25 than was provided in the similar, but simpler, graphic in Chapter 1.

These results were replicated in cross-sectional studies in Brazil and China. The Brazilian study included 447 participants ages 7–15, who were drawn from a wider spectrum of socioeconomic backgrounds than in the U.S. study. Once again, the centrality of the major hub regions in the default network increased with age, and the connectivity of the anterior and posterior regions of the network increased (Sato et al., 2014, p. 93). The resting-state fMRI study in the China study was based on 305 children between the ages of 6–12, who were studied twice within the space of a year. The results by age

12 were similar to those from a control group of 61 young adults ages 18–28 (F. Fan et al., 2021). As in the Brazilian study, it was concluded that it is the functional connectivity between the anterior and posterior regions in the default network that notably increases over this time period.

The four cross-sectional studies mentioned above are also extended and supported in a longitudinal fMRI study that included 45 participants (24 girls, 21 boys), who were scanned at ages 10 and 13. The investigators first of all found that "by age 10, the basic functional architecture of the default mode network is in place" (Sherman et al., 2014, pp. 151, 154). However, they also stress that the integration between the medial prefrontal cortex and posterior cingulate cortex increased between 10 and 13, which is consistent with the findings in the cross-sectional studies (Sherman et al., 2014).

The longitudinal and cross-section findings presented in this subsection demonstrate that the default network matures only gradually. These results raise the question of whether or not dreaming is possible before the neurocognitive network that gives rise to dreaming is sufficiently mature. Before that question can be addressed, the adequacy of the cognitive capacities that most likely are involved in dreaming has to be examined.

The Gradual Development of Four Waking Cognitive Capacities Relevant to Dreaming

In addition to the capacity to create visual imagery, it is likely that four other cognitive capacities are necessary for dreaming as well. They are the ability to form concepts, make use of narrative thinking, think imaginatively, and create and make use of personal memories. These capacities, along with the capacity to generate visual imagery, are the most plausible basis for the process of "simulation." As noted in Chapter 1, simulation is essential in rethinking the past and making plans for the future, but simulation is also the basis for mind-wandering, daydreaming, and dreaming as well (Domhoff, 2018, Chapter 5, 2022, Chapter 6, for more detailed overviews, but also see the many original developmental studies cited in subsequent paragraphs).

The ability to form concepts, which is a building block for the neurocognitive theory of dreaming, develops late in an infant's first year of life from the gradually developed capacity to create "image schemas." These image schemas, which are initially largely perceptual, if not entirely, provide the "raw material for conceptual thought" (Reznick & Bauer, 2008, p. 255). The earliest-formed concepts are usually very global and inclusive, but more specific categories then develop from them between late infancy and 30 months and provide the foundation for much of later cognitive development (Gelman, 2013; Mandler, 2004, 2008, 2012; Rakison & Lawson, 2013). They become "the basis for understanding ordinary life experience (i.e., knowing) as well as understanding the meaning of words" (Nelson, 2011, p. 100).

These conceptual systems, in turn, are at the core of the semantic network, which is primarily located in areas in the default network and is essential to dreaming. The semantic network is also important to waking consciousness and develops throughout the preschool years and beyond, a topic that is discussed in Chapter 9 (Binder & Desai, 2011; Duff et al., 2020; Sridhar et al., 2023, for the location of the semantic network within regions of the default network).

Within the general context provided by the gradual development of semantic memory, the ability to think narratively develops between ages 3 and 5, and by age 5 or 6, many children can tell a brief story that contains a beginning, middle, and end (Reese, 2013, pp. 197–198; Taylor, 2013, p. 803). By age 7 children can make use of three of the eight basic elements that are necessary for a well-developed narrative, and by age 11 they can include six of these elements, with girls including more elements than boys at each age (Bauer et al., 2007).

Similarly, the ability to imagine events, which is defined as "the capacity to mentally transcend time, place, and/or circumstance to think about what might have been, plan and anticipate the future, create fictional worlds, and consider remote and close alternatives to actual experiences," develops between ages 3 and 5 (Taylor, 2013, p. 791). In terms of imaginative thinking as it manifests in playing, "pretend dramatic play is typically delayed until age 4 or 5 in preschool environments" (Nelson, 2007, p 170). After age 5, though, children have the ability to create play scenarios in which they assign roles to their various playmates, and they are able to take the perspective of others (Nelson, 2007, p. 171).

However, children ages 5–7 have difficulties in simulating past episodic events, and all children have difficulties in simulating imagined future events through age 11 (Coughlin et al., 2019). These conclusions are based on a large-scale study of American children at ages 5–7, 7–9, and 9–11, along with an adult control group (n = 157 overall). Even more relevant in terms of the neurocognitive theory of dreaming, the children and adults were also asked to provide narratives of a make-believe event, which children at age 5 had difficulties in doing. They improved considerably between ages 7 and 9. However, the children were not proficient in developing imaginative narratives until age 9–10. These conclusions are consistent with the findings in two different longitudinal sleep-dream laboratory studies, discussed in the next section, which reveal that children do not dream in an adult-like manner until ages 9–11.

The capacity to remember and make use of personal memories is the final necessary ingredient that is needed for simulation. This capacity to form personal memories develops as one aspect of the ability to form episodic memories –memories for specific events. The development of episodic memory in general, and of personal memories more specifically, is facilitated by conversations between caretakers and their children. In addition, it is important to note that episodic memory does not develop until the semantic network is established. These topics are discussed more fully in Chapter 9 as part of a comparison of the parallel development of consciousness and dreaming.

For now, it is enough to say that the personal memory system is not adequately developed until ages 5–7 and continues its development for several more years (Fivush, 2020; Nelson, 2007, 2014; Nelson & Fivush, 2020). Further, personal memories are an essential factor in the development of the self-memory system, a concept that is examined in Chapter 9 as part of the discussion of the parallel development of waking consciousness and dreaming (Conway et al., 2019; Gopnik, 2009; Ross et al., 2024).

Most generally, the findings on the development of cognitive capacities that are briefly overviewed in this subsection suggest that preschool and elementary school children may lack the cognitive abilities to dream in an adult-like fashion.

Dreaming in Children and Adolescents Ages 3–16

Based on both the gradual maturation of the default network and the continuing development of cognitive capacities between late infancy and ages 9–11, the neurocognitive theory of dreaming leads to the expectation that dreaming is lacking or underdeveloped in children until ages 9–11. Allowing as always for large individual differences, this possibility can be examined in great detail on the basis of two longitudinal studies, one for ages 3–9 and the other for ages 9–15, along with a cross-sectional study of 80 children ages 5, 6, 7, and 8. All three of these studies were carried out by the same investigator and his graduate student co-workers (Foulkes, 1982, 1999; Foulkes et al., 1990). The expectation that there should be dreaming at ages 9–11 also can be further examined on the basis of a separate five-year longitudinal study of 24 participants, 12 girls and 12 boys—at ages 9–11, 11–13, and 13–15. This latter study was carried out over a decade later by a different investigator and her co-workers (Strauch, 2004, 2005; Strauch & Lederbogen, 1999).

The need for a mature neurocognitive network for dreaming is first of all demonstrated in an unanticipated way by the findings at ages 3–5 in the first phase of the five-year study of 14 young children (7 girls and 7 boys). Great care was taken to assure that these preschool participants, only four of whom had ever attended a nursery school, would feel completely at ease in the sleep-dream laboratory. After the attachment of the necessary EEG electrodes was completed in the half-hour to an hour before bedtime, the participants explored the several rooms in the sleep-dream laboratory, played in a nearby playroom, or read books in bed before the lights were turned out. Sometimes the main investigator, who made all of the awakenings over the five-year period, read books to the children before the lights were turned out, so they were well-acquainted with him (Foulkes, 1982, pp. 26–32, for the procedures involved in the study).

The children's levels of anxiety and stress were monitored during the pre-bedtime period, and through their sleep patterns. The young participants were rated as calm or relaxed on 79% of the nights and as extremely anxious on only 5.4% of the nights. Their median time to fall asleep was 20 minutes, which was subsequently shown to be very similar to the time it took them to fall asleep at ages 5–7 and 7–9. Furthermore, they seldom awakened spontaneously once they were asleep (Foulkes, 1982, pp. 32–34).

Since the default network was not discovered until nearly two decades after the longitudinal study of dreams was completed, the results were not biased by any knowledge of this network. Nor is it likely that the investigator's preconceived expectations influenced his descriptive empirical findings. In fact, he candidly stated that the results with the children ages 3–5 were initially "quite disappointing" because "neither prior theory or observation had prepared us for the results we obtained" (Foulkes, 1982, p. 44).

The results that the investigator found disappointing concerned the unexpected absence or near absence of dream reports from most of the children. The relatively few reports (median recall 15%) did not include anything more than brief, fragmentary content. The reports ranged in length from only 2 to 50 words, even though these children had normal verbal skills and memories when tested during waking. The dream reports consisted primarily of static imagery that included only one or two characters at most, a large plurality of which were animals. In addition, the dream reports rarely if ever included the dreamer as a character, and there were few or no social interactions among the few characters who did appear in their dream reports (Foulkes, 1982, Chapter 3, 1999, pp. 159–163, for the dream reports of one of the best recallers in the study at ages 3–5, 5–7, and 7–9). The preschool children had the same phasic bursts of rapid eye movements that adults do, but they had only static imagery in their few brief dream reports. As discussed earlier in the chapter, this finding provided further negative evidence concerning the claim that these random and jerky eye movements track the unfolding dream scenario.

By ages 5–7, the same 14 children had a median recall rate of 31% and provided longer dream reports, which by then included more characters and social interactions. The dream reports frequently dramatized positive social interactions and far less frequently included any hostile or aggressive interactions, unlike the large plurality of adult dream reports that are discussed in Chapters 3 and 4. However, the dreamers themselves were not frequent or central characters in their dreams. It was not until ages 7–9, when their median recall rate rose to 43% and the reports were longer, that the children began to include themselves, along with other human characters, in their dream reports (Foulkes, 1982, p. 104). This shift was accompanied by a continuing decline in the percentage of their dream reports that included an animal character (Domhoff, 2018, Figure 4.1, for a graphic summary of the decline in the percentage of dreams with at least one animal character between ages 3–5 and 9–11, when the frequency reaches adult-like levels).

The results for the 14 children at ages 5–7 and 7–9 were replicated in a cross-sectional study of 80 children, all of whom were within a month of their fifth, sixth, seventh, or eighth birthday. The median recall at each age was only 20%. However, as in the longitudinal study, there was an increase in characters and social interactions at each age level. At the same time, the participants' dream reports continued to lack adult-like cognitive complexity and the dreamers were primarily observers, not active participants (Foulkes et al., 1990, p. 460). Overall, these cross-sectional results provide an excellent conceptual replication of the longitudinal study of children of the same age.

The longitudinal study of participants ages 9–11, 11–13, and 13–15 produced results that were as surprising and unexpected as the paucity of dreaming at ages 3–5. The 16 children ages 9–11 (8 girls and 8 boys) dreamed with the same frequency and complexity as adult dreamers, a meaningful change from what was found in both the longitudinal and cross-sectional studies of children ages 7–9. They reported dreams after 65.8% of the 231 REM awakenings, which is close to what the same participants later reported at ages 11–13 and 13–15 (Foulkes, 1982).

In addition, there were gender differences and large individual differences within the overall results. The girls recalled a mean of 71.8% from REM awakenings and the boys only 60.0%, despite the fact that the median age of the girls was a little younger than that of the boys, 9.8 years as compared to 10.4 years. Then, too, there were also large individual differences. For example, two of the girls had mean recall rates of only 20% and 27%, far below the levels of most of the other girls, and two of the boys had rates of 27% and 25%, even though all four of these children were of at least average intelligence (Foulkes, 1982, pp. 150–151).

The dream reports provided by the participants at ages 9–11 had the same levels of cognitive complexity that they had at ages 11–13 and 13–15, which is further evidence that children at ages 9–11 have reached adult-like levels as far as their cognitive capacities for dreaming (Foulkes, 1982, p. 149). However, the rates of recall were nonetheless somewhat lower than the rates in studies of young adults, and there were differences in dream content compared to later adolescence as well, and in comparisons with findings from adult participants (Foulkes, 1982, pp. 74, 217).

The results for the children ages 9–15 were later supported in a direct replication and extension longitudinal study, based on 24 children (12 girls and 12 boys), at ages 9–11, 11–13, and 13–15 (Strauch, 2005). Most importantly, these 24 children had the same high recall rates and dream complexity at ages 9–11 as did the 16 participants in the first longitudinal study. Once again, these rates did not change significantly at ages 11–13 and 13–15. And, as in the first longitudinal study of participants at this age, there were gender and individual differences in dream recall.

In terms of individual differences in recall, three girls had 100% recall and another had 90.9%, but two other girls recalled only 54.5% and 45.5% of their dreams. The boys had an even wider range, with two participants who recalled 100% of their dreams, and four others who recalled only 36.4%, 33.3%, 25.0%, and 12.5% (Strauch, 2004, p. 223, Anhang 2). These findings await future studies to determine if and how the high and low recallers may differ in terms of the maturation of their default networks, and/or in the development of the waking cognitive skills that seem most likely to be involved in dreaming.

The 16 participants at ages 9–11 in the first longitudinal study of participants in this age group, when combined with the 24 participants at ages 9–11 in the second longitudinal study, add up to a total of 40 participants who were studied at this unexpectedly important age in the development of dreaming. Adding to the strength of these findings, these results were established in two independent sleep-dream laboratories in two different countries, the United States and Switzerland, in two different decades.

And these replicated results for ages 9–11 became all the more significant in light of the findings on the adult-like maturation of the default network at this same age by independent investigators many years later (Fair et al., 2007, 2008, 2009). Moreover, ages 9–11 are in the same age range that the cognitive capacities to think narratively and imaginatively during waking become adult-like. This generalization importantly includes the finding that the presence of abstract, psychological self-knowledge is not fully demonstrated until this age (Ross et al., 2024, p. 12). Taken together, these three sets of findings provide a completely unplanned, unexpected, and altogether remarkable triangulation of methods and results.

More generally, this chapter has used a triangulation of neuroimaging, lesion, and maturational/developmental studies to demonstrate that there is in fact a unique functional neurocognitive network that gives rise to dreaming. These results provide the neurocognitive theory of dreaming with the neurophysiological, neurocognitive, and behavioral levels that are necessary to establish the theory's plausibility and credibility as a basis for explaining dreaming, with verbal reports serving as the behavioral indicator that dreaming has occurred. The findings in this chapter also provide the basis for attempting to determine the theory's degree of compatibility with the adaptive inactivity theory of sleep and the multistate hierarchical model of consciousness, which are the topics of later chapters.

Conclusions, Implications, and Next Steps

The findings in this chapter fully establish the general contours and the main neural substrates that define the neurocognitive network that gives rise to dreaming. They also underscore the fact that the FPCN has to loosen its control of the default network if the dreaming network is going to reach relative ascendancy. The chapter also shows that the neural substrates that subserve dreaming have to be mature and intact, and that the cognitive capacities that support visual imagery, conceptualization, narrative skills, and imagination have to reach adult-like levels for dreaming to become similar to the dreaming in older teenagers and adults.

The impact of these discoveries is not as dramatic as the invention of, for example, the telescope. They are not even as dramatic as the "resolution revolution" in microscopy since the turn of the 21st century, which has made it possible "to zoom in on the minutest workings of the molecules of life in a more naturalistic setting—and to do so at speeds that would have astonished researchers a mere 20 years ago" (Weizmann, 2017). However, neuroimaging studies and the development of an extensive literature in waking-state cognitive neuroscience since the 1990s have given dream research a specific brain basis. These unexpected developments never could have been imagined by dream researchers before they unfolded.

Despite the potential for progress in outlining the neurocognitive basis of dreaming, further advances may be slow for two separate reasons. First, neurocognitive researchers interested in the functioning of the default network are rightly focused on many other issues, including the role of this network in social-affective cognition and in various neurodegenerative, neurodevelopmental, and psychiatric conditions, such as Alzheimer's, autism, and schizophrenia (Amft et al., 2015; Andrews-Hanna, 2012; Andrews-Hanna et al., 2014, for overviews). That said, two recent research articles based on longitudinal data from studies in several different countries nonetheless link self-reports of the lack of dream recall and disturbing dreams to the eventual development of Alzheimer's (Lipnicki, Valenti, et al., 2025; Lipnicki, Vella, et al., 2025).

Second, the type of studies of the default network and its relationship to ongoing cognitive activity that are needed (namely, combined EEG/neuroimaging studies) are more difficult to conduct during sleep because of the noise of traditional scanners and the near-impossibility of holding still and staying asleep for long periods of time within them. The difficulty of sleeping under these circumstances is usually mitigated by sleep-depriving the participants for as long as 24–36 hours, a procedure that can introduce confounds because sleep deprivation is highly stressful. Then, too, it generally takes one to two nights to adapt to sleeping in any laboratory in the best of circumstances, which means that results that have ecological validity are difficult to obtain in one-night studies (Tamaki et al., 2016; Wick et al., 2020). However, one methodological study suggests that participants can sleep reasonably well on the second consecutive night in an fMRI scanning study, but this approach has not been used widely as yet (Moehlman et al., 2018).

Although the pace of new neuroimaging research related to dreams will be slow, the existing neurocognitive findings are more than enough to raise serious doubts about many past assumptions and theoretical claims about dreaming. To begin with, several neuroimaging studies raise difficult questions about the frequent claim that dreaming is similar to a hallucinatory state. These studies demonstrate that hallucinations are the product of neurocognitive states in which the participants (hallucinating patients) have greater activation in both primary and secondary sensory regions, and in premotor and cerebellar areas as well (Allen et al., 2008; Ford et al., 2009; Hoffman & Hampson, 2012; Waters et al., 2016; Zmigrod et al., 2016, for a meta-analysis of several studies).

Moreover, it has been known for many decades from interview studies of psychiatric patients living in mental wards that they "easily differentiate their sleep and dream life from their waking life and hallucinating states," even though they cannot "effectively differentiate" their hallucinations "from their normal waking perceptions" (Kass et al., 1970, p. 496). Based on both neuroimaging studies and first-person testimony, it seems highly unlikely that dreams are similar to hallucinosis or psychosis, as is sometimes asserted by both clinically based and REM-based theories.

As for the drug-altered atypical states that are often claimed to be "dreamlike," such as those induced by psilocybin and LSD, they are in many ways the opposite of dreaming because they suppress and/or profoundly alter the default network (Avram et al., 2024; Berkovitch et al., 2025; dos Santos et al., 2016; Fox et al., 2018; Siegel et al., 2024). More generally, the default network is deactivated in all cases of "substance use disorder" (Zhang & Volkow, 2019). Then, too, the meditative states sometimes compared to dreaming are also characterized by the relative deactivation of the default network, so they are not at all like dreaming (Aguerre et al., 2023; Fox et al., 2016; Garrison et al., 2015).

Finally, there is the case of hypnosis, an intense waking-state relationship between two people, which is sometimes claimed to be useful in studying dreams by means of "hypnotic dreams." (Claims about the usefulness of hypnotic dreams in therapy and legal proceedings have led to serious harm by creating false memories (Hyman & Loftus, 2002; MacLean, 1993, for a book-length account of an unfounded murder trial and subsequent conviction, based on a hypnotic dream; Strange et al., 2007).) An assessment of the results of several neuroimaging studies of hypnosis concluded that this state leads to "the opposite pattern of brain engagement" that is found during dreaming (Abraham, 2016, p. 4206).

The neurocognitive networks underlying these putatively "dreamlike" waking states therefore differ from each other. Moreover, the neurocognitive network that creates dreaming is completely different from all of them and is normal, regular, and expectable, not at all atypical. Thus, any claims about the relationship between any "altered" state of conscious and dreaming have been out of date for many years by now.

In addition, developmental results in this chapter raise major questions about hypotheses relating to the adaptive function of dreaming that focus on dreams as having psychological functions in dealing with events from the previous day. They also lead to strong doubts about hypotheses claiming that dreams are rehearsals that prepare people for waking social interactions or for threatening situations that may occur in the future. More specifically, the finding that preschool children do not dream often or with any complexity, and that dreaming during the elementary school years is relatively infrequent and not adult-like until ages 9–11, is not easily explained by either of these two types of adaptive hypotheses. Instead, these findings suggest that such psychological adjustments must be carried out by waking cognitive processes until late childhood at the least. This fact further suggests that these waking cognitive processes very likely continue to occur throughout adulthood as well.

It therefore seems unlikely that any adaptive functions attributed to dreaming with regard to waking cognitive processing could add much, if anything, to what the waking cognitive processes have been carrying out with apparent success during the first decade of life. Although many human adaptations do not mature in the first few years of life, as seen most notably in the major changes that occur during puberty, no hypothesis concerning the adaptive function of dreaming has ever tried to explain how and why the adult-like frequency and complexity of dreaming would first develop at ages 9–11. Nor have they addressed the issue of how or why dreaming is needed at ages 9–11 and thereafter to supplement or replace the waking cognitive processes that have been carrying out these adaptive functions for the first decade of life.

The carefully controlled studies of dreaming in hospitalized schizophrenics, which showed that dreaming can be lost if the dorsomedial prefrontal subsystem in the default network is lesioned, also present difficulties for adaptive theories that stress the need for dreaming to deal with events of the previous day or to rehearse skills that will be needed in the future. This is because there is no evidence that these patients lost cognitive functioning as a result of losing the capacity to dream (Jus, Jus, Gautier, et al., 1973; Jus, Jus, Villeneuve, et al., 1973). Nor is there evidence that other patients who had this operation were cognitively impaired (Baker et al., 1970; Greenblatt & Solomon, 1952; Paul et al., 1956; Robinson, 1954).

Then, too, the finding that lesioned patients who lose dreaming nonetheless continue to sleep normally provides a refutation to Sigmund Freud's (1900, p. 180) assertion that dreams are "the guardians of sleep." According to this hypothesis, dreaming is essential to sleep because it allows sleep to continue uninterrupted in the face of urgent physiological needs. Dreaming purportedly transforms these physiological needs into wishes, which provide temporary hallucinatory satisfactions. Normal sleep without dreaming, as in the case of the lesioned patients, therefore provides a strong refutation to Freud's adaptive theory. More generally, the shortcomings of all pre-neuroimaging ideas about the possible adaptive function of dreaming are discussed more fully in Chapter 10.

The lesion results also raise problems for the various physiologically oriented theorists who focus on posterior areas of the brain—the temporoparietal junction—as the key to dreaming (e.g., Boly et al., 2017; Siclari et al., 2017). They stress that this area is activated during dreaming, and that lesions in this area lead to the loss of dreaming. However, they do not note that this area is part of the dorsomedial subsystem of the default network. Nor do they note that lesions in anterior areas of the dorsomedial subsystem also lead to the loss of dreaming, which negates their sole emphasis on the posterior "hot spot." Put another way, they do not think in terms of neurocognitive networks, which is a major shortcoming in their work on both dream and consciousness from the point of view of those researchers who theorize in network terms.

Back to the Future

Although progress may remain slow, the triangulation of findings presented in this chapter brings the study of dreaming full circle to the brief time between 1958 and 1965, when a majority of the early dream researchers thought that the previously marginal field of dream research had been brought to the center of the fledging field of neuroscience. They believed that dreaming provided the first strong example of a one-to-one relationship between a neurophysiological state, namely, REM sleep, and a cognitive process, namely, dreaming (Dement, 1968, for a detailed statement of this view; Dement, 1973, for a candid and scientifically admirable explanation for why he abandoned this psychoanalytically inspired view in which REM sleep was assumed to be essential for satisfying a hypothesized physiological drive state that is essential to life). This "REM = dreaming" conclusion originally had been doubted by the small minority of early laboratory dream researchers based in academic psychology, who tended to be at least somewhat cognitively oriented (e.g., Foulkes, 1962; Goodenough et al., 1959).

The REM = dreaming equation was sufficiently compelling that it led to widespread newspaper coverage, cover stories in several widely read popular magazines of the day, and a popular book by a science reporter, which captured all the excitement about *The Science of Dreams* (Diamond, 1962). The rise and fall of this failed equation, which in effect ignored what is now called the neurocognitive level, led to a decline in dream research by the early 1970s, with many researchers turning to a full focus on sleep, and still others turning to other fields of research (Domhoff, 2004, for an empirical critique of this Freudian-inspired idea; Foulkes, 1996, for a general account of the decline by one of the few laboratory dream researchers who was fully active in the field from the late 1950s to the early 1990s).

Starting in the late 1990s, however, the long-lost hope for a brain-based account of the cognitive process of dreaming has been haltingly revived due to the handful of neuroimaging studies of REM sleep in the 1990s. This hope was also fostered by the gradual realization that the REM sleep neuroimaging results had overlaps with the default network. Soon thereafter, it became more apparent that the lesion studies, along with the earlier developmental studies, also suggested that the relationships among (1) specific neural substrates; (2) the neurocognitive networks based in those neural substrates; and (3) dream reports after REM sleep awakenings were strong. This conclusion provides the basis for the neurocognitive theory of dreaming.

Most of all, though, the accumulating evidence that mind-wandering, daydreaming, and dreaming are all dependent upon the relative ascendancy of the default network made it possible to assert a causal relationship between a neurocognitive network and the process of dreaming. This time, however, there is no surprise to the hypothesis that such a relationship may exist for dreaming. By the turn of the 21st century at the latest, there was already strong evidence that focused waking thought is dependent upon the relative activation and ascendancy of another neurocognitive network, the FPCN.

Since then, it has been shown that there are several other relatively specific neurocognitive networks, as reflected, for example, in the seven-network framework for understanding perception and cognition (Yeo et al., 2011). There is even a neurocognitive network that involves tool-using. This network is activated by working with tools, or even simply viewing tools, with no intention of making use of any tools (MacDonald & Culham, 2015). Even more relevant to the focus of this book, there are two separate systems that involve comparisons of people, one for comparing oneself ("the self") to other people, and the other for comparing any two or more people to each other (Chavez et al., 2025).

After stating these strong conclusions, it is also essential to stress once again that the exact neural substrates that underlie the neurocognitive network that gives rise to dreaming have not been fully established, in part because this network has been studied at night far less than the waking networks involved in imagination, mind-wandering, and daydreaming. Further, much still needs to be learned about the contributions of each region within this neurocognitive network to its overall functioning.

More generally, there are ongoing debates and discoveries concerning exactly which brain regions, or specific areas within brain regions, are part of which waking network (e.g., Girn et al., 2024, for findings that suggest some areas thought to be in the limbic network are more likely in the default network). Such changes and debates, when they are based on new empirical findings, are an essential part of the development of any scientific community that can find enough shared agreement and agreed-upon rules of evidence to make further progress (Oreskes, 2019).

For now, though, there remain still other ways to assess the strength of the claims made in this chapter in relation to dreaming. Most immediately, what is known about the neurocognitive network that supports dreaming can be used to determine whether or not established findings concerning dream content are consistent with the expectations that follow from the theory.

If, for example, important areas of the self-system and the social brain are part of the neurocognitive network that supports dreaming, *then* quantitative studies of dream content should reveal that people are at the center of a very high percentage of their dreams, and also that there are many social interactions within these dreams. If, to provide another example, dreaming is an intensified form of mind-wandering and daydreaming, then dreams should be highly imaginative dramatizations, with many of these dramatizations including personal concerns that relate to important people and personal avocations in an individual's life. The presence of such personal concerns in daydreaming already has been documented for teenagers and adults (e.g., Gold & Henderson, 1990; Gold & Reilly, 1985/1986; Klinger, 1971, 2009; Singer, 1966; Singer & Singer, 2013). These and several further questions are addressed in the next chapter.

3

FINDINGS ON DREAM CONTENT IN LIGHT OF THE NEUROCOGNITIVE THEORY OF DREAMING

This chapter focuses on the degree to which replicated quantitative findings on dream content are consistent with the main tenets of the neurocognitive theory of dreaming. Although there are several useful findings on dream content that are based on rating scales, particularly in the study of children's dreams, this chapter relies on findings derived from the most comprehensive and highly detailed coding system that has been developed as yet. The Hall/Van de Castle coding system, which is named after the two dream researchers who created it, has been used for nearly 60 years in dozens of studies carried out by investigators in a wide range of countries (Hall & Van de Castle, 1966).

The Hall/Van de Castle Coding System

The Hall/Van de Castle coding system for dream content consists of ten general categories that are based on the categorical (nominal) level of measurement. This approach makes it possible to categorize every aspect of a dream report. For example, there are categories for characters (e.g., women, men, mothers, sons, strangers, celebrities, animals) and social interactions (e.g., aggressions, friendliness, and sexuality). There are also categories for activities (e.g., walking, talking); successes and failures; settings (e.g., indoor and outdoor, familiar and unfamiliar); and objects (e.g., books, furniture, and cars).

There is even a category for a frequent type of event in dreams called "misfortunes," which are defined as bad things that happen to a dream character "out of the blue," and without the intent of any other character. For example, losing a wallet or purse, or being hit by a falling tree limb, is a misfortune. Conversely, there are a few good fortunes in dreams in which a

DOI: 10.4324/9781003732969-3

character has a lucky break, such as finding money on the street or winning a raffle.

The findings based on these several categories, and still others that are not mentioned above, are organized, analyzed, and discussed in terms of a series of "content indicators." Content indicators link the results to meaningful aspects of waking life, such as the dreamer's personal concerns and avocational interests, as well as to gender and cultural context. For example, if the total number of animal characters found in a sample of dream reports is divided by the total number of characters (human, animal, and imaginary, the latter of which are very rare), then the content indicator called the "Animal Percent" can be used in studies with varying sample sizes that contain dream reports of varying lengths. Similarly, if the total number of aggressive interactions in a sample of dream reports is divided by the total number of aggressive and friendly interactions, the result is the "Aggressions/Friendliness Percent," which immediately provides an indication of the balance of aggressive and friendly interactions in a dream sample. Moreover, this "A/F%" can be calculated for the dreamer's interactions with specific characters in the dream reports, which may reveal striking differences between the interactions with mothers, fathers, sisters, brothers, and friends. (Specific useful findings using the Animal Percent will be presented shortly, and the A/F% will be used with regard to specific characters in the study of a dream series in Chapter 4.)

Methodologically, content indicators are highly useful because they provide an excellent control for the vexing issue of dream length. Table 3.1 provides a list of the most frequently used Hall/Van de Castle content indicators, most of which have to do with characters and social interactions. A full set of revised and updated content indicators can be found in other places (Domhoff, 1996; Schneider & Domhoff, 1995, in the "Resources for Scientists" section).

The statistical analyses of the findings using the content indicators in Table 3.1 are calculated by DreamSAT, a statistical analysis tool that is freely available on DreamResearch.net. DreamSAT compares any new findings with the results from the normative findings on dream content for either women or men, which are discussed below. The formulas for statistical significance used by DreamSAT have been verified using a powerful but computer-intensive statistical method called "approximate randomization," which is known as "permutation testing" by mathematicians.

Approximate randomization eliminates the need for random sampling, an underlying continuous distribution of scores, or normal distributions (see Craig & Fisher, 2019, for the usefulness of randomization-based statistical analyses; Domhoff, 2003, pp. 85–86, for an overview of the use of randomization in dream research; Domhoff & Schneider, 2008a, for the most recent randomization analysis of Hall/Van de Castle content indicators; Noreen, 1989, for an early overview of the value of using randomization-based

TABLE 3.1 The formulas for calculating 14 of the Hall/Van de Castle dream content indicators

Characters	
Male/Female Percent	Males ÷ (Males + Females)
Familiarity Percent	Familiar ÷ (Familiar + Unfamiliar)
Friends Percent	Friends ÷ All humans
Animal Percent	Animals ÷ All characters
Social Interactions	
Aggression/Characters Index	All aggressions ÷ All characters
Friendliness/Characters Index	All friendliness ÷ All characters
Aggression/Friendliness Percent	Dreamer-involved aggression ÷ (Dinv. aggression + Dinv. friendliness)
Aggressor Percent	Dreamer as Aggressor ÷ (D as Aggressor + D as Victim)
Befriender Percent	Dreamer as Befriender ÷ (D as Befriender + D as Befriended)
Physical Aggression Percent	Physical aggressions ÷ All aggressions
Dreams with at Least One:	
Aggression	Dreams with aggression ÷ Number of dreams
Friendliness	Dreams with friendliness ÷ Number of dreams
Sexuality	Dreams with sexuality ÷ Number of dreams
Misfortune	Dreams with misfortune ÷ Number of dreams

analyses). The only assumption underlying approximate randomization is that the shape of the two distributions is the same. In the case of dream studies using the Hall/Van de Castle coding system, the distributions are positively skewed, as illustrated in Figure 3.1.

For analyzing the size of the differences between two samples of dream reports, DreamSAT uses the effect-size statistic *h* for proportions, as well as the better-known effect-size statistic *d* for ratios. Both of these effect-size statistics were developed by the same psychologist, Jacob Cohen (1962, for his introduction of the *d* statistic into psychology; 1977, for the development of *h*; Domhoff, 1996, Appendix D; and Domhoff, 2022, for the most detailed discussions of *h* in the analysis of dream content).

In keeping with Cohen's (1977, p. 184) advice to determine the magnitude of effect sizes based on "theory or experience" related to each specific research field, past studies suggest that effect sizes in quantitative studies of dream content below .20 are "small," effect sizes between .20 and .40 are "moderate," and effect sizes over .40 are "large" (Domhoff, 1996, Appendix D). This conclusion is also consistent with the finding that the effect sizes in quantitative studies of dream content are larger than those in other types of psychological studies, including interview studies (.14) and reaction-time studies (.16), but smaller than those in learning and memory studies (.52) and

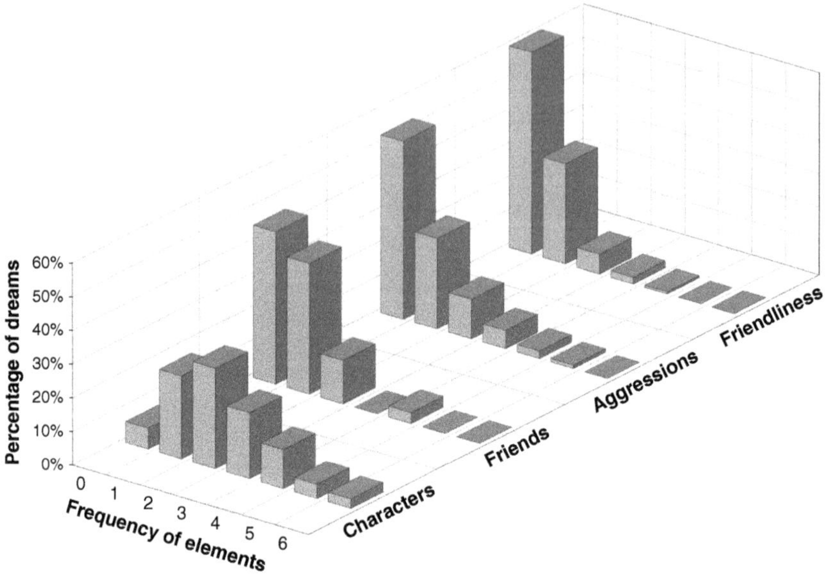

FIGURE 3.1 Positively skewed distributions of various elements in the Hall/Van de Castle male normative sample.

Source: Adapted with permission from Domhoff (2003, Figure 3.3).

person-perception studies (.54) (Domhoff, 2003, p. 89, Table 3.6; Rosnow & Rosenthal, 1997, p. 47).

The advantages of using the Hall/Van de Castle coding system, and the effect-size statistics *h* and *d* in the study of dream content, have been explained in several places (e.g., Domhoff, 2003, Chapter 3). The disadvantages of using rating scales in studying dream also have been discussed elsewhere (e.g., Domhoff, 2003, 53–66).

The main reasons that the Hall/Van de Castle system is not used more often—because it takes 10–15 hours to learn to use the coding system, and coding itself is time- and labor-intensive—may be ameliorated by the development of automated coding systems such as DreamCoder (Bongalon, 2025). DreamCoder makes use of Artificial Intelligence in the form of a Large Language Model (LLM), and it can perform Hall/Van de Castle coding of characters, social interactions, and emotions; more categories are likely in the future. It also can change the names of the people and places mentioned in the dream reports so that the reports are anonymous. At least two other developers have trained LLMs to use the Hall/Van de Castle system to code aspects of dream reports: one for characters and emotions, the other solely for emotions (Bertolini et al., 2024; Cortal, 2024).

The Animal Percent

As noted above, the Animal Percent—the total number of animal characters divided by the total number of human and animal characters—provides a good example of how informative content indicators are, starting with the fact that it can be used in studies with varying sample sizes that contain dream reports of varying lengths. If the Animal Percent is computed for the large normative samples that are discussed shortly, then the Animal Percent is 4% for women and 6% for men in a sample of 500 dream reports from 100 young adult American women and 500 dream reports from men. Substantively, this finding reveals that American adults dream relatively little about animals—that is, they have a low Animal Percent.

Moreover, these same low figures for the Animal Percent are found in several other countries. Thus, the Animal Percent, minor though it may at first seem to be, provides cross-gender and cross-national similarities that take on more theoretical interest when it is further noted that the Animal Percent is higher in indigenous societies not living on reservations than it is in any large industrialized society (Domhoff, 1996, Chapter 6, for both cross-national and cross-cultural findings). The fact that the Animal Percent is about the same for all adults who live in nation-states, but higher in indigenous societies, makes intuitive cultural sense.

The Animal Percent then becomes of greater psychological and theoretical interest because it is ten times higher—40%–50%—in both the dream reports and the made-up stories of American children ages 5–7. It does not decline to the adult level until ages 9–11, which is also the age when dreaming becomes more adult-like, as discussed in Chapter 2 (Domhoff, 1996, pp. 89–90, Tables 5.3 and 5.4). This result makes intuitive psychological sense in terms of how much children like animals, zoos, and children's books with animal characters.

Moreover, in adults a high Animal Percent predicts a greater personal concern with animals, as was the case of an individual dream series that has been fully analyzed using Hall/Van de Castle content indicators (e.g., Domhoff, 2018, pp. 119–121, for a summary). This dream series with 234 dreams reports in it was kept in the summer of 1939 out of scientific curiosity by a man in his mid-40s. The dreamer, who never made use of the dream series or showed it to anyone, was later identified as an entomologist by means of an obituary in a scientific journal. In addition to his highly detailed work with beetles, he also enjoyed hunting by virtue of being raised on a farm in Iowa, to which he often returned from his job in the Department of Agriculture in Washington, DC, during the summer. His Animal Percent of 11% is significantly higher than the norm at the .0001 level of confidence, and the effect size of .20 is a moderate one (Domhoff, 2022, pp. 119–121).

The findings on the dreams of this entomologist show that two of his main waking interests, classifying insects and hunting animals, are enacted in his dreams. His dreams thereby provide empirical support for the emphasis in the neurocognitive theory of dreaming on the continuity between waking personal concerns and the nature of dream content. The entomologist's dream reports are available for searching or downloading on the DreamBank, an open website for researchers that includes 34,000 dream reports and various utilities for searching and analyzing them (Domhoff, 2003, Chapter 4; Domhoff & Schneider, 2008b; Domhoff, 2022, pp. 103–105; Schneider & Domhoff, 1999).

With the usefulness of content indicators fully demonstrated, it is now possible to determine the extent to which dream content fits with the expectations created by the neurocognitive theory of dreaming. These expectations concern the importance of imagination, conceptions of self and others, waking personal concerns, and waking avocational interests.

The Miami Lab Studies: The Road to Replicated Findings on Dream Content

With a reliable and valid quantitative coding system for studying dream content in hand, the quest for the kind of rigorous, laboratory-based findings on dream content that would later become of great relevance to a neurocognitive theory of dreaming began in a large, Spanish-style suburban home in a laid-back neighborhood in Miami, about 10 minutes from the University of Miami. The house was partly converted into a sleep-dream laboratory in order to collect ecologically valid rapid eye movement (REM) dream reports from 11 young adult male participants. Each of the participants lived in what would be his own bedroom for one month. The participants were also asked to write down any dreams they recalled over the space of two weeks, either before or after their month of sleeping in the sleep-dream lab. These two-week dream diaries made a lab/non-lab comparison possible (Domhoff & Schneider, 1999, for an overview and further analysis of the findings; Hall, 1966b for the original unpublished study, which is now available as a freely downloadable pdf).

The concern with ecological validity first arose in part because the 1953 discovery of a large amount of dreaming each night might mean that previously collected samples from outside of a lab were unrepresentative of people's dream lives. Then, too, there was also a concern that dreams collected in a sleep-dream lab might provide distorted samples because the participants might feel uncomfortable and on guard. In fact, early studies had found that a significant minority of dream reports—as many as 30%–32%—included the laboratory setting and/or the researchers themselves (Domhoff & Kamiya, 1964, p. 526; Whitman et al., 1962, for evidence concerning the impact of the laboratory setting on dream content).

To ensure to the greatest degree possible that the participants were comfortable in the Miami sleep-dream lab, they slept undisturbed on their first night in the lab bedroom. Electroencephalogram (EEG) electrodes were attached on the second night, but the EEG machine was not turned on, and there were no awakenings. On the third night, the EEG machine was turned on, but there again were no awakenings. From the fourth through seventh nights, the participants were awakened once each night from a REM period to provide a voice-recorded dream report, but these trial dream reports were not part of the dataset (Hall, 1966b, p. 8). As this recounting of the step-by-step procedure shows, the researchers proceeded with an abundance of caution.

During the formal data-collection phase of the study, the participants were awakened once each night until they had provided four dream reports from each of the first four REM periods of the night. Then they were awakened from all four of those REM periods during each night to obtain a minimum of 16 dreams reports from each participant (Hall, 1966b, pp. 8–9). In addition, 57 dream reports were voice-recorded after unexpected spontaneous awakenings. All 11 participants had at least one spontaneous awakening during the course of the study, a finding that will become relevant in the discussion of dream recall in Chapter 8. (Most of the dream reports collected in this study—274 laboratory dream reports and 171 non-laboratory dream reports—are available on the DreamBank under the title "Miami dreams.")

The first important methodological finding from the Miami study is that the participants had very little difficulty adjusting to the laboratory setting. Beginning with the first night, the EEG machine was turned on, which was the third adjustment night, it took them no longer to fall asleep than it did on later nights (Hall, 1966b, p. 38, Table 9). Then, too, from the first night they were awakened—the fourth night—to the end of the study, only 10.6% of the dream reports included any mention of the experimental situation, far lower than in previous studies. Moreover, most of these inclusions of the laboratory setting were benign and showed an interest in the study, which suggests that the participants did not find the experimental setting to be threatening (Hall, 1966b, p. 32, 1967, pp. 200, 202). Finally, a later comparison of the 37 trial dream reports collected on the fourth through seventh nights of the adjustment period found that they did not differ from those in the larger dataset that provided the basis for the systematic analyses (Hall, 1966b, pp. 32–34).

These reassuring findings are consistent with those in another early study of the possible influence of the experimental situation on dream content, based on 695 dream reports from 77 participants, which also showed a decline in mentions of the experimental setting (Dement et al., 1965, p. 121). They also make sense in terms of a later neuroimaging study, which found that portions of the left hemisphere are atypically more alert—more vigilant—on the first night in a sleep lab than they are on the second night (Tamaki et al., 2016). Still other neuroimaging studies show the need for at least one adjustment night, with a few studies suggesting that two adjustment nights are needed to obtain normal sleep patterns in a sleep-dream laboratory (Wick et al., 2020, p. 1). Thus, the results of these several other studies, which were carried out before and after the Miami study, suggest that the Miami researchers' concerns about the ecological validity of their results were well founded. However, the possible confounds are not insurmountable if one or two adjustment nights are included in the research design.

The second important methodological finding from the Miami lab study is that dream reports from nights during which there were multiple awakenings did not differ from dream reports collected on nights when there was only one awakening. This null finding reduces or eliminates concerns about the impact of multiple awakenings on normal dream content. The third general methodological finding is that there are no differences among the REM dream reports collected from different REM periods. This conclusion is important because it suggests that dream samples based on morning recall, and recall later in the day, are representative samples of a person's dream life during REM sleep (Hall, 1966b, pp. 19–23). Nor did the 57 spontaneously recalled dreams differ in their content from dreams from scheduled awakenings (Hall, 1966b, pp. 26). (The similarity between REM dream reports and dream reports collected in sleep-dream labs from N2 awakenings in the early morning hours is discussed in Chapter 8.)

The Comparison of Lab and Non-Lab Dream Content

The comparisons of the lab and non-lab dream reports collected in the Miami study are first of all of great importance in terms of evaluating the usefulness of non-lab samples in the study of dream content. However, the lab/non-lab comparisons were not as tightly controlled as the within-laboratory comparisons because the participants provided uneven numbers of dream reports to each sample, and the length of both their laboratory and non-laboratory reports varied widely. Nor were the content indicators in Table 3.1 used to analyze and discuss the results, which means there were no controls for either dream length or the number of characters in the lab and non-lab dream reports. Finally, more precise statistical methods are now available, including the effect sizes that were discussed above, as well as approximate randomization (Domhoff & Schneider, 1999, pp. 145, 147–148, for a commentary on the original lab/non-lab comparisons).

Due to these shortcomings, along with the highly general nature of the original findings, which made them less useful for specific purposes, the original codings were re-analyzed using DreamSAT. To provide the tightest possible comparison, the re-analysis is based on the eight young adult males who could each provide 15 non-lab dreams and 24 lab dreams, a total of 120 non-lab reports and 272 lab dreams (Domhoff & Schneider, 1999, p. 144, for explanatory details). This re-analysis found that there were two statistically significant differences between the two samples, both of which related to aggressions. There is a higher rate of aggressions per character (.18 vs. .31) and a higher percentage of dreams with at least one aggression (42% vs. 56%) in the non-lab dreams. These findings are consistent with the importance of aggression in differentiating many different samples of dream reports, as discussed at various points in the rest of the chapter. These findings are presented in Table 3.2.

With this larger context in mind, the findings in Table 3.2 provide a baseline for comparing the non-lab findings in the Miami study with the earlier-mentioned Hall/Van de Castle non-lab normative samples for men and women. The two normative samples are based on 500 dream reports from 100 men and 500 dream reports from 100 women, with each person contributing five dream reports. These large samples were drawn randomly from over 1000 semester-long dream diaries.

TABLE 3.2 Miami non-lab dreams vs. lab dreams

	Miami lab (n = 272)	*Miami non-lab (n = 120)*	*Effect size*
Characters			
Male/Female Percent	72%	67%	−.11
Familiarity Percent	44%	39%	−.11
Friends Percent	31%	28%	−.07
Animal Percent	3%	6%	+.13
Social Interactions			
A/C Index	.18	.31	−.29**
F/C Index	.14	.17	−.10
Aggression/Friendliness Percent	53%	61%	+.16
Aggressor Percent	46%	51%	−.08
Befriender Percent	56%	59%	+.06
Physical Aggression Percent	28%	48%	+.43
Dreams with at Least One:			
Aggression	42%	56%	+.28*
Friendliness	36%	33%	−.05
Sexuality	5%	9%	+.17
Misfortune	18%	20%	+.04

Notes:
* $p < .05$. ** $p < .01$.
Effect size is given in Cohen's h for percent-based indicators, and Cohen's d for ratios/indexes. The p values were determined via approximate randomization. It is notable that the two samples differ only in terms of two aggression indicators.

The dream diaries from which the samples were drawn contained 19–25 dream reports, which were kept by students in classes at Case Western Reserve University and Baldwin-Wallace College in Cleveland, Ohio, from 1947 through 1950, a four-year span. Only dream reports that were 50–300 words in length were randomly chosen from each student's portfolio (Hall & Van de Castle, 1966, p. 158. for a discussion of how the dream reports were collected and how a subset of them was drawn for use in developing the normative samples for men and women).

As a later study showed, the length of dream reports that contain at least 50 words is not an issue when the content indicators are used. First, dream reports with 50–175 words do not differ from dream reports with 175–300 words. Second, the content indicators did equally well in controlling for length with dream reports of any length above 300–400 words, with one exception. The "At Least One Indicators" (e.g., there is at least one aggressive interaction, or at least one friendly interaction, in a dream report) are not useful for dream reports with more than 400 words because they do not contain a control for reports of varying lengths (Domhoff, 2003, pp. 79–83). Moreover, this same study found that dream reports with less than 50 words cannot yield reliable and useful results using the content indicators. This conclusion lends further support to Hall and Van de Castle's decision to eliminate these brief reports from the normative samples.

When the Miami non-lab dreams are compared with the men's normative sample, the results reveal that the Miami non-lab reports and the normative sample of non-lab dream reports differ very little from each other. The full results are provided in Table 3.3.

The similarity of the two sets of non-lab dream reports collected from men provides an empirical rationale for using the non-lab normative sample for men for a substantive comparison with the normative women of 500 dreams reports collected at Case Western University and Baldwin-Wallace College. The results are presented in Table 3.4. Once again, the largest differences concern aggression indicators, but there are numerous other large differences as well.

In addition, several of the differences found in these dreams are consistent with findings on differences in behavior and experiences between genders in waking life. This is especially the case with the differences on aggression. Meta-analyses demonstrate that American men's greater involvement in aggressive interactions is the largest of the relatively few gender differences that have been found, with an effect size of .55 (Hyde, 2014, p. 385; Leaper & Farkas, 2015). On the other hand, in waking life women are more likely to be involved in "relational aggression," which includes the same kind of non-physical aggressions—such as exclusion, rejection, and criticism—that are found more frequently in women's dreams, although this difference is not

TABLE 3.3 Miami non-lab dreams vs. the male norms

	Male norms (n = 500)	*Miami non-lab (n = 120)*	*Effect size*
Characters			
Male/Female Percent	68%	67%	–.01
Familiarity Percent	45%	39%	–.13*
Friends Percent	31%	28%	–.07
Animal Percent	06%	06%	–.01
Social Interactions			
A/C Index	.34	.31	–.06
F/C Index	.21	.17	–.12
Aggression/Friendliness Percent	59%	61%	+.04
Aggressor Percent	40%	51%	+.23
Befriender Percent	50%	59%	+.17
Physical Aggression Percent	50%	48%	–.04
Dreams with at Least One:			
Aggression	47%	56%	+.18
Friendliness	38%	33%	–.10
Sexuality	12%	09%	–.08
Misfortune	36%	20%	–.36**

Notes:
* $p < .05$. ** $p < .01$.
Effect size is given in Cohen's *h* for percent-based indicators, and Cohen's *d* for ratios/indexes. The *p* values were determined via approximate randomization.

as large in waking life (Bussey, 2013, pp. 87–88; Leaper & Farkas, 2015, p. 830).

About half of the human characters in women's dreams are other women (48% women, 52% men), which seems only natural in that there are about the same number of women and men in all societies. So it comes as a surprise that two-thirds of the human characters in men's dreams are other men. This unexpected difference leads to a moderate effect size ($h = .39$, $p < .001$). In addition, similar results have been reported in studies in several different countries, as well as in indigenous societies (Hall, 1984, for worldwide findings, with a few exceptions).

According to one analysis of this difference on the Male/Female Percent (M/F%)—a content indicator based on dividing the total number of male characters by the total number of male and female characters—it may be due to men's strong personal concerns about competing with other men, combined with their wariness and fear when encountering unknown men (Domhoff, 2022, pp. 88–93). The few exceptions include a sample of German college students in which the men had a M/F% closer of that of women (Domhoff et al., 2005–2006, for a direct replication study of German students as an

TABLE 3.4 The Hall/Van de Castle female norms vs. the male norms

	Male norms (n = 500)	*Female norms (n = 491)*	*Effect size*
Characters			
Male/Female Percent	68%	48%	–.41**
Familiarity Percent	45%	58%	+.27**
Friends Percent	31%	37%	+.12*
Animal Percent	06%	04%	–.08
Social Interactions			
A/C Index	.34	.23	–.21**
F/C Index	.21	.21	+.01
Aggression/Friendliness Percent	59%	51%	–.16*
Aggressor Percent	39%	34%	–.12
Befriender Percent	50%	49%	–.03
Physical Aggression Percent	50%	34%	–.34**
Rejection Percent #	17%	36%	+.43**
Dreams with at Least One:			
Aggression	47%	44%	–.07
Friendliness	38%	41%	+.06
Sexuality	12%	03%	–.32**
Misfortune	36%	33%	–.07
Good Fortune	07%	06%	–.04
Success	15%	07%	–.28**
Failure	16%	09%	–.22**

Notes: * $p < .05$. ** $p < .01$. † Rejection Percent is the number of A3 aggression codings divided by the total number of aggressions; A3 is defined as "an attempt by one character to reject, exploit, control, or verbally coerce another character."

Effect size is given in Cohen's *h* for percent-based indicators, and Cohen's *d* for ratios/indexes. The *p* values were determined via approximate randomization. The women's sample size is nine less than the men's because nine of the women's dreams and coding cards were lost when Hall and Van de Castle were mailing materials back and forth between California and Virginia after they both left Miami in 1966. Comparisons of the original results using all 500 of the women's dreams show that they do not differ significantly from the results based on 491 dream reports.

exception; Schredl et al., 2003, for the original findings on a sample of dream reports from German students as an exception).

Although there are differences between the Miami lab and non-lab dreams on aggressions, and also prominent differences on some aggression indicators between women and men, it is important to add that aggression is always more frequent than friendliness in all four sets of dream reports that have been discussed up to this point in the chapter. This point is best seen by a simple comparison of the findings using the Aggression per Character Index (the A/C ratio) with the findings using the Friendliness per Character Index (the F/C ratio), as displayed in Table 3.5. This finding shows once again that

TABLE 3.5 In both lab-collected and normative dream reports, aggression is more common than friendliness in four different samples

	A/C index	*F/C index*
Miami Lab	.18	.14
Miami Home	.31	.17
Male Norms	.34	.21
Female Norms	.23	.21

differences in aggressions on one or more of the content indicators are often the most important differences in a wide range of dream samples, as will be seen later in this chapter and in Chapter 4.

Providing further evidence for the validity and usefulness of the normative findings for women and men, the Hall/Van de Castle normative findings have been replicated twice in two separate decades. They were first replicated using 340 dream reports from 69 women and 263 dream reports from 53 men at the University of Richmond (Hall et al., 1982). The normative findings for women were then replicated again in a sophisticated methodological study that included several safeguards to ensure a high-quality sample. It is based on 500 dream reports collected from 100 women in the late 1980s at the University of California, Berkeley (Tonay, 1990/1991). These results also reveal that the dream life of Americans remained consistent from the late 1940s to the late 1980s, a span of 40 years.

These results lead to the conclusion that large samples of dream reports collected outside the laboratory setting can provide representative samples of dream content *if* they are collected carefully, without introducing any of the demand characteristics and other biasing effects that haunt all psychological studies (Corneille & Lush, 2023; Incelli & Gallagher, 2022; Rosenthal & Rosnow, 2009; Rosnow & Rosenthal, 1997, for ongoing evidence of how frequently seemingly systematic studies lead to questionable results). However, achieving these results is more easily said than done (Domhoff, 2003, pp. 46–52, for a critical evaluation of the frequently used methods of collecting samples of dream reports).

For example, asking any group of people, such as students in a classroom, or friends and acquaintances of the researcher, to keep a dream diary for one to three weeks often leads to a large minority of participants who lose interest and drop out, which is easy to do if participation is voluntary and anonymous. Then, too, samples collected by means of one- to three-week dream diaries often consist of widely varying numbers of reports from each participant. This imbalance leads to difficulties in mitigating the impact of the few participants who provide a large percentage of the dream reports, which often requires a large reduction in the size of the sample. On the other hand, if researchers have to prod unmotivated participants one or more times to write down their dreams, then these requests can lead to hasty or made-up dream reports due to what are known as "demand characteristics" (Corneille, 2023).

This point was demonstrated in a classroom survey of 206 women students that was part of the replication study at the University of California, Berkeley. When asked if they might turn in made-up dream reports if they were required to turn in dreams, 43% said they would do so (Tonay, 1990/1991, p. 89). When the 104 women who had voluntarily turned in five dreams were asked if they had made up any of the dreams, four of them said they had made up at least one of the dreams they submitted. All of the five dreams that these four students submitted were then dropped from that dataset (Tonay, 1990/1991, p. 88). More generally, this study provides a prototype of what a rigorous study of non-lab dreams looks like.

Collecting dreams from large samples of volunteers by means of the Internet also has major drawbacks (Domhoff, 2022, pp. 128–129, for an overview; Incelli & Gallagher, 2022, for a critique that is supported by a methodological study of Internet responses). More generally, there are a growing number of problems in using online volunteers in any form of psychological research, including detecting people who use bots to make money and accumulate gift cards (Falk et al., 2025; Webb & Tangney, 2022).

Within this context, the findings from the Miami lab study provide the rock that the neurocognitive theory of dreaming stands upon in the sea of uncertainty surrounding the study of dream content. They can be that rock, that starting point for understanding dream content, because of the methodological rigor of both the Hall/Van de Castle coding system and the Miami study. Put another way, what people say they dream about in surveys and interviews, and what they report in one- to three-week dream diaries kept at the request of investigators, cannot provide an adequate starting point. These approaches have too many unresolved methodological issues attached to them to be a rock for anyone to stand on, as shown in a variety of excellent studies (e.g., Beaulieu-Prévost & Zadra, 2007; Beaulieu-Prévost & Zadra, 2015; Bernstein & Belicki, 1995–1996; Blagrove, 2007; Tonay, 1990/1991, pp. 88–89).

Instead, the other methods of dream collection have to be judged against the standard set by the Miami lab/non-lab study, including on the crucial issue of necessary sample sizes. And, as already noted, the Berkeley replication study provides an excellent starting point for obtaining large and solid non-lab samples of dream reports (Tonay, 1990/1991).

The "Most Recent Dream" Method for Collecting Large Representative Samples

Due to the many problems involved in collecting large representative samples of non-lab dream reports that are not confounded by one or more biasing factors, the current best method for collecting dream reports outside of a laboratory setting is to ask anonymous volunteers to write down the Most Recent Dream (MRD) they can remember. This simple and straightforward method, which was first developed in the early 1990s (Hartmann, 1991), has been used with college students in Canada and the United States to create samples that lead to results that are similar to those for the Hall/Van de Castle normative system (Dale et al., 2016; Domhoff, 1996). It also has been used to collect normative samples of dream reports from young women and men in Iran, which differed from the Hall/Van de Castle normative samples only in terms of two or three coding categories that make sense culturally (Mazandarani et al., 2013). In addition, the MRD method has been used to study threatening dreams in South Africa and Wales (Malcolm-Smith & Solms, 2004; Malcolm-Smith et al., 2008) and the dreams of animal rights activists in the United States (Lewis, 2008).

To increase the possibility that the dream that is provided is the most recent one the participants can recall, they are further primed for recency by asking them to write down the date for the collection day and also the date on which they think the dream occurred, along with the time during the day that they think they recalled the dream. Moreover, dreams that are stated to have occurred two or more weeks before the date on which the dreams are collected should be discarded. This is due to the results of a study revealing that such reports may be compromised by memory problems, including false memories of dreams that never occurred (Beaulieu-Prévost & Zadra, 2015).

This approach also makes it possible to eliminate dream reports in which it is indicated that the report the participant is about to write is a recurrent dream, a dream from childhood, or a particularly memorable or frightening dream. Finally, it is essential to set aside dream reports containing less than 50 words, so that the findings can be compared with the Hall/Van de Castle normative samples (see Domhoff, 2016, for a discussion of methodological issues with regard to MRDs).

The MRD method also has proven to be useful in Hall/Van de Castle studies of the development of dreaming in children and adolescents from the fifth grade (ages 10–11) through high school, by means of several different studies in the United States (Avila-White et al., 1999; Saline, 1999), Spain (Oberst et al., 2005), and Italy (Crugnola et al., 2008). In the largest and best-controlled study of MRDs that had been carried out as of 2025, researchers in Greece were able to study 756 participants ages 8–18 from all socioeconomic regions within a school district (Karagianni et al., 2013). The results replicate and extend the previous studies with regard to several age and gender differences. These various studies of children and adolescents have been synthesized and then compared with developmental findings in studies that used other methodologies for collecting dream reports (Domhoff, 2022, Chapter 7).

Taking the Importance of Large Sample Sizes More Seriously

The large sample sizes used in the Hall/Van de Castle normative studies for women and men made it possible to do three different methodological studies, using increasingly sophisticated methods of analysis, to determine the number of dream reports that are necessary to replicate the original findings. First, any 250 dream reports from either normative sample provide the same results as were obtained with the 500 dream reports. Second, samples of 125 dream reports still replicate the norms within 2–5 percentage points for most content indicators, but the differences from the norms grow large with sample sizes of 100 dream reports or less (Domhoff, 1996, pp. 64–66, Table 4.7, 2003, pp. 92–94).

Approximate randomization was then used to determine the exact sample sizes that are needed to detect the six largest gender differences in the normative samples of women and men at the .05 confidence level. Overall, it takes 125 dream reports to replicate most of findings with 250 or 500 dream reports at the .05 level of confidence (Domhoff & Schneider, 2008a). For example, the Indoor Setting Percent and the Physical Aggression Percent are significant only half the time at the .05 level of confidence with 100 dream reports, and the differences on the Familiarity Percent and the Aggressions Per Character Ratio (the A/C Index) are lost with 60 or less reports (Domhoff & Schneider, 2008a, pp. 1263–1264, including Table 2 and Table 3).

When we looked at the five largest differences between the female norms and the 250 dream reports drawn from the Barb Sanders series, an individual dream series that will be discussed in detail in Chapter 4, all five of these differences could be replicated at the .05 level of confidence with 125 dream reports. However, two of the five differences were not detectable when 100 reports from each sample were compared, and three of the five differences were not significant with sample sizes of 75. It therefore once again takes 125 dream reports to detect the full range of differences found with larger samples, as was the case when comparing the female and male normative samples (Domhoff & Schneider, 2008a, pp. 1263–1264). It is also important to note that these necessary sample sizes could be anticipated on the basis of statistical estimations alone (Cohen, 1977, pp. 192–195, Tables 6.3.4 and 6.3.5; Domhoff, 1996, Appendix D, p. 317, Table D3).

The need for large sample sizes is due to two issues that are endemic to any study of dream content that goes beyond global ratings of one or more of the few dimensions of a dream report that have been found to be reliably rated: e.g., activity levels and degree of vividness (Cohen, 1979). First, most elements of dream content, including specific characters, such as mother or father, appear in less than half of all dream reports, so the actual sample size for any one content indicator is always far smaller than it first appears to be on the basis of the total number of dream reports. Second, the sizes of the substantive differences between samples of dream reports are not large. This second point also can be stated in statistical terms: effect sizes are small in dreams, so large samples are needed to find these small but psychologically meaningful differences (Domhoff, 1996, Appendix D).

The need for large sample sizes also may help explain why many seemingly new discoveries concerning dream content cannot be replicated. Nor is this emphasis on the importance of large sample sizes unique to the study of dream content. In fact, a good part of the "replication crisis" in psychological science, neuroscience, and medicine is due to small sample sizes (e.g., Bogdan, 2025; Replication Crisis, 2025; Open Science Collaboration, 2015).

Substantive Findings on Gender, Cultural, and Age Differences

The previous section was methodological in nature and meant to establish a solid foundation for turning to the detailed substantive results that have been produced by the Hall/Van de Castle system. However, the substantive findings on gender similarities and differences presented as part of this methodological presentation should not go unremarked because gender differences have long been a topic of great interest in the biological and social sciences. Then, too, as shown in this section of the chapter, the different personal conceptions and concerns of men and women during waking are consistent with expectations based on the neurocognitive theory of dreaming (Domhoff, 2022, pp. 83–85, 88–93).

As mentioned earlier, the most salient of these differences, which concern aggression, are consistent with what has been found in waking life. In observational studies of children ages 4–5 in pre-school play settings, the boys are rougher, take things from girls as well as boys, and tend to establish dominance hierarchies among themselves very quickly (Maccoby, 1998, pp. 36–43 and Chapter 5). These differences are also found in the dreams of boys and girls by early adolescence (Domhoff, 2022, Chapter 7, for Hall/Van de Castle findings on the dream content of preadolescent and adolescent girls and boys; Strauch, 2004, 2005, for detailed Hall/Van de Castle findings in a longitudinal laboratory study of 12 girls and 12 boys between ages 9–11 and 14–15).

It is also the case that there is more physical aggression in men's dreams, as measured by dividing the number of physical aggressions by the total of both physical and non-physical aggressions, which provides the content indicator called the Physical Aggression Percent. The effect size h is .34 and $p = .000$. This difference is punctuated by the finding that 3.0% of men's dreams contain a murder, as compared to only .6% in women's dreams. On the other hand, women's dreams contain far more relational forms of aggression, such as rejection (36% vs. 18%), which leads to the largest gender difference that is found in dreams ($h = .44$, $p = .0001$).

The use of the Hall/Van de Castle coding system in studies of young adults in six Western countries has led to several cross-national similarities in addition to the Animal Percent that was discussed earlier in the chapter (Domhoff, 1996, pp. 100–107). These studies show that there are generally more aggressions than friendliness, more misfortunes than good fortunes, and more failures than successes in the dreams of women and men in these countries.

Dream reports collected from adults in ten indigenous societies have been analyzed using Hall/Van de Castle categories. Two of the societies were based on hunting and gathering economies, and the rest relied primarily on one or another type of agriculture. These dream reports were collected under many different conditions, and many were relatively brief, so the most important conclusions are somewhat general (Domhoff, 1996, pp. 99, 115–120, for a more detailed discussion). Most impressively in terms of characters, the men in all ten of the indigenous societies have the same M/F% that is found in the American normative dream reports. In addition, women in four of the six indigenous societies for which there is information have M/F%'s that are similar to those in the United States (Domhoff, 1996, pp. 119, Table 6.17).

As is the case with the American normative findings, the A/C ratio is higher than the F/C ratio in these societies, with the exception of Hopi women. The findings from dreamers in indigenous societies are also similar to the American normative findings in that they have more familiar than unfamiliar characters, and they are more often the victims of aggression, with two exceptions. There is usually more physical than non-physical aggression as well. Moreover, the Physical Aggression Percent is higher than it is in the United States in all but one of the indigenous societies, namely, the Hopi in the American Southwest, who had been forced to live on reservations almost 100 years before their dream reports were collected (Domhoff, 1996, pp. 119–120, Tables 6.17 and 6.18, and p. 128). These findings are also supported by studies of the nonviolent Mehinaku society in the Amazon and in a Zapotec Indian village in Mexico (Gregor, 1981a; O'Nell & O'Nell, 1977). More generally, the results on social interactions in the indigenous societies that have been studied once again suggest that aggression is a key variable in differentiating among both industrialized nations and indigenous societies (Domhoff & Schneider, 2008a, p. 1260, Table 1).

Turning to age differences in dreams in three Western societies, it is striking that there are few age differences once people reach young adulthood. Using an earlier version of the Hall/Van de Castle coding system, which varied only slightly from its final form in terms of the categories for characters, aggressions, and friendly interactions, two cross-sectional studies of 281 dream reports from women and 281 reports from men, who ranged in age from 30 to 80, showed small declines in aggression and friendliness when compared with younger dreamers (Hall & Domhoff, 1963, p. 260, Table 2, 1964, p. 310, Table 1).

The most rigorous study of age changes in dream content between young adulthood and the mid-50s used a longitudinal design in which the researchers collected two-week, follow-up dream diaries from French–Canadian women who had originally written down their dreams 10, 15, or 17 years earlier. At the time they were asked if they would keep a second dream diary, seven of the women were between ages 30 and 39, ten were between 40 and 49, and four were between 50 and 55. Using a large number of Hall/Van de Castle content indicators, the researchers found no statistically significant differences (Lortie-Lussier et al., 2000, pp. 71–72, Tables 1, 2, and 3).

Two large-scale and well-controlled studies of the elderly were carried out at the University of Zurich using samples that were analyzed with Hall/Van de Castle coding categories. In the first of the two Swiss studies, 15 women and 9 men between ages 66 and 78, with a mean age of 70, first served in a sleep-dream laboratory study and then voice-recorded their dreams at home for two weeks, which led to a sample of 253 dream reports. The reports were coded for characters, settings, social interactions, and activities. The only two differences from a sample of dream reports from younger Swiss adults were a higher percentage of unfamiliar characters and unfamiliar settings (Strauch, 2003).

In the second study, 45 men and 106 women, ranging in age from 65 to 89, who attended two different lectures in a series of lectures for senior citizens in Zurich, wrote down the "Most Recent Dream" they could recall. As explained earlier in this chapter, the MRD method provides a fast and simple way to collect large representative samples of dream reports from participants aged 9–11 to adulthood. As in the first study of elderly people in Zurich, the dream reports were compared with dream reports from younger Swiss adults and once again there was a higher percentage of unfamiliar characters and unfamiliar settings in the elderly sample. There was also less aggression in the elderly sample (Strauch, 2014). The fact that the MRDs method led a replication of the first Zurich study provides further validation for this method of dream collection.

The Self-System and Social Interactions in Dreams

If, as suggested at the end of Chapter 2, the self-system and the social brain—both of which are supported in good part by regions in the default network—are also part of the unique neurocognitive network that gives rise to dreaming, then quantitative studies should reveal that people are at the center of a very high percentage of their dreams. Such studies should also find that the dreamer is often interacting with other people, whether as part of social interactions (aggressive, friendly, or sexual) or as part of shared activities, such as discussing a topic together or lifting a heavy object. These expectations are supported by several new analyses of the combined normative findings for men and women, some of which were carried out for the purposes of this book. These analyses are then supplemented on the basis of earlier findings in a somewhat similar study (Domhoff & Schneider, 2018).

Overall, the dreamer is the center of activity in 86.7% of dreams. In most of these dreams, the dreamer is involved in social interactions with other human characters or engaged in various activities with other human characters (80.3%). In still others, the dreamer is doing something while alone, such as working with a piece of equipment, driving a car, or taking a walk, so is of necessity at the center of the dream (4.3%). In another small subset (2.1%), only the dreamer and one or more animals are present. In the remaining 13.3% of dreams, the dreamer is either observing other people engaged in social interactions or social activities (6.6%) or thinking about or perceiving a group of human characters who are not engaged in social interactions or social activities (6.7%). (See Domhoff & Schneider, 2018, pp. 10, 13, for findings on this issue.) The findings on the percentage of dreams in which the dreamer is an observer are similar to those for young adults in a large-scale study of "observer dreams," which made use of a newly created and more detailed scale with three categories in order to study the frequency of such dreams in children and the elderly as well as young adults (Lipnicki, 2025).

The small percentage of dreamer-only and animal-only dream reports have unique characteristics, which are useful in demonstrating the emphasis on personal concerns in the neurocognitive theory of dreaming. In dreamer-only dream reports, misfortunes are almost twice as likely to occur than in the remainder of the normative sample, which leads to a large effect size (62.8% vs. 33.5%; $h = .59$, $p = .001$). For example, the dreamers are not simply driving alone, they are also facing possible car failure. They are not only walking in the forest, they are also becoming lost. Or they are not only shaving, they also see blood from a cut (Domhoff & Schneider, 2018, pp. 9–10, 13).

The animal-only dreams are distinctive in that the dreamers are often physically attacked or chased by an animal or dangerous insect. The Physical Aggression Percent in animal-only dream reports is 72.2%, compared to 42.4 in the rest of the dream reports, which leads to an unusually large effect size ($h = .62$, $p = .001$). These dreams dramatize the great fear that people have about being attacked by animals, especially animals that are not their pets (Domhoff & Schneider, 2018, pp. 8–10, 13, for details).

The findings on high misfortunes in the dreamer-only dreams and high aggressions in the animal-only dreams lead to another set of findings that support the neurocognitive claim that dreaming is an intensified form of mind-wandering. These findings suggest that dream content is more negative than positive, a claim that is consistent with the finding that there is a "negativity bias" to thoughts during waking (see Johnston & Madson, 2022, for the finding that the negativity bias does not differ between liberals and conservatives; Norris, 2021, for an overview from a neurocognitive point of view; Sparks & Ledgerwood, 2019, for a large-scale study showing the robustness of the negativity bias and its attenuation with age).

The possibility that dream content has a negativity bias can be examined by comparing the percentage of dream reports with at least one aggression, misfortune, or failure with the percentage of dream reports with at least one friendliness, good fortune, or success. By this metric, women's dreams have a negativity bias of 68.2%/48.7%, which can be expressed as a negativity ratio of 1.40. For men, the negativity bias is 73.6%/51.2%, a ratio of 1.65. It is likely that dreaming has a larger negativity bias than waking thought, as reflected by the popular characterization of dreams as "worst-case scenarios."

Overall, the wide range of findings in this section support the neurocognitive theory of dreaming by showing that dreams frequently dramatize the age, gender, cross-national, and cross-cultural similarities and differences that are known to exist in the mental lives of people while they are awake. However, there is a substantial minority of dreams—most likely 10%–30%,—that do not appear to dramatize personal conceptions and concerns. Such dreams are called "adventure dreams" by one of the other researchers who has made note of such dreams (Foulkes, 1999, p. 136). Adventure dreams may draw upon semantic memories that are shared by many people as a result of growing up in the same culture.

Adventure Dreams May Not Dramatize Specific Personal Concerns

A comparison of dreams that have only familiar characters with dreams that have only unfamiliar characters provides a starting point for studying the frequency and nature of adventure dreams. As can be seen in Table 3.6, this comparison shows that there is a sizable minority of dreams that may not have any relation to personal conceptions and concerns. In addition, Table 3.6 reveals a large gender difference on this issue, with only 16.5% of women's dreams containing only unfamiliar characters, compared to 32.6% for men.

TABLE 3.6 The frequency of "familiar" and "unfamiliar" dreams in the Hall/Van de Castle normative samples of women's and men's dreams

	Female norms (n = 491)	*Male norms (n = 500)*
Dreams with only familiar characters	34.8%	24.8%
Dreams with only unfamiliar characters	16.5%	32.6%

TABLE 3.7 The difference between the content of "familiar" and "unfamiliar" dreams

	Female norms			*Male norms*		
	Familiar (n = 171)	*Unfamiliar (n = 81)*	*h*	*Familiar (n = 124)*	*Unfamiliar (n = 163)*	*h*
Male/Female Percent	44%	55%	+.24	55%	70%	+.31**
Aggressor Percent	43%	17%	–.59*	48%	34%	–.27
Physical Aggression Percent	13%	48%	+.78**	30%	62%	+.64**
At Least One Aggression	39%	37%	–.04	40%	53%	+.27*
At Least One Friendliness	43%	33%	–.20	43%	30%	–.26*

Note : ** $p < .01$. * $p < .05$. The p values were determined via approximate randomization.

Moreover, the atypical nature of dreams that lack familiar characters is further evidenced by the other differences in their content. Table 3.7 reveals that such dreams are more dangerous than dreams with familiar characters. These results suggest that these dreams are more like sagas or adventures than the enactments of personal concerns, especially in the case of men.

The distinction between dream reports that express personal conceptions and concerns on the one hand and adventurous dream reports on the other also was examined from a slightly different angle using four general categories of activities that were created for studying this issue. They provide a more substantive, qualitative idea of the everyday activities that occur in a majority of dreams. The first general category concerns familiar characters, who were classified in terms of four subcategories: parents or siblings; spouses, boyfriends, or girlfriends; other family members; and friends. The second category concerned familiar activities, which included five subcategories for commonplace leisure activities—travelling or vacationing; watching or playing sports; going to parties, cafes, or bars; watching entertainers or shows; and shopping. There was also a category for activities that related to school, work, or politics, which had no subcategories. The fourth category, "nothing familiar," was defined by having no instances of any topic in the first three general categories. The nothing-familiar dreams were considered to be instances of adventure dreams.

The first four analyses using these categories were carried out on random samples drawn from four sets of dream reports that were discussed earlier in the chapter on the basis of the Hall/Van de Castle analyses of the full samples. They included 100 normative dream reports from women and 100 from men, along with 100 Miami lab dream reports and 100 Miami non-lab dream reports from nine young male participants, which is an ample sample size for this type of analysis (Domhoff, 2018, p. 66, Table 2.4, 2022, p. 85, Table 3.4, for earlier versions of this analysis; Domhoff et al., 2005–2006, p. 272). In addition, two sets of dream reports from German students—which were mentioned in the earlier discussion of differences in the M/F%—were examined by the bilingual dream researcher who was part of the earlier study, Katrin Meyer-Gomes (Domhoff et al., 2005–2006). The German women contributed 246 dream reports and the German men contributed 95 dream reports. In each of the six examples, the percentage of dream reports that included one or more of the characters and activities in the three main categories—familiar characters, familiar activities, and school/work/politics—was 70% or higher.

Since the figures for the three general "everyday" categories are not mutually exclusive, Table 3.8 compares the percentage of dreams with any familiar element and the percentage with no familiar elements. The results support the distinction between everyday dreams and adventure dreams and once again show the same gender difference, with women having fewer dreams with no familiar people or activities. The fact that the percentage of adventure dreams from both German women and German men is lower than for the American women and men may suggest that cross-national differences might be found in future studies as well.

The results presented in Tables 3.6, 3.7, and 3.8 provide evidence that as many as 16%–18% of women's dreams and 30%–32.8% of men's dream reports may be adventure dreams. However, due to the lack of in-depth information about the participants in most studies of large representative

TABLE 3.8 Number of dream reports that were judged to have at least one familiar element, vs. dream reports containing nothing familiar

	One or more familiar characters or activities	*Nothing familiar: no familiar characters or activities*
Female Norms (100 randomly selected dreams)	82%	18%
Male Norms (100 randomly selected dreams)	74%	26%
Miami non-lab (n = 100)	71%	29%
Miami lab (n = 100)	70%	30%
German women (n = 246)	87%	13%
German men (n = 95)	80%	20%

samples, these results can take us only so far. There is thus a need for in-depth studies of a large number of dream reports from each of several people with widely different backgrounds and interests. One such study is discussed in the next chapter.

Conclusion

The findings on dream content that have been presented in this chapter are consistent with what would be expected on the basis of the imaginative capabilities of the neurocognitive network that gives rise to dreaming. These findings show that this neurocognitive network, based in large part in portions of the default network, can draw on the vast semantic network that it has at its disposal in order to produce dramatizations of the dreamer's conceptions, personal concerns, and personal avocations, whether they involve family or friends, their favorite sports activity, or some of their biggest failures and disappointments. And the combination of a large semantic memory and a capacity to generate spontaneous imaginative thought also leads to a sizable minority of adventure dreams that may not express personal conceptions and concerns.

These many replicated findings are due to the creation of a large number of coding categories that are based on the categorical/nominal level of measurement, the Hall/Van de Castle coding system. Such categories make it possible to make use of virtually every piece of information that is provided in a dream report. The findings are analyzed using percentages and ratios, which do not risk violating any of the assumptions that underlie more complex statistics. Moreover, the statistical results can be checked using approximate randomization, which was recognized many decades ago as the strongest possible method by many of the mathematicians and statisticians who created modern-day statistics—but who did not, at the time, have access to the necessary computing power.

It also bears repeating that the many findings on dream content using the Hall/Van de Castle coding system cannot be replicated with samples with less than 125 dream reports. Even a carefully collected sample with 60–100 dream reports leads to different outcomes, as shown through the earlier-mentioned systematic studies of sample sizes (Domhoff, 1996, pp. 64–67, 2003, pp. 85–86; Domhoff & Schneider, 2008a). To repeat a conclusion from earlier in the chapter, large samples are necessary because (1) the most relevant elements in dreams, such as parents, friends, and children, or aggression, friendliness, sexuality, and misfortunes, appear in less than half of any dream sample; and (2) the substantive differences between dream samples can be small and therefore difficult to detect with samples that contain less than 125 dream reports.

In the case of laboratory-collected dreams, there may be differences from the normative findings if the dream reports are collected on the first or second of several consecutive nights in the sleep-dream laboratory. This is because the vigilance factor in new sleep settings may have impacts on the neurocognitive network that produces dreaming in ways that are as yet unknown in terms of dream content (Tamaki et al., 2016; Wick et al., 2020). Any reported differences from the norms therefore should be replicated before substantive or theoretical claims based on the results of one small study are made.

In addition, the lawful nature of dreams with regard to memory, including the fact that the frequency of appearance reveals the intensity of a personal concern, provides evidence for the conclusion that dreams can be useful. Dreams provide a starting point for people to talk about their personal conceptions and concerns in counseling, clinical, and group-discussion sessions. When given their choice among several topics to discuss, systematic studies suggest that the participants chose talking about their dreams most frequently; furthermore, there is evidence that such discussions in counseling sessions are productive (Hill et al., 1997; Hill & Spangler, 2007). There is also evidence that new personal insights can arise from discussing a dream in a dream group (Blagrove et al., 2019; Edwards et al., 2013).

In order to be more specific concerning many of the substantive issues discussed in this chapter, it is necessary to turn to the excellent databases that arise from a seemingly unlikely source: personal dream journals that have been kept by a very small number of women and men of all ages and from all walks of life, over the course of months, years, or decades. The "dream series" that are written down in dream journals, when made anonymous, digitized, and studied with quantitative methods, are in many ways the polar opposite of the MRDs method. However, they yield overlapping and complementary results when they are studied using either word strings, which are based on a reading of many of the dreams in the dream journal, or Hall/Van de Castle coding categories (Domhoff, 2016, for information on evaluating and analyzing a dream series; Domhoff & Schneider, 2008, for the use of word strings to study some of the many dream series on the DreamBank; Domhoff & Schneider, 2020, for information on the creation of personalized word strings).

Then, too, the explanations that people provide for why they keep a dream journal show that their reasons for developing an interest in dreaming are varied. The entomologist, whose dream series from the summer of 1939 was mentioned early in this chapter, was motivated by scientific curiosity about Freud's widely known claims about dreams. But he also reported that he had experienced some frightening dreams when he was younger (Domhoff, 2022, pp. 119–121). A steel worker, who was convinced that his dreams gave him good clues for betting on upcoming horse races, wrote down 1093 dreams between 1949 and 1964. He sent them to Calvin S. Hall in the mid-1960s after reading about Hall's work in a city newspaper. These dreams are available on DreamBank.net under the pseudonym "Pegasus" (Hall, 1980, for a quantitative analysis of specific aspects of the dreams, which accompanies the full dream series).

A widower wrote down every dream he had about his deceased wife over the course of 22 years—143 dreams in all—because his first several dreams about her after her death, including two in which she seemed to be alive again, had a big impact on him (Domhoff, 2015). A very shy young teenager began writing down her dreams at age 12 because she enjoyed recalling and remembering the dreams she had about the various movie stars on whom she developed a "crush." As a result, she entered 4329 dream reports into a Microsoft Word document between that early age and her mid-20s. Still another young teenager, legally blind since birth, began to tape-record her dreams at age 12 at the suggestion of her mother, who noticed that she appeared to enjoy talking about her dreams in the morning (Domhoff, 2022, pp. 195–206; Domhoff & Schneider, 2020).

The penchant to keep a dream journal is not merely a result of the increased media attention to dreams that resulted from the clinical theories developed by Freud, Jung, and others at the turn of the 20th century. Seven dream journals, stretching back to a well-born and highly educated man living in the Roman Empire about 900 years ago, have been studied in detail using a digital word-search methodology based on standardized word strings (Bulkeley, 2023). Another dream researcher has provided a catalog of still other dreams series from the past, which appears in the context of his quantitative study of his own dream series (Schredl, 2024, Chapter 2). To provide a scientifically inspired example from two years before Sigmund Freud's *The Interpretation of Dreams* (1900) appeared, a physiology graduate student at MIT, who later became a professor at Harvard, wrote down every dream he remembered over the space of six weeks in the winter of late 1897 and early 1898 (see Stiles, 1897–1898, for the dream series and the dreamer's perceptive reflections on what he learned by examining his dream series once he had completed it).

The findings based on quantitative studies of individual dream series, and their theoretical implications, are presented in the next chapter.

4

FURTHER INSIGHTS ABOUT DREAM CONTENT BASED ON STUDIES OF INDIVIDUAL DREAM SERIES

A series of dreams provided by one person has methodological standing in psychology as a type of "personal document." Such personal documents have been recognized by psychologists for many decades as possessing the potential to provide new insights (e.g., Allport, 1942; Webb et al., 1966/1981/2000). They are called "unobtrusive" and "nonreactive" measures, which are valuable precisely because they have not been influenced by the demand characteristics and expectancy effects that can be confounding factors in many types of experiments in the psychological and health sciences (e.g., Corneille & Lush, 2023; Kihlstrom, 2002; Orne, 1962; Rosenthal & Ambady, 1995). Most types of dream research are not immune from these potentially confounding factors.

Therefore, asking friends, the friends of friends, or online volunteers to keep a dream journal for a month or more undercuts the advantages that are inherent in self-motivated individual dream series. Such requests re-introduce all the issues related to demand characteristics and expectancy effects that can potentially compromise experiments and questionnaires. Similarly, scientifically useful dream series cannot come from Internet postings by individuals because posting them is a form of public communication with others for possibly self-serving reasons.

The findings with individual dream series are most rigorous and convincing when they are analyzed without any information about the dreamer. Such blind analyses are necessary even when carefully defined coding categories are used because anything known about the dreamer might influence the coding process. This approach is most convincing when the results of the content analysis of a dream series are used to make specific predictions about a person's conceptions, personal concerns, and avocational interests.

DOI: 10.4324/9781003732969-4

Studies of individual dream series are not simply an accumulation of case studies because coding them with the Hall/Van de Castle coding system turns them into comparable, systematic quantitative data. Second, they can be compared to the Hall/Van de Castle normative samples for women or men, which is similar to comparing an individual's scores on a personality test to the normative findings with that test. Third, individual dream series coded with the Hall/Van de Castle categories can be compared with each other. Fourth, different segments of an individual dream journal—e.g., the first 125 dream reports, the middle 125 reports, and last 125 reports in dream series with 600 for more dreams—can be compared for possible age-related changes on one or more content indicators. The dreams in individual dream series also can be compared from before and after a significant event in the dreamer's life.

In addition, the same statistical analyses, including approximate randomization, can be used in studying individual dream series (e.g., Franklin et al., 1997). Then, too, since dream series are similar to other forms of time-series data, and therefore potentially susceptible to autocorrelation, they can be checked for autocorrelation with a statistical test that is compatible with the nominal/categorical level of measurement. Using this statistical tool, which is available through DreamResearch.net, there was no evidence for autocorrelation in a study of 10 subsets of dream reports, which provided the basis for the 125 separate runs that were used for detecting autocorrelations. These ten subsets were drawn from four different dream series, which showed there was no evidence of autocorrelation (Domhoff & Schneider, 2015).

In keeping with what would be expected by the neurocognitive theory of dreaming, inferences based on blind analyses of dream series—which are then corroborated or rejected on the basis of printed sources, or through interviews with the dreamers and their close friends—reveal that a large majority of dream reports contain content that is continuous with waking conceptions, personal concerns, and avocational interests. At the same time, such an analysis makes it possible to assess the frequency and nature of the adventure dreams that do not appear to dramatize the dreamer's personal concerns.

These conclusions, which are derived from studies of roughly a dozen different dream journals, are revealed most clearly in terms of the frequency with which the main people in the dreamer's life appear, and the way in which they are portrayed in social interactions (e.g., as being aggressive or friendly). There are also clear indications of the dreamer's primary waking avocational interests—e.g., music, sports, traveling (Domhoff, 1996, Chapter 8; 2003, Chapter 5; 2018, Chapter 3; 2022, Chapter 4; Domhoff & Schneider, 2020; Markert & Schredl, 2024). Similar findings are reported in quantitative content analyses of dream series that are found in the dairies kept by well-known novelists (Barrett et al., 2024; Hall & Lind, 1970).

This inference-and-response methodology, which allows the questions to be tailored to the individual case, has proven to be far more successful than attempts that began in the 1950s to correlate dream findings with the results of personality tests (Blagrove, 2007; Domhoff, 1996, pp. 154–156; Hall, 1956, for evidence that personality tests have not proven to be very useful for studies of dream content). In instances in which the dreamer disagrees with the researcher's inferences, interviews with third persons who are friends of the dreamer can serve as the final arbitrator. This is possible because people usually have a very accurate understanding of their friends (e.g., Jackson et al., 2015; Körner & Schütz, 2023, for the most recent evidence on this point).

Building on this methodology, quantitative content analyses of nearly two dozen individual adult dream journals since the late 1940s also reveal that dream content is generally consistent for most individuals over months, years, and decades, but only to the degree that their personal concerns remain consistent (Domhoff, 1996, Chapter 7; 2003, Chapter 5; 2018, Chapter 3; 2022, Chapter 4; Domhoff & Schneider, 2020; Smith & Hall, 1964). This past research reveals that there are three types of consistency: absolute, relative, and developmental. (Many of these dream series are available to one and all for further study on DreamBank, the online research tool mentioned several times in Chapter 3 (Schneider & Domhoff, 1999).)

"Absolute consistency," which also can be called "constancy," means that the frequency of a dream element varies very little over time periods of several months or years. It is this form of consistency that is reported most frequently in the remainder of this chapter, so the general term "consistency" will be used to describe this type of finding unless stated otherwise. "Relative consistency," on the other hand, is defined in terms of one or another dream element always exceeding the frequency of a related element, although one or both of them may increase or decrease in frequency. Finally, "developmental consistency" is defined as a continuous increase or decrease in any dream element (Domhoff, 1996, pp. 133–143, for an overview of the first detailed study of all three types of consistency; 2022, Chapter 4, for a summary of the major studies of consistency in adult dream series; Domhoff & Schneider, 2020, for a study of developmental consistency and absolute constancy in the dream series of two young women from their teenage years to mid-20s).

Rather than trying to demonstrate the usefulness of individual dream series by overviewing numerous different studies, the next subsection will demonstrate the considerable personal detail that can be learned about a person whose dream series has been extensively studied by three different sets of researchers. This focus also makes it possible to demonstrate two of the methods that can be deployed for such an analysis—codings using the Hall and Van de Castle coding system, and word strings that make possible extremely fast searches of a large sample of dream reports for specific names, events, or activities (Domhoff & Schneider, 2008b).

Then, in a briefer section that follows, a person's daytime diary is used in conjunction with their dream series to show in week-by-week detail how intense new personal concerns became prominent in a person's dreams about a week after they were articulated in waking life. However, these new personal concerns disappeared almost entirely from the dream series when they were no longer a part of the dreamer's waking thoughts.

Continuity, Consistency, and Change in a Long Dream Series

"Barb Sanders" was in her early 50s when she attended a panel session on the study of dream content at a meeting of dream researchers in the late 1990s, out of her own curiosity. Following the panel presentations, she introduced herself to the author and offered her ongoing, 20-year dream series for possible future studies.

It later emerged that she had been interested in her dreams since she was in her 20s and had written down several dozen dreams at various times in her early adulthood. Shortly after she divorced her husband of about ten years at age 30, she returned to her home state. She entered graduate school to earn an M.A. degree in a helping profession, which led to a job as a disability counselor at a community college in a Western state. (She left their three daughters, ages 7, 4.5, and 2.5, in the care of her ex-husband during the nine months of the school year.)

At the same time as she was earning her M.A. degree, she also began to keep a dream journal, with the thought that it might help her deal with her post-divorce thoughts and emotions. By this point, her rheumatoid arthritis, which had first caused pain in her feet a week before her wedding at about age 20, had progressed to the point that she often used a pair of canes to walk. Soon thereafter she began to use a wheelchair. Despite this painful disability (which only occasionally appeared in her dreams over the next 20 years), she was involved as an actress, singer, and director in local theatrical productions.

After I satisfied myself that her dream series was authentic through an examination of the files and other written material she provided, I hired five research assistants. All were recent graduates of the University of California at Santa Cruz, who had taken my course on dreams and had done excellent work in carrying out their individual class research projects on a topic of their own choosing. They were therefore ideally suited to work for varying lengths of time on a multi-year study that has led to research projects by two additional independent groups of researchers over a 25-year period (Domhoff, 2003, Chapter 5; 2018, pp. 100–115; 2022, pp. 112–119; Han, 2014; Han et al., 2015; Markert & Schredl, 2024, 2025; Schweickert, 2007b, 2007c;

Schweickert et al., 2020). All of Barb Sanders' dream reports are available on DreamBank for use by interested researchers.

The first study began with a random sample of 250 dream reports that contained between 50 and 300 words, all drawn from the initial sample of 3116 dream reports provided by Barb Sanders. This representative sample became the basis for many subsequent analyses using a variety of methods. Several of these subsequent analyses also made use of the additional 1138 dream reports that Barb Sanders later provided, a total of 4254 dream reports. All but 89 of them were documented between early 1980 and mid-December, 2001. At the same time, one of the research assistants on the Barb Sanders project, Adam Schneider, used his expertise with spreadsheets and websites to create the DreamBank, along with tools on it that make quantitative analyses possible (Schneider & Domhoff, 1999).

Based on many dozens of iterations using the approximate randomization program available through DreamResearch.net and the DreamBank, the first important finding from this study is a methodological one that was first mentioned in Chapter 3. The codings from any 125 of the 250 dreams in the normative Barb Sanders sample replicate the overall results almost exactly. However, as also was the case with the group norms, there are many deviations from the overall results with subsamples of 100 dream reports, and the drop-off is large at 75 and 50, demonstrating once again how risky it is to accept or reject hypotheses based on inadequate sample sizes. To add a new example to those provided in Chapter 3, her Aggressions Per Character Ratio (the A/C index) of .33 with the full sample of 250 dream reports is usually between .30 and .35 with approximate randomization samples containing 125 dream reports, but it ranges from .27 to .39 with samples of 75 (Domhoff, 2003, pp. 113–114).

The first substantive finding (among the many summarized in Table 4.1) concerns the fact that Barb Sanders' dream reports contain both more aggression and more friendliness than the women's normative sample. This result is first of all demonstrated by the Aggressions Per Character Ratio (A/C Index) of .33 that was mentioned in the previous paragraph, which is substantially higher than the normative figure of .23 ($p < .01$). Secondly, Barb Sanders' friendliness per character ratio (the F/C Index) is .32, almost the same as her A/C Index, but higher than the normative figure of .21 for women ($p < .01$) (Domhoff, 2003, Table 5.3).

Barb Sanders' balanced Aggression/Friendliness Percent (49%) is very close to the female normative figure (51%). Despite high levels of both types of interactions, her ratio of aggression to friendliness is therefore not unusual. Moreover, her Physical Aggression Percent is not high; most of the aggressive interactions in her dreams involve angry thoughts toward a person, critical comments, or rejections. In friendly interactions, Barb Sanders' tendency to

TABLE 4.1 The Barb Sanders "baseline" series compared to the Hall/Van de Castle female normative sample

	Female norms	*Barb sanders*	*Effect size*
Characters			
Male/Female Percent	48%	53%	+.11
Familiarity Percent	58%	36%	–.45**
Friends Percent	37%	16%	–.50**
Animal Percent	4%	7%	+.10
Social Interactions			
A/C Index	.23	.33	+.19**
F/C Index	.21	.32	+.22**
Aggression/Friendliness Percent	51%	49%	–.05
Aggressor Percent	34%	50%	+.34**
Befriender Percent	49%	53%	+.07
Physical Aggression Percent	34%	31%	–.05
At Least One:			
Aggression	44%	54%	+.21*
Friendliness	41%	53%	+.24**
Sexuality	3%	20%	+.55**
Misfortune	33%	43%	+.20*

Effect size is given in Cohen's *h* for percent-based indicators, and Cohen's *d* for ratios/indexes. The *p* values were determined via approximate randomization.

Note
* $p < .05$. ** $p < .01$.

be the initiator (the Befriender Percent) is close to average: 53%, vs. 49% for the female norms. But in aggressive interactions, she is the initiator 50% of the time; her Aggressor Percent is well above the female normative figure of 34% ($p < .01$).

These general findings on Barb Sanders' social interaction patterns now can be used to provide profiles of how differently she conceives of the most important people in her life. This analysis is based on codings of all of her social interactions with seven of the most important people in her life in the first 3116 dream reports (Domhoff, 2003, p. 116). All of the inferences that were drawn from the interaction patterns that follow were corroborated by Barb Sanders in the interview with her, and also by those among her four friends who had knowledge about her relationships with one or more of these people. The results have been presented in previous publications (e.g., Domhoff, 2003, Table 5.5), so only three striking contrasts that highlight important theoretical points will be presented here.

First, the coding results suggest that the person of greatest personal concern to Barb Sanders is her mother, who appears more frequently than any other known characters. The analysis reveals that their relationship is a tense one. A graduate of a small denominational college, Barb Sanders' mother worked as a high-school music teacher while raising her four children. Barb Sanders' A/C ratio with her mother (.70) is more than double her baseline for all characters (.33). Similarly, the A/F% between them is 72%, which is much higher than Barb Sanders' normative figure of 49%. In addition, this A/F% is consistent over the entire series, which suggests that her conceptions of her mother did not change over a 20-year period. Barb Sanders described her mother as follows:

> My mother is an angry, isolating person, and she also has good things too, don't get me wrong. But she and I have had a personality clash as long as I can remember. I feel that she keeps herself so distant that I didn't feel I was getting nurturing mother love. I told one of my women friends that the love of my mother is like carrying a barbed blue baby blanket, you know, with barbs in it. It's supposed to be soft and cuddly and loving, but in fact, she was sharp and critical and negative and physically distant.

Barb Sanders' relationship with her father is very different. The A/C ratio with him is .36, which is almost half of what it is with her mother, and not far above her normative figure with all characters. Her F/C ratio with her father is .37, which is slightly above her normative figure of .32, and 10 *h* points higher than it is with her mother. The A/F% with him is 50%, which is far more positive than the A/F% of 72% with her mother. Clearly, her relationship with her father, who taught music in the same school system as her mother did, differs greatly from her relationship with her mother. This contrast provides an excellent example of how specific Hall/Van de Castle studies of dream content can be in portraying a person's conceptions and personal concerns. This contrast is made very clear in Table 4.2.

Barb Sanders' middle daughter, who was 4.5 years old at the time of the divorce, is even more difficult for Barb Sanders than her mother. She ran away from her father's home when she was 14 and came to live with Barb Sanders. She did poorly in school, could not hold a job, and suffered from severe psychological problems. She had a daughter when she was a teenager and left her for Barb Sanders to raise. Barb Sanders worries about this daughter constantly and there is great tension between them.

TABLE 4.2 Aggressive and friendly interactions in Barb Sanders' dreams that include her mother and father

	A/C index	*F/C index*	*A/F%*
Mother	.70	.27	72%
Father	.36	.37	50%

Barb Sanders' A/C ratio with her middle daughter is .92, which is even higher than with her mother, but the F/C ratio (.52) is very high as well, primarily because Barb Sanders is helping her in one way or another. Taken together, these two ratios show that there is a high rate of interaction between them. The A/F% is 64, with Sanders initiating 79% of the aggressive interactions and 70% of the friendly interactions, far above her averages for all characters. These indicators provide an accurate summary of how Sanders conceives of their relationship.

By contrast, Sanders dreams only half as often of her oldest and youngest daughters, both of whom adjusted to the divorce better, went to school in their father's adopted home town, saw their mother regularly during summer vacations, and led normal adult lives. The F/C ratios with both of them are double the normative baseline or more. The positive nature of her relationships with both of them is seen in her A/F % of 44% with the older daughter and 31% with her youngest daughter. As is the case with her middle daughter, Barb Sanders is much more likely to be the initiator of both aggressive and friendly interactions (Domhoff, 2003, p. 116, Table 5.5).

As a final example of how much is revealed about personal conceptions and concerns in a dream series, Barb Sanders' positive relationships with two of her closest friends are apparent in her dreams. However, there are slight differences on some content indicators, which reflect her different patterns of interaction with each of them. Sanders met her closest friend of long standing, Ginny, when she returned to college for her M.A. degree. Ginny's husband and children are also friendly with Barb Sanders, who frequently visited them at their home 90 miles to the north of where she lives. The A/F% of 23 with Ginny is by far the most positive balance with any character. The comradely nature of their relationship is seen in the fact that they are equally likely to initiate friendly or aggressive interactions.

Sanders met another close friend, Lucy, when Lucy was a student at the community college where Sanders was employed and later worked with her in helping disabled students. Lucy, who is partially blind, is outgoing and dramatic, and she and Sanders soon ended up working together in musicals and other theatrical productions. Sanders is the big sister in this relationship, giving Lucy instructions, helping her, and becoming annoyed when Lucy is late or resists direction. This pattern is reflected in the fact that Sanders initiates 78% of the many friendly interactions between them as well as 78% of the relatively few aggressive interactions. The findings for all seven of these important people in Barb Sanders' life are summarized in Table 4.3.

The frequency with which various people appear in the Barb Sanders series has an unexpected lawfulness that is expressed through a mathematical power law—Zipf's Law. This power law is of special interest because it characterizes

TABLE 4.3 Barb Sanders' aggressive and friendly interactions with seven significant people in her life, compared to the codings of the baseline 250 sample

	Number of interactions	*A/C Index*	*F/C Index*	*A/F Percent*	*Aggressor Percent*	*Befriender Percent*
Baseline 250		.33	.32	49%	50%	53%
Mother	239	.70	.27	72%	46%	48%
Father	213	.36	.37	50%	47%	42%
Middle daughter	165	.92	.52	64%	79%	70%
Youngest daughter	83	.36	.81	31%	63%	61%
Oldest daughter	81	.51	.65	44%	73%	77%
Friend Ginny	96	.26	.89	23%	52%	53%
Friend Lucy	59	.39	.63	38%	78%	78%

a wide range of rankings in many different aspects of waking life, such as the frequency with which words are used in the English language or the size of cities throughout the world. This law is expressed as a proportional relationship between two variables by means of an exponent, such as squaring or cubing, although most exponents are *less than one* in networks of dream characters (Schweickert, 2007a, 2007b, pp. 287–289; 2007c).

The striking degree to which the frequency distribution of characters in the Barb Sanders series is mathematically lawful is demonstrated very clearly by the *r*-squared of .91, which quantifies how closely the distribution approximates a straight line. This *r*-squared approaches the perfect fit that is expressed by a correlation of 1.0. This point is shown very clearly in Figure 4.1, which provides a graphic display of the shape of this type of frequency distribution for the eight most-frequent characters in the Barb Sanders series.

In non-mathematical terms, the drop-off in the frequency of appearances from the most frequent dream character to the second-most frequent character is very great, and the drop-off from the second to the third character is almost as large, and so on for a few more characters, until the decline becomes very gradual for the large number of characters that appear relatively infrequently in the dream reports. These findings, which include high frequencies for all three of her children, provide strong evidence for a key concept in the neurocognitive theory of dreaming. There is *continuity* between dream content and the dreamer's waking conceptions and personal concerns with regard to the most important people in her life.

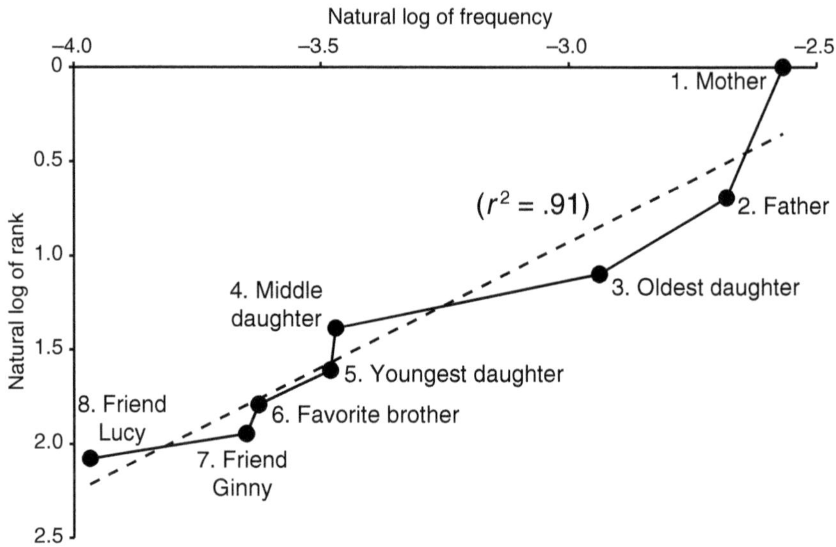

FIGURE 4.1 The eight most frequent characters in Barb Sanders' dreams follow Zipf's Law, which describes the relationship between rank order and frequency.

Source: Adapted with permission from Domhoff (2018, Figure 3.4).

Consistencies in the Barb Sanders Series

The Barb Sanders dream series also provides an excellent platform for studying the issue of "consistency" in a lengthy individual dream series. To begin with, a comparison of the first 125 dream reports in the baseline 250 sample with the second 125 reports determined that her dreams were consistent within 5 or 6 percentage points in all but two or three categories. Her Male/Female Percent fell from 58/42 to 49/51, placing her very close to the female norms of 48/52. It is also interesting that she dreamed less frequently about friends and more about family members, perhaps due to her tensions with her middle daughter and her granddaughter, in the second half of the series, but the Familiarity Percent remained more consistent.

The issue of consistency was also studied by a search of 4146 of her dream reports using a word string in the DreamBank's search utility (Domhoff & Schneider, 2008b; Schneider, 1999; Schneider & Domhoff, 1999); the results were split into five chronological segments of equal size. The word string consisted of the names of 13 people who were important figures in her life—her mother, father, ex-husband, 3 siblings, 3 children, granddaughter, and 3 best women friends. Based on this word search, one or more of these 13 people appeared in 34% of Barb Sanders' dreams; the results for the lowest

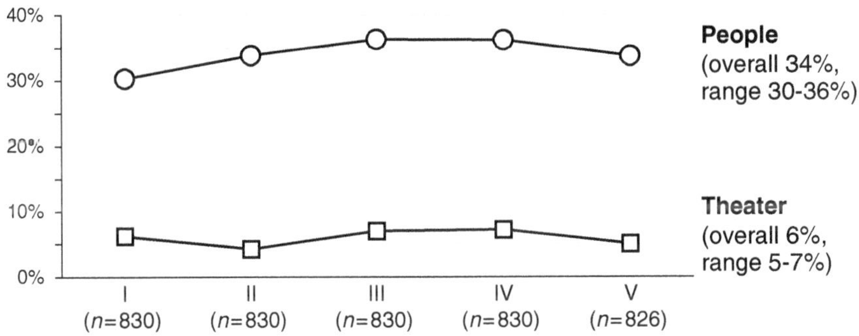

FIGURE 4.2 Consistency in the Barb Sanders series with regard to dreams including significant people in her life, and theater-related dreams.

and highest quintiles were 30% and 36%, respectively, which suggests the great consistency with which these people appear in her dreams.

In addition to the consistency with which the main people in her life appear in her dreams, her dreams are also consistent in portraying her interest in theatrical productions, as a producer, actor, and/or singer. The dreams that concern directing or acting include equal amounts of success and failure. They often include misfortunes as well, which involve just about everything that can go wrong for a producer or actor. Her friend Lucy attests to the fact that Barb Sanders worries constantly about forgetting her lines or being ignored (Domhoff, 2003, pp. 126–128). The consistency over time about the important people in her life and her interest in theatrical productions are presented in more detail in Figure 4.2.

Although the three instances of consistency presented in this subsection demonstrate that Barb Sanders' dream life shows the same kinds of patterns that are found in numerous dreams series, it is nevertheless the case that changes in conceptions and personal concerns can lead to changes in dream content. That is, changing conceptions can lead to changes that can be characterized as "developmental consistencies." This concept also can be demonstrated in detail in the case of Barb Sanders.

Changing Conceptions of Her Granddaughter Lead to Changes in Dream Content

Barb Sanders had a very large role in raising her granddaughter due to the many psychological problems experienced by her middle daughter, as discussed earlier (Domhoff, 2018, pp. 102–103, for the original analysis of her relationship with her granddaughter). Her changing conceptions of this granddaughter from infancy to her mid-teens therefore provide a simple and excellent example of how changing conceptions and personal concerns lead to changes in dream content—a developmental form of consistency. During the granddaughter's infancy, the 14 dreams that included her granddaughter had high frequencies of friendliness and very low frequencies of aggression, which is reflected in an A/F% of 29%, well below her normative figures. And, as might be expected, she initiated 100% of the friendly interactions with her granddaughter at this time.

There were even more friendly interactions in the 33 dream reports that included her granddaughter when she was a young child, as shown by the even lower A/F% (20%) during this period, with Barb Sanders initiating 88% of these interactions. However, when her granddaughter became a preadolescent and then a teenager, Barb Sanders became increasingly frustrated with her due to her deficiencies as a person and student. This frustration led to more aggressive interactions, which were usually initiated by Barb Sanders in the form of angry thoughts, criticisms, and physical punishments. There were also fewer friendly interactions. As a result, her A/F% with her granddaughter rose to 69% in the 93 dream reports during her late childhood, and to 75% in the 65 dream reports during her adolescent years, which are very large changes from when she was a baby (A/F% = 29%) and a young child (A/F% = 20%) (Domhoff, 2018, p. 103, Table 3.4). These later conceptions of her granddaughter—a mixture of anger, disappointment, and exasperation—were strongly expressed by Barb Sanders in our interview.

Changing Conceptions of Her Former Husband

Barb Sanders' 164 dream reports involving her former husband in the first 15 years after they were divorced reveal her conception and dramatization of the negative interactions with him during their marriage. The consistency of this conception over the 15-year period is best reflected in the A/F percentages of 57%, 59%, and 61%, in the first three segments of this subseries. All of these figures are above her baseline with all characters, which is 49%.

However, her conception of her ex-husband began to change at the beginning of the fourth segment. Within a few months after this segment began, he unexpectedly died of a heart attack in his early 50s, without any history of serious illness. At this point the dream reports that include him become more reflective and sometimes include the awareness he is dead, even though she is interacting with him in the dream. The changes in this fourth segment are captured in the dramatic decline of the A/F% from 61% in the third segment to 34% (Domhoff, 2003, pp. 118–122, for a detailed account of her relationship with her ex-husband, including many of the dream reports that dramatize her conception of their relationship, as well as the softening of her relationship with him in the final set of dreams about him).

However, the general change that occurred in the final segment of her dreams about her former husband does not mean that every dream during that time period was a benign one. For example, in a dream that occurred about two years after he died, he came to her house, insisted on sex, and then tried to rape her. She knocked him unconscious and escaped in a car (Domhoff, 2003, p. 121).

The Appearance and Disappearance of a Secret Romantic Infatuation

It is also possible for a new person to come into someone's life and soon thereafter appear in their dreams. Moreover, such a person can disappear from an individual's dreams if she loses interest in them. This important point is demonstrated by the rise and decline of a romantic infatuation that Barb Sanders developed in the fall of 1994, several years after she had dated anyone regularly. She met this much younger, wheelchair-bound man, whom she found very attractive, at a party. She saw him several times at public events due to the fact that they had a mutual interest in the theater and shared some friends in common. Later they were in a dream-sharing group. She quickly became infatuated with "Derek" and expressed her hopes for a romantic relationship with him to her friends, even though he was 12 years younger and did not seem interested in more than a friendship, which Barb Sanders seemed to clearly understand.

Her friends were certain from the outset that she would end up disappointed and worried about her, as they frankly told me in the separate interviews with each of them. At the same time, some of these friends thought that this romantic crush would be reinvigorating for her even if it did not work out. As they feared, Barb Sanders became very upset when Derek showed romantic interest in another woman in her presence. Shortly thereafter, when he came to a meeting of the dream group with a date, Barb Sanders expressed her annoyance to him and ended her friendship with him. After that, she only saw him around town once or twice in passing.

Derek appears in 43 dream reports during the time period in which she hoped a relationship might develop, and then in another four dreams after that. The first dream occurred on October 7, 1994, just a few days after she met him. From that point on, the frequency and content of the dream reports reflect the rise and fall of her romantic hope. Fully 13 of the first 16 dreams she had about him, which occurred before she knew him very well, included intimate physical interactions or sexual relations with him. Although these early dreams are primarily positive in nature, they sometimes dramatized her fear that he did not really care about her (Domhoff, 2003, pp. 122–126 for details, including the text of several dream reports).

The sexual dreams became less frequent as Barb Sanders came to realize that a relationship with him was not going to develop. In addition, her dreams about him portray her as jealous because she learns through the grapevine—in her dream, not in waking life—that he is having sexual intercourse with another woman and becomes very angry. Then, about a month after she had ended their friendship in waking life, she had dreams on two consecutive nights during which she is upset because he is with another woman. One of these dreams included a dramatization in which she says "I am sobbing. My heart is broken. Derek has betrayed *our* relationship with another woman..." (Domhoff, 2003, pp. 124–125, italics added).

Despite these negatively toned dreams at the time when her infatuation is ending in despair, the 43 dreams that include Derek nonetheless have a high rate of friendly and sexual interactions overall, and a low rate of aggressions. They are especially low in physical aggressions compared to the results in the representative sample of 250 of her dream reports, but the size of the Derek sample is too small for statistically significant differences to emerge.

After a five-month period in which Barb Sanders documented 72 dream reports, none of which included Derek, she had a dream in which she told him that she had forgiven him for the many ways in which he had mistreated her. One week later, she had a dream that suggests they were still friends, although she had not seen him during waking life in several months. At that point, Derek had been a character in 43 of the 334 dream reports (12.9%) during the time when her infatuation grew increasingly intense and then declined.

Strikingly, he then essentially disappeared from her dream life. He appeared in only 4 of the following 461 dream reports (0.9%) and did not appear at all in the final 654 dream reports. This disappearance contrasts greatly with the continuing presence of her former husband about 20 years after her divorce. She could let go of her romantic thoughts about Derek, but not of her angry feelings about her marriage. It is therefore noteworthy by way of contrast that she still dreamt about her ex-husband in 8% of the final 100 reports in her dream series in 2001, whereas she had not dreamt about Derek since June, 1998.

In addition to showing that new personal concerns can appear in dreams and then disappear when the personal concerns dissipate, the dreams about Derek also have additional theoretical relevance. They highlight the fact that dreaming is not a reflection or incorporation of waking events. Instead, dreams are a product of our imaginations in that they dramatize events that may or may not have occurred in waking life. This distinction between dreaming as imagination and dreaming as an incorporation of waking events is discussed in Chapter 10, when various dream theories are assessed. At that point several other dream series in addition to Derek's, which also include events that did not happen in the dreamer's waking life, will be discussed briefly in demonstrating the inadequacy of theories that claim dreams are based on the incorporation of waking events.

Character Networks in the Barb Sanders Series

Both consistency and change in Barb Sanders' dream series are strikingly revealed in an innovative study of the social networks in Barb Sanders' full dream series of 4254 dream reports (Han, 2014; Han & Schweickert, 2016). The study is also unique because it examined her waking social network in detail. The study began with the assumption that the characters that appear in the same dream report are linked in the dreamer's waking cognitive social network. Her waking social network was constructed from a questionnaire in which she rated how well each possible pair of people actually knew each other in waking life, and how personally close they were to each other on a 1 (low) to 5 (high) scale (Han, 2014, p. 36). She also rated how close she was to each person on the same five-point scale.

Taken together, there were 120 characters in her dreams whom she knew—9 immediate family members, 55 other relatives, 28 friends, 14 co-workers, 9 boyfriends, and 5 miscellaneous characters. The study found that the pairs of people who appeared together frequently in dream reports were more likely to be connected to each other in waking life. For example, 80% of the 138 pairs of characters who appeared together in at least four dream reports actually knew each other in waking life (Han, 2014, p. 50). The "density" of the networks, defined as the percentage of all possible connections that actually appeared, was .16 in the waking network and .14 in the dreaming network (Han, 2014, p. 47).

These results also reveal that both the waking and dreaming social networks are "small-world networks." This is an important discovery because small-world networks have special properties and are found elsewhere in nature, including the five association networks in the human brain (e.g., Bassett & Bullmore, 2017; Bullmore & Sporns, 2009; Watts & Strogatz, 1998). For example, they differ from random networks in that they include short paths to other people by means of shared connections, and a tendency for the people who appear frequently to appear together (clustering). Then, too, both waking and dreaming social networks have a few characters who are more central to the overall network than others and are connected to each other by a large "general component" (Han, 2014, p. 83; Schweickert, 2007c; Schweickert & Xi, 2010, 2011). Moreover, similar social networks during dreaming were found in a study of five other dream series by the same team of researchers (Han et al., 2015). These findings were also replicated in a study of 696 dream reports that were documented in the year 2015 (Schredl

& Schweickert, 2022). These findings show that dreams are far more lawful than is often assumed.

A centrality measure based on how connected a person is to other well-connected people revealed a high correlation between the dream and waking-life networks in the Barb Sanders series. Her immediate family members were the ten most central characters in both networks, and her mother and father had the highest centrality scores in both networks. Very significantly in terms of the neurocognitive theory of dreaming, her network of dream characters more often brought together immediate family members, other relatives, and friends than was the case in waking life (Han, 2014, pp. 48–49, Figures 5 and 6). That is, the people that Barb Sanders cared about the most in waking life tended to appear together in dreams, even though they were not in the same social networks in waking life (Han, 2014, pp. 50, 67).

These co-appearances support a key tenet of the neurocognitive theory of dreaming—the frequency of appearances in dream reports reveals the intensity of personal concerns in waking life. This is because the people she thought about the most in waking life were brought together in dreams even though they were often in her different—non-overlapping—social networks in waking life—e.g., her family network, her network of friends, and her network of co-workers. Put another way, she tended to bring together in her dreams the people about whom she expressed the closest connections, even though they were in different social networks in waking life.

The study also discovered yet another consistency in the Barb Sanders dream series by breaking it into four separate parts. The density of the network and the degree of clustering of characters were the same over time, and the people who appeared frequently at the start of the series were the most likely to persist over time, including family members and women friends (57 of the 120 people appeared in all four subsets) (Han, 2014, p. 68). In addition, the persisting characters tended to be connected to the same people that they were connected to in the first of the four subsets, although the number of these connections diminished over time and some new ones appeared (Han, 2014, p. 96). Then, too, the centrality of characters sometimes shifted to some extent, but her mother and father were the most central figures in the first three subsets. Her granddaughter, as might be expected on the basis of the earlier analysis of Barb Sanders' dreams about her, gradually rose in centrality from the first to the third subset and became the most central figure in the fourth subset (Han, 2014, p. 83).

In all, this overview of several of the main findings on continuity, consistency, and change in the Barb Sanders series provides excellent evidence that the neurocognitive theory of dreaming is on solid ground in emphasizing the importance of these three features of dreaming. The findings with her dream series support in great detail the many past studies that led to this emphasis, an emphasis that has not been incorporated into other theories of dreaming (Bell & Hall, 1971; Domhoff, 1996, pp. 133–145, for detailed summaries of Hall's first two major studies of consistency in dream series; Hall & Lind, 1970; Smith & Hall, 1964).

Barb Sanders' High Percentage of Adventure Dreams

For all the detailed evidence on the ways in which Barb Sanders' dreams consistently portray her main personal conceptions and concerns, her dream series is nonetheless distinctive for the degree to which it also includes adventure dreams. As shown in Table 4.1 earlier in the chapter, her Familiarity Percent is 22 percentage points below the women's norms, an h of $-.45$ that is significant at the .01 level. Since her baseline 250 dreams have a typical Family Percent, it can be inferred that her lower Familiarity Percent is driven by a lower Friends Percent, an unexpected conclusion in that she has several close friends. Moreover, her dreams with no familiar characters are higher than her dreams with familiar characters on Animal Percent ($h = +.21$, $p = .01$) and Physical Aggression Percent ($h = +.41$, $p = .01$), and lower on Aggressor Percent ($h = -.41$, $p = .01$), which means she is a victim of aggression in her adventure dreams far more often than she is the aggressor.

Due to the fact that the overall Barb Sanders series includes over 4000 dream reports, it was possible to make more specific studies of adventure dreams that had similar content. To take one extensive example, there are 33 dream reports in the overall series in which she is holding or shooting a gun. In these dreams she also fixes and reloads guns, kills dangerous animals, and even fights off human attackers. In one dramatic dream, she captures seven men at gunpoint. In still another, she takes a woman's gun away from her and then kills her with it. Although these dreams seem to suggest she has an interest in guns and is proficient with them, she said that she did not like guns and had rarely shot one. She had done some target shooting at a range to be companionable with her then-husband, but that was the extent of her involvement with guns (Domhoff, 2003, p. 130).

There are also 24 dreams in the overall series in which Barb Sanders is riding a horse and sometimes wielding a gun as well. However, contrary to any suggestion that any aspect of these dreams dramatize any waking interest in horses, she explained during extensive questioning that she had only been on a horse a few times in her younger days, usually when a horse trainer led the horse around a ring:

> It's not, it's not a real-life experience. I think I have ridden horses max eight times in my whole life, you know, and I can remember the specific incidences. Somebody else held the horse, one had a tendency to bite and I was very afraid of him, and we sort of walked slowly around the pasture.

Another one, that one was okay, but it got spooked by another horse that started running, so I was just hanging on for dear life.

(Domhoff, 2003, p. 129)

Although the Barb Sanders series is the only series that has been studied systematically in terms of adventure dreams, it provides support for the conclusion that a significant minority of dream reports do *not* dramatize personal conceptions and concerns—perhaps in the range of 13%–35%, if the figures for both women and men are included in this estimate. Then, too, Barb Sanders' adventure dreams provide further evidence that dreams are fundamentally imaginative in their nature. Adventure dreams do not simply incorporate or reflect elements of the culture that surrounds us from the early years of life. It is our individual imaginations that determine which few elements in the boundless possibilities that culture provides are sometimes the basis for adventure dreams.

Beverly: The Rise and Fall of a New Personal Concern

Beverly, a divorced woman in her 60s, who has an M.A. in Early Childhood Studies and is retired in a Sunbelt state, has kept a record of her dreams for over 35 years. Happily, she also kept a brief daily dairy as well, which is what makes this analysis possible. Recent aspects of her dream series are relevant to the theoretical concerns of this chapter because they provide good evidence that a new personal concern begins to appear in dream reports shortly after the new personal concern is expressed during waking life and then gradually disappears after the new waking concern begins to decline. This analysis occurs within the context of earlier findings developed on the Beverly series by another dream researcher, who used 17 generic word strings to discover that her main personal concerns have persisted in her dream series for several decades (Bulkeley, 2018).

The recent aspects of Beverly's dream series that are relevant to the purposes of this chapter focus on her personal concern with helping people to deal with the COVID-19 pandemic in 2020, and in particular with helping lower-income people to obtain face masks to protect themselves and others. The fact that she also kept the aforementioned daytime diary makes this example highly useful in tracing the relationship between a sudden new waking personal concern and its subsequent appearance in her dreams. (I did not receive any of the information in the following paragraphs until I sent an email to her on November 5, 2020.)

Beverly first mentions COVID-19 in her daytime journal on February 22, 2020, and then discusses it more fully on February 28, when she calls the coronavirus a "threat" and writes that she worries because "lots of people could die." She expresses concerns about flu-like symptoms on March 1 and wakes up "with her head spinning" and a runny nose on March 3. However, she soon realized she did not have the virus. Beverly documented 11 dream reports between March 1 and March 9 but did not recall a dream related to the pandemic until March 10, which is over two weeks after she first mentioned COVID-19 in her daytime diary, and nine days after she developed flu-like symptoms.

This first dream is of interest because it did not directly express the personal fears she had concerning the dangers of being sick with COVID-19. In the dream she was wearing mittens to pick weeds because they would “help stop the spread” of the disease. The tangential way in which COVID-19 appeared in this dream is in fact similar to what was also found in the ongoing dream series of five other women, ranging in age from 18 to 19 to their mid-30s (see Domhoff, 2022, pp. 129–133, for an analysis of each of these dream series). (As was the case with Beverly, I did not ask these five women for their dream series until early November, 2020.) In a combined total of 382 dreams in the first ten months of 2020, only 18 (4.7%) of their dreams included a mention of the virus or the pandemic, and often in a peripheral way, unlike what has been found in online surveys. (See Domhoff, 2022, and Incelli & Gallagher, 2022, for methodological critiques of the online studies of the frequency of dreams about COVID-19; it is likely that they greatly overestimate the frequency and bizarreness of dreams about the virus.)

A day after documenting her first pandemic-related dream, Beverly wrote in her diary that COVID-19 is “really scary” and expressed her fear that she might “get the bad virus if I don’t have it already.” She continued to comment on COVID-19 in her diary over the next several days and recorded 11 more dreams before she wrote down her second pandemic-related dream on March 18. In this dream she was helping the police at a “crime scene” to figure out what to do with boxes that might have been in some way infected by the virus. This helping theme then persisted in her dreams related to COVID-19 over the next 7.5 months. For example, from March through August, she had 47 dreams mentioning the virus, 79.8% of which portrayed her helping people in one of several ways (Domhoff, 2022, pp. 133–135, for further details and dream excerpts).

In April, Beverly decided to contribute to the effort to mitigate the impact of the pandemic by making masks that would be distributed to people through various nonprofit organizations. Her increasing involvement in this effort from April through September, and the decline in her focus on this project in October and early November, continued to appear in her daytime diary from April through September. Then she mentions mask-making only twice in October—once early in the month, and then again on the last day of the month.

The concern with COVID-19 and making masks follows the same pattern in her dream series. In April when she was just getting into a rhythm on her sewing work, only one of her 25 dreams was about sewing masks, and another 6 were pandemic-related, with the other 18 dreams focusing on other personal concerns. More generally, 36 of her 159 dream reports from

May through September involved the coronavirus in one way or another, which is 22.6% of the total number of dreams she documented in this time period. Fourteen of those 36 (39.9%) relate to her concern about making and distributing masks. In October and early November, she documented 27 dreams, only 4 of which (14.8%) related to the pandemic in any way, and even fewer, 2, related to making and distributing masks.

Beverly's declining interest in mask-making during October is discussed in her diary entry for October 30. Reflecting on the past several months, she noted how much her "priorities had changed" when the pandemic hit, and that she had been making 100 masks or more each week for several months. She further noted that she only had made 100 masks in the month of October—which was only 25% of her production level of the previous several months. Three days later she wrote that "maybe it's time to hit pause" because "everyone has a mask."

Nor did the deep personal concerns that Beverly developed about the pandemic and about making masks have any lasting impact on her dream life. An examination of her dreams from 2021 through 2023, based on the relevant records obtained from her in November, 2024, showed that mentions of protective masks or the disease itself appeared in only 4.5% of the 381 dream reports she wrote down in 2021. This figure declined even further, to 0.7% of 398 dreams in 2022 and 0.9% of 337 dream reports in 2023. This analysis of the rise, decline, and near-disappearance of COVID-19 and mask-making from Beverly's dreams suggests that events, and activities related to those events, can decline in dreams, or disappear altogether, if they are no longer a waking personal concern.

This analysis of the rise, decline, and near-disappearance of COVID-19 and mask-making from Beverly's dreams, when combined with the disappearance of Barb Sanders' romantic crush, Derek, from her dreams, suggests that events and activities, as well as people, can decline, or disappear altogether, in dreams if they are no longer a waking personal concern. Once again, it can be concluded that there is continuity and consistency in dream content only to the degree that the dreamer continues to have the same personal concerns during waking life. And once again, these analyses demonstrate the validity of a key axiom in the neurocognitive theory of dreaming: the frequency of a topic or person in a set or series of dream reports reveals the intensity of a personal concern in the waking mind.

Conclusion

When the many normative, cross-national, and indigenous societal similarities presented in Chapter 3 are combined with the individual differences revealed by the studies of personal dream journals in this chapter, the results suggest that dreams are best characterized by their several pan-human similarities on the one side, and by their substantial individual differences on the other. The relatively few gender differences, although very real and often replicated, and the several cross-national and indigenous differences, seem to be secondary to the dreaming mind.

In the case of the Barb Sanders series, this chapter shows in considerable detail that it is possible to draw many correct inferences about a dreamer's specific relationships with the characters that appear most frequently. The analysis of her dream reports demonstrates once again that the frequency of the appearance of any given character, or of a personal avocation, reveals the intensity of the dreamer's concern with that character or avocation. In addition, the large number of dreams in the Barb Sanders made it possible to demonstrate with greater certainty than was possible in Chapter 3 that there are a significant minority of adventure dreams in addition to the many dreams that express personal concerns. It also seems likely that Barb Sanders has a higher percentage of adventure dreams than was found in the group data for women in Chapter 3. If so, it may be possible to add that there are individual differences in the frequency of adventure dreams as well as gender and possible cross-national differences.

At the same time, the striking findings on the lawfulness of character networks in dream series, in terms of both Zipf's power law and small-world networks, suggest that dreaming is based on many of the same principles that govern waking memory to a greater extent than was realized in the past. This emphasis on the similarities with the findings on several aspects of waking memory is shown once again in Chapter 8 when the factors involved in dream recall are discussed.

Most generally, the findings in this and the previous chapter document the discoveries and successes of the quantitative analysis of dream content over a period of nearly 70 years. Moreover, this labor-intensive work over seven decades may be only a starting point: it is likely that Artificial Intelligence (AI)-based tools (e.g., Bongalon, 2025) will be able to carry out Hall/Van de Castle codings much faster than humans. Although several of the more complex codings carried out by the DreamCoder would have to be checked for accuracy by a trained human coder, the savings in time and money would still be extremely large, and therefore well worth the extra human effort.

Chapter 2 demonstrated that the neurocognitive theory of dreaming is consistent with basic findings on visual imagery, imagination, and the development of an autobiographical self in waking academic studies in psychology and the neurosciences. Chapter 3 and this present chapter have shown that the neurocognitive theory of dreaming readily encompasses solid empirical findings on dream content that go back to the early 1950s. It therefore becomes of interest to determine exactly when, how, and why the unique neurocognitive network specified in Chapter 2 becomes activated and relatively ascendant over the frontoparietal control network. The appearance of this neurocognitive network in the sleep-onset process, long before REM sleep occurs, is demonstrated in the next chapter.

5

DREAMING DURING THE SLEEP-ONSET PROCESS

The sleep-onset process provides a challenging initial setting for examining the relationship between the frontoparietal control network (FPCN) and the neurocognitive network that gives rise to dreaming. The likelihood that a person is dreaming, not simply thinking about the events of the day or mind-wandering, increases gradually throughout the first few minutes of the sleep-onset process—which can be as short as 7–9 minutes or as long as 16–20 minutes. The early phase is initially indicated by the appearance of the first of the two electroencephalogram (EEG) rhythms discussed in Chapter 2, alpha waves. Dreaming then makes a small jump in frequency and complexity with the arrival of theta waves. The frequency of dreaming during the sleep-onset process then gradually declines for a minute or two, for reasons that are not known, until sleep formally begins.

Although the dreams during the sleep-onset process are less frequent, shorter, and sometimes less internally coherent than dreams during rapid eye movement (REM) sleep and are almost always forgotten, dreaming during sleep onset is important for theoretical reasons. First, it demonstrates that dreaming can occur outside of sleep, and without any preceding REM sleep. Second, it demonstrates in a step-by-step fashion how the neurocognitive network that produces dreaming gradually ascends over the space of a few minutes, at the same time as the relative deactivation of the FPCN is occurring. Moreover, in one study that will be discussed later in the chapter, researchers could not accurately separate the sleep-onset dreams from the REM dreams collected from the same participants.

In addition to including brief moments of dreaming, sleep onset is also a time when, "quite simply, everything changes," according to a synthesis of 35 years of sleep-onset research that appeared at the beginning of the 21st

DOI: 10.4324/9781003732969-5

century. "*There is not a single human physiological, cognitive, subjective, or behavioral system which is unaltered by the process of falling asleep*" (Ogilvie, 2001, p. 259, italics in the original). Twenty-three years later, on the basis of a thorough analysis that included more recent research, another team of sleep dream researchers similarly concluded that the sleep-onset process involves numerous changes in neurophysiological and neurocognitive processes as "brain activity slows down, muscles relax, heart rate lowers, consciousness and responsiveness to the environment fluctuate ..." (Lacaux et al., 2024, p. 273).

The complex changes during the sleep-onset process also include a decline in information flow from posterior to frontal areas of the brain, as indexed by a decrease in alpha waves in posterior areas and a concomitant increase in alpha waves in frontal areas. Thus, changes in the anterior/posterior ratio in alpha (the A/P ratio) become a good indicator of these changes, as does an increase in theta waves (De Gennaro et al., 2004; Gorgoni et al., 2019; Hori et al., 1994; Vecchio et al., 2017). These findings set the stage for the neurophysiological and neuroimaging studies of the sleep-onset process, which are discussed in the next section.

The Neurophysiology of the Sleep-Onset Process

Although the phrase "falling asleep" suggests that the sleep-onset process is one of gradual deactivation as people become "tired," in fact the transition into sleep involves an "active process of inhibition of the multiple arousals circuits" that are "essential for wakefulness" (Jones, 2020, p. 6). The initiatory points for this inhibitory process are located in two very specific areas in the brainstem: the lateral pons and the midbrain, which were shown in Figure 1.2. They are supported in these efforts by areas within the basal forebrain, which reduce their release of the neurochemicals that support brain activation.

The pons/midbrain portion of the sleep-onset network also propagates its signals to an area just above—"dorsal to"—the midbrain, called the hypothalamus. The hypothalamus is important in the sleep-onset process because it includes an area—the ventrolateral preoptic area—that is highly active in promoting sleep onset. It also includes the timers and clocks of the brain, which are in the suprachiasmatic nucleus. These timers and clocks have a major role in controlling several bodily rhythms, including the circadian rhythms that are essential to the wake/sleep cycle. The hypothalamus has the further capacity to propagate messages to many other areas in the brain, as well as to send messages back to the midbrain and lateral pons. In that regard, the hypothalamus is more than a way station. It is a subcortical control room that has an important role in the transition into sleep.

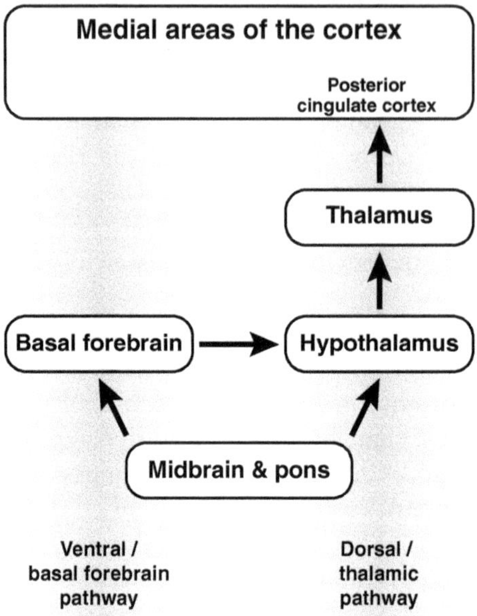

FIGURE 5.1 A schematic diagram of the subcortical neural substrates that work together to bring about sleep onset.

Note: The actual locations of the subcortical brain regions in this diagram were shown in Figure 1.3.

As important as the hypothalamus is to the transition into sleep, the thalamus stands at the pinnacle of this process because it is in close communication with the cortical regions just above and surrounding it. More exactly, the anterior region of the thalamus is connected to portions of the posterior cingulate cortex, a relationship that was discussed in Chapter 2 with regard to the feeling of drowsiness. In effect, this and the previous two paragraphs outline the subcortical regions that are involved in the feeling of drowsiness (McGinty & Szymusiak, 2022). The thalamus also has a role in regulating the sleep-wake cycle, based in part on the information it receives from the suprachiasmatic nucleus in the hypothalamus. The main areas in the wake-suppression/sleep-promoting network that are involved in the sleep-onset process are shown in the schematic in Figure 5.1.

The Sleep-Onset Process at the Neurocognitive Level

The decreasing activation levels in the forebrain lead to an accompanying symphony of changes at the neurocognitive level. As readers may recall from the discussion of drowsiness in Chapter 2, the sleep-onset process includes a gradual disconnection of the posterior cingulate cortex from the dorsal attention network, which aids the frontoparietal control network in regulating the default network during waking. This gradual disconnection is accompanied by an increasing connectivity and relative ascendancy within the anterior portions of the default network, as also noted in Chapter 2 (Chang et al., 2013; Dixon et al., 2017). This increasing connectivity and the relative ascendancy of areas within the default network are essential to dreaming.

It is at this juncture that the FPCN consistently shows "reduced activity in the frontoparietal cortices and thalamus" (Lacaux et al., 2024, p. 276). This reduced activation—in both the FPCN and the thalamus—is an important step, not only in the sleep-onset process, but in terms of the neurocognitive theory of dreaming. This is because, to recall the more detailed analysis in Chapter 2, the posterior areas in the thalamus are part of the salience/ventral network—a network that is essential in aiding the FPCN in constraining the default network during waking. Since the salience/ventral network is also critical in preparing the body for immediate action in response to both internal and external alerting signals relating to danger, this decline in its activation levels indicates that there is less attention and vigilance with regard to the monitoring of sensory input (Chang et al., 2013, p. 230; Menon & Uddin, 2010; Seeley et al., 2007). This decline is therefore a factor in making it possible for the activated portions of the default network to produce dreaming during the sleep-onset process.

Neuroimaging studies of the sleep-onset process, several of which were combined EEG/fMRI studies, conclude that the subcortical neurophysiological changes discussed above are accompanied by the relative deactivation of the FPCN and the two attention networks, while at the same time the default network remains relatively activated (e.g., Horovitz et al., 2009; Picchioni et al., 2008; Sämann et al., 2011). In fact, one of these studies determined that the relative activation level of the default network increased within the first 30 seconds of the sleep-onset process (Picchioni et al., 2008, p. 81). Still another study with a large sample size (57 participants, 39 of whom were women) made use of a different method for analyzing the neuroimaging data. The research team concluded that the default network might "serve a gate-function..." (Stevner et al., 2019, p. 12). The idea that the default network might serve a gateway function provides an ideal image from the perspective of the neurocognitive of dreaming. It is likely that these are the processes that are also captured by the detailed EEG studies revealing a decline in information flow from posterior to frontal areas of the brain and by the frontalization of alpha. This transition is indexed by the aforementioned increase in the A/P ratio (De Gennaro et al., 2004; Gorgoni et al., 2019; Hori et al., 1994; Vecchio et al., 2017).

EEG Studies of Dreaming during the Sleep-Onset Process

The fMRI studies that also included EEG recordings further support the use of alpha and theta waves as useful indicators for studying mind-wandering and dreaming. Their appearances parallel the unfolding neurocognitive transition process, with the frequency of alpha waves gradually declining and the frequency of theta waves gradually increasing, as the FPCN deactivates and portions of the default network become ascendant. In addition to the alpha and theta rhythms, there are two other EEG indicators related to sleep onset and sleep that are relevant to these analyses. "Vertex waves," which are sharp, saw-toothed waves of relatively high amplitude (12–13 Hz), often intermingle with theta waves. (They derive their name from the area in the center of the brain, the "vertex," where the frontal, parietal, and temporal lobes meet.)

The other new sleep-related EEG indicator introduced in this chapter, "sleep spindles," are bursts of high-amplitude waves (12–14 Hz.). They are relevant here because their appearance marks the fact that the sleep-onset process has ended and sleep has begun, as formally defined in a set of definitions relating to sleep, which were created by members of the Association for the Psychophysiological Study of Sleep in 1968 (Rechtschaffen & Kales, 1968). This standardized scoring system for EEG records has been updated several times since 1968 because of the advent of machine scoring and the use of automated algorithms, but sleep spindles maintain their traditional definitional role (de Chazal et al., 2022). Table 5.1 contains an overview of the four sleep-related EEG indicators that are mentioned in this chapter—alpha waves, theta waves, vertex waves, and sleep spindles.

Building on the knowledge that alpha and theta rhythms are useful as biomarkers in studying dreaming, the next subsection discusses two sets of studies from two different research groups that focused on dreaming and dream content. These two sets of studies were carried out in the pre-neuroimaging era in two different countries—the United States and Japan—a decade or more apart. Taken together, these several studies provide a replicated set of findings that can be used for drawing conclusions about the degree to which dreaming occurs during the sleep-onset process. (To reduce confusion in comparing these two sets of studies, they will be referred to as the "Foulkes studies" and the "Hori studies," based on the lead roles played by these two researchers.)

The first set of studies from the pre-neuroimaging era, three separate studies in all, included a total of 64 participants, 40 women, and 24 men (Foulkes & Schmidt, 1983; Foulkes et al., 1966; Foulkes & Vogel, 1965). The researchers began with four EEG stages—two based primarily on alpha, one based on the appearance of theta, and one based on the appearance of sleep spindles, which it will be recalled mark the beginning of sleep. In the

TABLE 5.1 Four EEG waveforms/rhythms that relate to mind-wandering, drowsiness, and the sleep-onset process

Name of pattern	*Frequency*	*Description*	*Illustration*
Alpha	8–13 Hz	Alpha waves are often present in drifting waking thought. They are also found in the sleep-onset process and sometimes in REM.	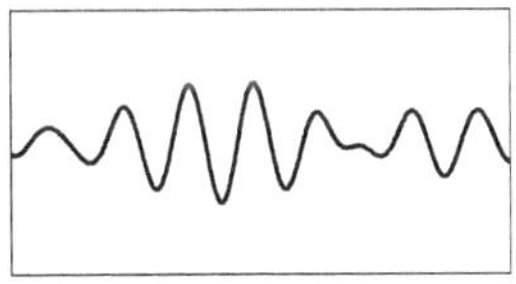
Theta	4–8 Hz	Theta waves are sometimes present in drifting waking thought, are present in the later half of the sleep-onset process, and are prominent in REM sleep.	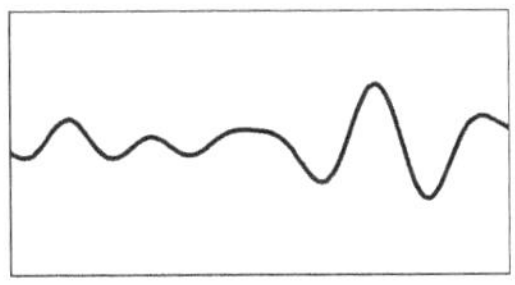
Vertex	n/a	Vertex waves (V waves) are brief, sharp, V-shaped waves that can be detected in some parts of the brain during sleep onset.	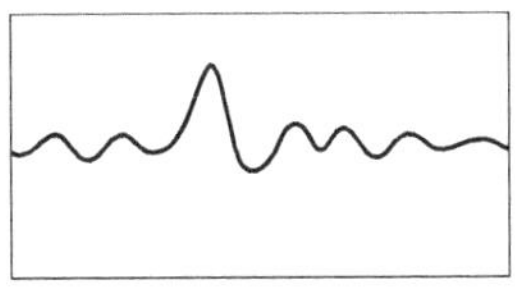
Sleep spindles	12–15 Hz	Sleep spindles (sometimes called Sigma waves) occur in half-second bursts, at sleep-onset and in N2, early in the sleep process.	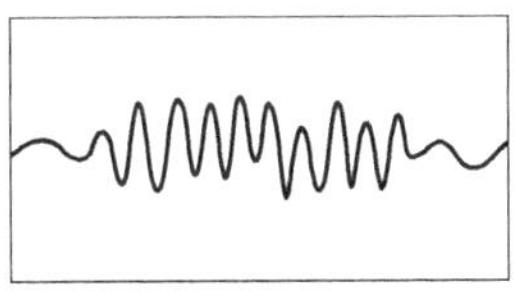

initial study, the participants arrived to the sleep laboratory close to their normal bedtimes and were randomly contacted within each of the four sleep-onset intervals by calling out their names. They were then asked "what were you experiencing just before I called you?" (Foulkes & Vogel, 1965, p. 232). The nine participants, one woman and eight men, were then asked a series of questions, starting with the degree to which they felt awake and the degree to which they felt in control of their thoughts. They were also asked subsequent questions concerning the nature of the experience they had reported.

This procedure led to 212 successful sleep-onset calls over the space of four separate sessions with each participant. The participants invariably reported some form of cognitive activity, which mostly consisted of what is now called mind-wandering. The researchers concluded that all of the participants went through the same general process of increasing drowsiness and a declining sense of volitional control. Once participants no longer subjectively felt they were awake and in control of their thoughts, an increasing number of their

TABLE 5.2 The main findings on dreaming and dream content during various EEG patterns associated with the sleep-onset process

	Alpha 1	*Alpha 2*	*Theta*	*Sleep spindles*
Are you controlling your thoughts?	60%	33%	0%	0%
Are you aware that you are in the laboratory?	67%	33%	17%	0%
Percent of reports that are dreams	31%	43%	76%	71%
Self as character	62%	78%	83%	97%
Other characters	69%	83%	100%	81%

Source: These findings are drawn from Foulkes and Vogel (1965).

reports could be classified as dreams, which were defined in this study as dramatic episodes that the participants experienced as "really" happening (Foulkes & Vogel, 1965, p. 239). In addition, the participants appeared more frequently as characters in their dream reports as the sleep-onset process unfolded, as did other characters. The specific findings related to these generalizations are presented in Table 5.2.

However, there were significant individual differences in the frequency with which the participants reported dreamlike content in the different stages. For example, five of the nine participants had "frequent dreams" when in one of the two alpha stages and the other four participants only reported dreams when they were in the theta and sleep-spindle stages and did so far less frequently than the other five participants (Foulkes & Vogel, 1965, p. 238). This finding at least in part reflects the fact that alpha and theta are not perfect indicators of the relative ascendancy of the neurocognitive network that produces dreaming. However, it also very likely expresses individual differences that are not well understood.

The investigators concluded that the "typical" dream report during the sleep-onset period is "no less well organized than its REM-period counterpart," which they drew from an earlier REM-awakening study based on other participants. However, there are more "fleeting progressions of visual imagery or dissociated images and thoughts" in sleep-onset reports than there are in REM dream reports (Foulkes & Vogel, 1965, p. 238). The researchers also noted that there were few or no instances of the several striking imagistic phenomena that are alleged to occur during the sleep-onset process. Claims about these imagistic phenomena, including spectacular light shows, large bodily distortions, a sense of falling, and abstract thoughts turning into imagery, have been made repeatedly in popular accounts based on questionnaire surveys, clinically based case studies, or anecdotal reports in one or another media story (Foulkes & Vogel, 1965, p. 242).

In an immediate follow-up study, 32 participants, 16 women and 16 men, were studied for one night by means of four separate calls to them. The calls were made at various points in the first two of the four categories that these investigators used to analyze the sleep-onset process (Foulkes et al., 1966, p. 281 and footnote 2). The participants were also called during the second, third, and fourth REM periods, which provided the basis for close comparisons of sleep-onset reports and the REM reports from the same participants. They were also given a battery of personality tests that are not relevant to the purposes of this book and in any case led to tentative and meager results that were not pursued in further studies.

The rate of dream recall from the 128 calls during the first two stages of the sleep-onset process was 39.1%, which is not very different from the range of recall rates for those two stages in the initial study (31%–44%), as presented in Table 4.3. On the other hand, this 39.1% recall rate from sleep-onset calls is far below the recall rate of 69.1% for the successful 78 awakenings from REM periods for the same participants (Foulkes et al., 1966, p. 282).

Although there were fewer reports of dreaming during sleep onset to analyze in this study, the dream reports from sleep onset and REM sleep did not differ in their dreamlike quality according to two independent raters who did not know whether the reports they were judging were from sleep onset or REM arousals (Foulkes et al., 1966, p. 282). As in the initial study, there were large individual differences in the frequency of reports from sleep-onset calls, with no recall at all for eight of the participants, and 100% recall for two others. The other 22 participants had overall response rates ranging from 25% to 75% (Foulkes et al., 1966, p. 283).

The third study, which took place over the course of three non-consecutive nights, was primarily focused on a very detailed analysis of dream reports from REM and non-REM sleep. However, the 23 participants, all women, were first of all called by vocalizing their names four different times when theta waves appeared in the later portions of the sleep-onset process (Foulkes & Schmidt, 1983, p. 267). This focus on contacting them during theta bursts provided a contrast with the focus on alpha awakenings in the second study. Overall, the calls from the experimenters when theta rhythms were appearing resulted in dream reports from 88% of the 92 sleep-onset calls to the 23 participants in the course of the three experimental nights, which is not a statistically difference from the 93% recall of dreams from REM awakenings by the same participants (Foulkes & Schmidt, 1983, p. 268).

While it is possible that the high percentage of dream reports from both sleep onset and REM sleep in this study may be inflated by the frequency and length of the arousals that were made, it is noteworthy that the participants nonetheless were characters in only half of their sleep-onset reports, compared to the appearance of the dreamer herself in virtually all of the REM reports.

The sleep-onset reports also had a lower overall character density than the REM reports, and the narrative flow of the sleep-onset reports was not as smooth. The sleep-onset reports had a "jumpier" quality according to two independent judges, who did not know whether they were rating a sleep-onset report or a REM report (Foulkes & Schmidt, 1983, p. 272). In the end, then, the sleep-onset reports in this study differed from REM reports in the same ways as they did in the first two studies in this series.

However, obtaining detailed information on the content of what the participants were experiencing also meant that the sleep-onset process was interrupted for relatively long periods of time in these three studies. These periods of wakefulness may have inflated the findings by keeping the brain at higher activation levels than is usual for the sleep-onset process. As the main investigator in these studies later noted, the timing and frequency in such studies may be "overestimated" because the participants "have been awakened again and again as they fall asleep..." (Foulkes, 1985, p. 69). They therefore may become "somewhat self-conscious about falling off to sleep..." and "the results may be a prolongation of the sleep-onset process, and a consequently greater than usual opportunity to dream a REM-like dream" (Foulkes, 1985, p. 69). (The length of the sleep-onset process was not mentioned in the three Foulkes studies.)

The greater detail and rigor in the second set of studies thereby can serve as both a control group and conceptual replication study in relation to the first set of studies. The first study in this second set of studies—"the Hori studies"—began by examining the appearance of alpha and theta during 5-second epochs throughout the 16–20-minute sleep-onset process that was typical for this study. This extremely fine-grained analysis was based on "1,996 artifact-free EEG datasets" obtained from 26 participants, 12 women and 14 men, aged 21–24, which were collected on two non-consecutive nights from 2340 trials (Hori et al., 1994 pp. 239, 245).

The participants were called by means of a bell tone and asked two brief questions: (1) did you feel awake or asleep at the moment you were called, and (2) what were you experiencing? Due to the brevity of the questions and answers, the sleep-onset process in this study was likely shorter than in the case of the Foulkes studies. (In a later study by the Hori group in which the 11 participants were allowed to fall asleep normally over the space of three consecutive nights, the sleep-onset process lasted only 7–9 minutes on the second and third nights, so there is once again evidence of vigilance on the first night in a sleep-dream lab (Tamaki et al., 2005, p. 197, Figure 1).)

The analysis of the 5-second intervals led to nine stages in this initial study, which were defined by the changing EEG rhythms during the sleep-onset process. The first three stages were defined by varying degrees of alpha. They were followed by a very brief "flattening stage," which lasted for as little as 4–6 seconds; it was characterized by a very low-voltage EEG wave that is not usually found during waking or sleeping (Hori et al., 1994, pp. 240–241). The next four stages were based primarily on varying amounts of theta, but they often included intrusions of the small, sharp vertex waves that were shown in Table 4.1. On further analysis, however, the researchers concluded that the vertex waves "have a secondary or enhancing role, instead of independent characteristics" (Tanaka et al., 1996, p. 731). The vertex waves therefore can be ignored for the purposes of dream-oriented studies. The final stage in this nine-stage analysis was defined by the appearance of sleep spindles, as in the case of the Foulkes studies.

When the participants' verbal reports from the brief arousals were linked to one of the nine stages, the results showed that the presence of what these researchers called "dreamlike imagery" increases from 23% to 34% during the three alpha stages, and then to 46% in the first theta stage, followed by gradual declines to 32% when sleep spindles appear. These findings, along with (1) the mean number of minutes in each sleep-onset stage, (2) the declining percentage of contacts that led to reports of subjectively feeling awake, and (3) the percentage of the dream reports that contained visual imagery, are presented in Table 5.3.

The results presented in Table 5.3 show the same pattern of dream recall as the earlier set of Foulkes studies, but with lower frequencies in the theta stages. Moreover, the Hori group later replicated its initial set of findings. This direct replication was based on a one-night study of seven participants (four women and three men), who were called at 1-minute

TABLE 5.3 Detailed findings on dreaming and visual imagery during the sleep-onset process

EEG category	*Mean time (minutes)*	*Awake*	*Dream-like imagery*	*Visual imagery as a % of dream-like imagery*
Alpha 1	2.1	83%	23%	74%
Alpha 2	3.4	82%	26%	75%
Alpha 3	1.9	77%	34%	77%
Low-voltage flattening stage	0.9	65%	38%	82%
Theta 1	1.9	51%	46%	91%
Theta 2	0.8	50%	40%	95%
Theta 3	1.3	46%	39%	93%
Theta 4	1.4	42%	35%	93%
Sleep spindles	3.9	26%	32%	91%
Total time spent in sleep-onset process	17.6			

Source: From Hori, Hayashi and Morikawa (1994) and Tanaka, Hayashi and Hori (1996).

TABLE 5.4 The presence of dreamlike imagery during the sleep-onset process in two separate studies

Study	*Alpha*	*Flattening*	*Theta A*	*Theta B*	*Sleep spindles*
Hori et al. (1994)	27.5%	37.7%	42.8% (Hori 5+6)	36.7% (Hori 7+8)	31.9%
Hayashi et al. (1999)	29.8%	33.3%	36.2% (Theta)	34.2% (Theta)	22.8%

Notes: The figures for the original study are based on (1) the mean dreamlike-imagery percent in the three alpha stages; (2) the mean of the first two theta stages, and (3) the mean of the last two theta stages in Table 5.3. The figures for flattening and sleep spindles for the original Hori study are the same as they appeared in Table 5.3 (Hori, Hayashi, & Morikawa, 1994). The replication figures are drawn from Hayashi et al. (1999).

intervals throughout the sleep-onset process. Since a further analysis of the original nine stages had found that they could be collapsed into four stages, a four-stage analysis was used in the replication study (Hayashi et al., 1999, p. 677; Hori et al., 1994, p. 245, for the collapse of the nine stages into four stages). The three alpha stages were grouped into one alpha stage, and the four theta stages were grouped into two catch-all theta stages, with the "flattening" stage in between them and the spindles category at the end. As shown in Table 5.4, the results are very similar to the results in their original study.

These two different sets of results, one set from the original Hori et al. (1994) study, one from the replication study by Hayashi et al. (1999), provide the basis for a comparison with the results from the first set of three studies by Foulkes et al. (1965, 1966; Foulkes & Schmidt, 1983). This comparison shows that dreaming occurred in alpha stages in both sets of studies but was more frequent when theta was present. However, the comparison also shows that the percentages for dream recall are 10–15 percentage points higher during alpha in the Foulkes studies than the Hori studies, and roughly twice as high during theta.

This disparity in frequencies between the Foulkes and Hori studies supports the earlier-mentioned possibility that brain activation levels remained higher in the first set of studies due to the longer time periods it took to question the participants (Foulkes, 1985, p. 69, for a discussion of the possibility of higher activation levels in his three co-authored studies of the sleep-onset process). The Hori studies therefore provide a conceptual replication of how the process of dreaming unfolds. But they also contribute a corrective concerning the likely frequency of dreaming during the sleep-onset process.

More generally, the Foulkes and Hori studies discussed in this section, the first set of which were carried out in the mid-1960s and early 1980s, and the second set in the 1990s, establish that dreaming can and does occur at varying points during the sleep-onset process. This finding fits well with the neuroimaging evidence presented earlier in the chapter, which shows that the anterior portions of the default network gradually become functionally connected and ascendant at the same time as the FPCN and the two attention networks become relatively deactivated. However, as some of the defects in the dream reports from the sleep-onset process suggest, the relative deactivation of the FPCN and the attention networks, and the concomitant ascendancy of the dream-relevant portions of the default network, may be an uneven one during the sleep-onset process, and perhaps even more so in some individuals than others.

In addition to demonstrating that dreams occur during the sleep-onset process, the two sets of studies discussed in this section demonstrate from a new vantage point that theta waves are the most useful single EEG indicator of dreaming. As readers may recall from Chapter 2, theta waves also became increasingly frequent in anterior portions of the default network when the posterior cingulate cortex decouples from the dorsal attention network and posterior areas of the thalamus during drowsiness (Chang et al., 2013, p. 230). Furthermore, theta is usually present during REM sleep, and sometimes during N2 as well, which are the two sleep stages in which dreaming occurs (e.g., Armitage, 1995, pp. 336–338).

But Why Do Mammals Sleep?

Much is known about the sleep-onset process from the neurophysiological to the neurocognitive levels, and also about the extent and nature of the dreaming that occurs at various points in this process. As stressed at the outset of the chapter, and as underscored here, the dreaming that does occur in the sleep-onset process is important for theoretical reasons, even though it is less frequent, briefer, and sometimes less coherent than REM dreams, and is almost always forgotten.

The combination of neuroimaging and EEG-based awakening studies used in this chapter to study dreaming during the sleep-onset process also provides close-in evidence that the neurocognitive network that supports dreaming becomes relatively ascendant at the same time as the frontoparietal control network becomes relatively deactivated. Further, the discovery of dreaming during the sleep-onset process reveals that sleep, as formally and conventionally defined, does not have to be present for dreaming to occur. In that sense, the sleep-onset process demonstrates that dreaming is a world unto itself, even though it occurs far more frequently and for much longer periods of time during sleep.

At the same time, the large individual differences in when dreaming is recalled during the course of the sleep-onset process, if any dreaming is recalled at all, suggest that the process of falling asleep is an uneven one. Moreover, falling asleep may be more difficult for some people than it is for others, as a large amount of anecdotal evidence suggests. The ease of falling asleep also may vary nightly based on stress levels, which would mean that the attention networks may remain more active on those nights than they usually are.

For all that is known about the sleep-onset process and its unevenness, however, the reasons why there is a small subcortical network that suppresses waking activation, and thereby leads into the inactive, relatively non-responsive, and non-conscious state called "sleep," are not known. "Sleep remains a scientific enigma" according to a comprehensive review of the major theories concerning the function of sleep. In fact, sleep is "the last major physiological process for which there is a lack of consensus concerning its function" (Krueger et al., 2016, p. 1). It is to this unresolved mystery that the book now turns to in the next two chapters, through a new set of findings and analyses concerning (1) the evolutionary origins of sleep; (2) the uniqueness of human sleep; and (3) the sources for the activation levels during sleep that are necessary for dreaming to occur.

6

THE ADAPTIVE INACTIVITY THEORY OF SLEEP

As the detailed neuroimaging, lesion, and developmental evidence presented in Chapter 2 demonstrated, much is known about four of the five conditions that are necessary for dreaming to occur. The neural substrates that support dreaming have to be mature and intact, external stimuli have to be occluded, the cognitive capacities that give rise to dreaming, such as simulation and imagination, must be at adult-like levels, and the frontoparietal control network (FPCN) and the two attention networks have to be relatively deactivated.

However, there is as yet no one parsimonious and widely accepted theory, drawing upon uncontested systematic empirical studies, that can fully explain the activation patterns that make dreaming possible in three different states: (1) during the sleep-onset process; (2) during the 4–6 REM periods; and (3) in the 1.5–2.5 hours of N2 sleep before the morning awakening. It is therefore the purpose of this chapter to suggest that a recent theory of sleep, the adaptive inactivity theory of sleep, can provide a general explanation for the activation patterns that are the essential final causative factor in leading to the functional connectivity of the neurocognitive network that gives rise to dreaming.

As part of this analysis, it is first of all shown that the adaptive inactivity theory of sleep provides an account of the origins of rapid eye movement (REM) sleep as a brain-heating mechanism, which periodically restores the brain to waking-level brain temperatures. The theory thereby can explain why REM sleep predominates in the sleep of monotremes (e.g., the platypus and the short-beaked echidna) but is nearly or completely absent from the sleep of dolphins and porpoises. The most detailed evidence for these claims includes comparative brain-temperature studies, experimental studies of two

DOI: 10.4324/9781003732969-6

different aquatic mammals with little or no REM sleep, and an experimental lesion study involving cats. As also discussed in this chapter, the adaptive inactivity theory of sleep can explain the very wide variations in the amount of time that various mammals sleep, ranging from 19 to 20 hours to no hours at all.

The adaptive inactivity theory of sleep also can explain dreaming during the sleep-onset process because brain temperatures are still at or close to waking levels during this transitional process. Then, too, it can explain dreaming during N2 sleep in the 1.5–2.5 hours before morning on the basis of the 24-hour circadian rhythms that gradually raise brain temperatures in preparation for full functioning shortly after waking up in the morning.

Then, in the next chapter, the conclusions drawn from the analyses of mammalian sleep in general provide the basis for applying the adaptive inactivity theory of sleep to findings from field studies of people living in three small hunting-gathering and hunting-horticultural societies located in Africa and South America. These three groups live without electricity in conditions at least somewhat resembling those in which anatomically and cognitively modern humans first appeared in the southern half of Africa 70,000–250,000 years ago (Hallett et al., 2025).

The findings from the field study of the three small-scale societies are then used to illuminate and lend ecological validity to several findings from laboratory studies of sleep and dreaming over the past 70 years. To the degree that this analysis is found to be a solid one, then to that degree the adaptive inactivity theory of sleep can augment the neurocognitive theory of dreaming, and perhaps other theories of dreaming. More specifically, the findings related to the adaptive inactivity theory of sleep lead to the conclusion that *wake-like brain temperatures* provide the basis for the activation levels that are necessary for dreaming to occur during the sleep-onset process, N2 sleep, and REM sleep.

This conclusion concerning the wake-like level of brain temperatures at sleep onset, during REM sleep, and before the morning awakening is based on established empirical findings. It therefore stands *even if* the explanations for these high activation levels that are offered by the adaptive inactivity theory are met with skepticism. However, rejecting the hypothesis that REM sleep provides a brain-warming function means that dreaming during REM sleep cannot be explained, at least as yet, by any adaptive theory of sleep that has been proposed as of 2025.

An Overview of the Adaptive Inactivity Theory of Sleep

Adaptive inactivity, which is best characterized by reduced metabolism and a decrease in energy consumption, has been found to be pervasive in the long evolutionary histories of both plants and the earliest animals, well before mammals and birds first appeared (Siegel, 2022b, 2022d). For example, the seeds of many plants can lie dormant for as long as 1300–2000 years before they germinate; deciduous trees lose their leaves in winter and become dormant; parasites can be dormant in animal tissue until the animal's immune system is compromised; many insects experience seasonal dormancy, and the internal gas exchanges on which their metabolism is based often stop for several seconds or more throughout the course of the day. Reptiles become dormant when the ambient (surrounding) air temperature falls to specific trigger points (Siegel, 2022d, p. 944).

As for mammals and birds, which are the two kinds of warm-blooded animals (homeotherms), they have an evolutionarily new form of adaptive inactivity that was given the name "sleep." Sleep is most readily defined by several behavioral criteria, including reduced activity, reduced responsiveness to stimuli, and a loss of consciousness, and it is easily reversible (Siegel, 2022a, pp. 52–53, for the complexities of defining sleep in more detail for research purposes). Sleep first of all conserves energy by limiting the search for energy supplies to the most propitious and safest hours within a species' ecological niche. This hypothesis leads to a more general, multi-variable formulation: the sleep patterns and total sleep time of every species of homeotherms varies in terms of the energy-acquisition, predator-avoidance, and energy-conservation strategies that are necessary for survival within a specific ecological niche.

The adaptive inactivity theory of sleep can explain why homeotherms sleep instead of going into pre-mammalian forms of dormancy, and why they have two kinds of sleep—REM sleep and non-REM sleep. It can explain the variations in the amount of REM sleep among mammals, as well as why birds have very small amounts of REM sleep. Further, the theory can explain why REM sleep always occurs after periods of non-REM sleep, and why in humans the REM periods become longer in the hours before awakening. Then, too, the theory can explain why there are increasing amounts of N2 sleep toward morning. Moreover, the theory can explain the shorter sleep times that some mammals experience in the wild as compared to the longer stretches of sleep they have when they are held in captivity. Finally, the adaptive inactivity theory of sleep can explain the seasonal variations in total sleep time that some mammals experience, including humans living in hunting-gathering and hunting-horticultural societies.

The emphasis on energy conservation in the adaptive inactivity theory of sleep also can explain why slow-wave N3 sleep leads into and out of the two homeothermic versions of dormancy that everyone agrees are energy saving: the daily state of torpor in some small mammals and birds, a state in which the metabolic rate declines precipitously for several hours, and hibernation during winter in some mammals, which continues for as long as four to five months in ground squirrels (Siegel, 2022b, pp. 93–94; 2022d, p. 938; von der Ohe et al., 2006; Walker et al., 1979).

Although the adaptive inactivity theory of sleep hypothesizes that energy conservation is the first and primary adaptive value of sleep, the theory is compatible with the possibility that other, cellular-level adaptive processes have been incorporated into sleep in many different mammals during the course of their evolution. In humans, for example, sleep may provide the context for the removal of toxic metabolites from the brain ("neural detoxification"); for the replenishment of the brain's energy supplies; for the enhancement of the immune system; and for the promotion of "synaptic plasticity," which improves the brain's ability to modify connections among neurons during the waking period through synaptic pruning (Frank, 2012, 2021; Krueger et al., 2016, for overviews and critiques of the major theories that address the adaptive function of sleep). Still another set of studies suggests that sleep, and perhaps preferentially non-REM sleep, provides the occasion for the consolidation of new memories that were acquired during the previous day or two (e.g., Chen & Wilson, 2017; Hudachek & Wamsley, 2023; Kaida et al., 2015; Rasch & Born, 2015; Wilson & McNaughton, 1994).

However, based on numerous comparative studies, which discovered that some land mammals sleep for as little as 2–5 hours, and that some species of dolphins and porpoises have little or no sleep, it seems likely that these processes of removal, restoration, enhancement, pruning, and consolidation can be carried out in waking. Even more generally, it is likely that at least some of these processes occur during both sleeping and waking in some species, as is the case for memory consolidation in humans, to take one highly relevant instance (Cordi & Rasch, 2021a; Siegel, 2021; Tucker et al., 2020; Wamsley & Summer, 2020; Wang et al., 2021).

The idea that sleep serves the adaptive function of energy conservation is not new and has been suggested in past studies on the basis of empirical findings (e.g., Allison & Van Twyver, 1970a; Berger & Phillips, 1995; Lesku & Schmidt, 2022; Schmidt, 2014; Snyder, 1969; Walker et al., 1979; Wehr, 1992). However, the importance of energy conservation in understanding sleep has been until recently considered to be a secondary factor, if relevant at all, because the energy savings were thought to be very small (Zepelin et al., 2005, p. 95, for a summary of past critical arguments). The amount of energy conservation as an evolutionary adaptation seemed especially meager to some researchers when the energy expended during REM sleep—which has brain activation levels very similar to those during waking—is taken into consideration. (See Lesku & Schmidt, 2022, and Schmidt, 2014, for important exceptions, based on their well-established findings on energy conservation during sleep in birds.)

Then, too, the high levels of brain activation during REM sleep, along with the frequent twitching limb movements, the irregular breathing patterns, and the jerky eye movements that occur during REM sleep, were sometimes seen as a refutation of the idea that any significant amount of energy could be saved during sleeping. Sleep was also thought by some researchers to be a time when mammals are especially vulnerable to attack by predators. If the seeming danger of being asleep is taken into consideration, it did not make sense that such a risky adaptation would survive for so little energy savings. Most sleep researchers therefore reasoned that sleep must have a more important primordial purpose than energy conservation.

Contrary to these earlier concerns, the considerable amount of energy that is *not* expended in fruitless and perhaps dangerous searches for energy supplies at times when they are not likely to be available has to be taken into consideration. Nor is REM sleep as energy-intensive in terms of brain activation levels as the resting waking state it resembles. This is due to the fact that a large percentage of waking human energy consumption is still needed to maintain normal brain temperatures and muscle tone while in the resting state. And the waking brain during states of rest still accounts for 20%–25% of human energy consumption.

On the other hand, REM sleep consumes a little less energy than a quiescent waking state because the musculature is deactivated during REM sleep via complex neurochemical processes that have been carefully traced, leading to a state called "atonia." In addition, as discussed in more detail shortly, parts of the brain have slightly lower temperatures during REM sleep than during waking (Siegel, 2022d, p. 643, and especially Panel 3, for a summary and references on these energy savings). Still, the fact remains that the main energy savings are during N3 sleep, not REM sleep.

Further, there is little reason to believe that sleep is a time of unusual danger for most mammals now that the places in which most mammals sleep are better understood via intensive field research (Siegel, 2022b, p. 93). For example, some mammals burrow into the ground, others hide under rocks, and still others slip into crevices or hollow tree trunks. Still others retreat into caves or climb into trees. Moreover, most mammals sleep during the day and thus at the same time, so they cannot be hunting each other. That is, fully 70% of all mammals, and especially the small mammals that evolved early in mammalian history, are nocturnal creatures. Then, too, most birds of prey hunt during the day, not at night. The exceptions are owls and nighthawks, but they feed on nocturnal mammals, such as mice and rats, not on sleeping mammals. More generally, animals are in the greatest danger when they are moving about, feeding, or taking care of their offspring, or when they are very young or very old and do not have the capacities to escape or fight back.

One of the most important aspects of sleep is often overlooked when the possible dangers of being asleep are highlighted. The transition from sleep back to waking can be very fast. Most adult mammals are alert and able to run or fight within seconds of awakening if they sense danger, which would not be possible for animals that have gone into dormancy. In the case of giraffes and other herbivores that live in large groups, which are indeed in danger of predation by lions or tigers at night, they sleep more lightly and for shorter times (3–5 hours) and awaken often. Then, too, the animals on the outer perimeter of the group tend to sleep even more lightly than those closer to the center, and a few of those on the perimeter are always awake at one point or another (Burger et al., 2020). (However, it needs to be added that giraffes and other herbivores sleep less primarily because they need more time for foraging, as explained shortly.)

There is also evidence that the energy savings during sleep are not trivial even for those present-day humans who live in a world of electricity, heating furnaces, and warm buildings. In one carefully controlled study, the sleep of two women and five men, each of whom separately spent three days in a chamber equipped with sophisticated technologies (a "whole-room indirect calorimeter"), was carefully monitored and recorded in order to measure energy expenditures in a very precise fashion. The study concluded that the nightly energy savings are a "physiologically meaningful amount of whole-body total daily energy expenditure" because they provide enough energy for a 150-pound adult to walk 1.9 miles "at a moderate pace" (Jung et al., 2011, p. 241).

This figure becomes even more significant if the amount of energy conserved over the course of weeks or months is taken into consideration in the context of likely limits on energy resources in any given ecological niche. In addition, it is frequently the case that very small adaptations add up to major advantages for the establishment of a new species over the course of many thousands of generations or more. And, as discussed later in the chapter, the energy savings are likely larger for other mammals. Then, too, the sleep of people living in hunting-gathering and hunting-horticultural societies is impacted very directly by daily and seasonal temperature changes, as discussed in the next chapter.

REM Sleep Keeps Brain Temperature Near a Set-Point

Due to the fact that all mammals and birds are homeotherms, sleep as an energy-conservation strategy is complicated by the need to maintain an adequate brain temperature. The forms of dormancy and other types of inactivity that are used by pre-mammalian organisms and animals are not feasible ways for mammals and birds to conserve energy because their higher level of brain metabolism, and the more complex and energy-intensive mechanisms involved in maintaining their very fast processing, are needed for alert functioning shortly after they awaken.

More specifically, as shown by the evidence discussed below from comparative studies, case studies of atypical mammals, and experimental lesion studies of cats, the periodic recurrences of REM sleep "suggest that REM sleep has a thermoregulatory role for the brain, which is triggered by decreases in *brainstem temperature* during Non-REM sleep, and ceases when the target temperature is reached, in a repeating cycle" (Siegel, 2022d, p. 942, italics added).

The fact that REM sleep is accompanied by a rise in brain temperature, as well as an increase in cerebral blood flow (CBF), was first discovered in the mid-1960s in a study of 12 cats with surgically implanted thermistors. The researchers found temperature increases between 0.1°C and 0.7°C (0.2°F and 1.3°F) in 670 of 689 REM periods. Sixteen of the 19 REM periods with no temperature change came from one or two electrodes in one cat. Three other cats had one REM period each in which no temperature change occurred (Rechtschaffen et al., 1965, Table 1; 1966).

The researchers interpreted the temperature increases and the increases in CBF during REM sleep as being "the result of increased cerebral metabolism" (Rechtschaffen et al., 1965). Their findings on the relationship between the increases in cerebral metabolism, the rise in brain temperatures during REM sleep, and the occurrence of dreaming anticipate the general thrust of the adaptive inactivity of sleep, but the researchers did not suggest any adaptive function for their findings.

Although this line of research was not pursued and fell by the wayside, similar findings on cerebral metabolism, CBF, and brain temperature were discovered independently in a pioneering series of studies of rats. These studies added the puzzling fact that body temperature is deregulated during REM sleep, and therefore usually declines, at the same time as brain temperature is rising (Parmeggiani, 1977, 2011). These later findings have been supported by two of Parmeggiani's former co-workers, who also state as part of their overview of the possible functions of thermoregulation during sleep that "the autonomic outflow and the activity of the endocrine system, the respiratory system, the cardiovascular system, and the thermoregulatory system" during non-REM sleep "seem to be directed at increasing energy saving" (Cerri & Amici, 2021). They also note that body temperature is deregulated and can fall during REM sleep.

As part of still another study of changes in brain temperature throughout the sleep period, other researchers note the fact that the regulation of body temperature "switches off during REM" in cats, rabbits, and fur seals, which allows body temperature to fall, even while brain temperature nonetheless increases during REM sleep (Csernai et al., 2019). Based on these various findings from several independent research teams, there is some degree of agreement among sleep researchers that brain temperature rises during REM sleep. However, there is as yet no agreement about the idea that REM sleep has a thermoregulatory role for the brain (Siegel, 2022d).

Initially approaching these issues on the basis of both comparative and lesion studies, the adaptive inactivity theory of sleep suggests that the essential problem is the maintenance of the necessary brain temperatures during sleep, while at the same time conserving energy. It further suggests that this problem was solved at the outset of mammalian evolutionary history by the selection for REM sleep and non-REM sleep in near tandem. The comparative evidence for the role of REM sleep in heating the brain is first of all found in studies of two of the three extant *monotremes*, which are thought to share the most genes with the original ancestral mammal (Flannery et al., 2022). The platypus and the short-beaked echidna are distinctive as egg-laying mammals that nonetheless also produce milk to nourish their young after they hatch (Siegel, 2022b, 2022d; Siegel et al., 1996, 1999).

Detailed studies of sleep in the platypus, which is even more genetically similar to the original mammalian ancestor than the two echidna species, discovered that it has more REM sleep (8.0 hours) than any other mammal that has been studied (Siegel, 2022b, pp. 93–94). These 8 hours of REM sleep per day account for 57.1% of the platypus' 14 hours of total sleep time, a far higher percentage of REM sleep than for any other mammal, as shown shortly. These findings lead to the hypothesis that "the REM sleep state might be the phylogenetically oldest sleep state in mammals" (Siegel, 2022d, p. 941).

The platypus and other monotremes are not only distinctive among mammals in that they have long periods of REM sleep. At the same time that REM sleep is occurring in their brainstems, they simultaneously have slow-wave high-voltage patterns of N3 slow-wave sleep in their cortex. This is highly unusual in that N3 slow-wave sleep is only found in the cortex in all other adult mammals when they are not in REM sleep. Moreover, the mixture of REM and N3 sleep patterns that occurs at the same time in monotremes is also found in the "active" or "dissociation" stage of sleep that is present in newborn placental mammals, including humans. However, this pattern differentiates into REM sleep and N3 sleep within a few days or weeks, with variations in the timing from species to species. When clearly defined sleep stages appear in human neonates, they spend as much as 50% of their sleep time in REM sleep, which is reminiscent of what is known about REM sleep in the platypus, followed by a steady decline to adult-like levels by ages 3–4 (Frank, 2020, for a comprehensive analysis and overview; Siegel, 2022d, p. 941).

It is important to stress that the platypus and other monotremes also have the lowest brain temperature among mammals (31°C/88°F, as compared to about 37°C/99°F in humans and other placental mammals). This large difference leads to the inference that they have more REM sleep because their brain temperatures quickly reach the lower limit during sleep that is viable for homeotherm brains (Siegel, 2022d, p. 942). It therefore can be argued that "REM sleep might have initially evolved to maintain brainstem function during sleep in mammals that had relatively low body temperatures and metabolic rates..." (Siegel, 2022d, p. 942).

This analysis is further supported by detailed studies of the opossum, a representative of the *marsupial* family, which branched off from the common ancestor of all mammals later than the monotremes did. Marsupials, which also include kangaroos and koalas, among others, are distinctive in that they carry their young in pouches. They have a brain temperature of around 35°C (95°F), which is 4°C higher than that of monotremes, but slightly lower than that of placental mammals. The common opossum, for example, which sleeps 19 hours a day and has 4.4 hours of REM sleep, is second only to the monotremes in terms of both the amount of REM sleep and the percentage of total sleep time spent in REM sleep (30.5%) (Siegel, 2022b, p. 942). (The sleep of the common opossum is discussed in more detail later in the chapter.)

As noted above, brain temperature is higher in placental animals than in monotremes and marsupials, which is due to adaptations that caused them to have a very useful higher metabolic rate. Placental mammals also have a lower mean number of hours of REM sleep (2 hours per night), which may be a result of beginning sleep further from their tolerable lower-bound brain-temperature limits. These differences, along with the comparable figure for birds, are shown in Table 6.1, which is based on more than 70 species of monotremes, marsupials, and placental mammals (Siegel, 2022d, p. 942, Figure 4). Moreover, the range in the number of hours of REM sleep is somewhat wider in placental mammals (0 to 3–4 hours), for ecological reasons that are discussed in the next section of the chapter. Further, the percentage of total sleep time spent in REM sleep varies as well, once again for ecological reasons addressed in the next section.

It is important to note that the findings in Table 6.1 are based on core body temperatures, which can serve as a good proxy for *waking* brain temperature because they are closely related under normal conditions (e.g., Kiyatkin,

TABLE 6.1 The inverse relationship between core temperature and hours spent in REM sleep in homeotherms

		Typical core temperature	*Time in REM sleep*
Monotremes	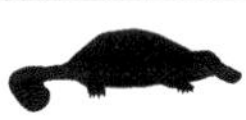	31°C	7.5 hours
Marsupials	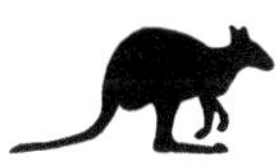	35°C	4.4 hours
Placentals	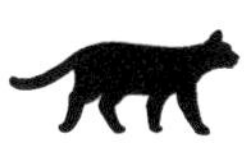	37°C	2.0 hours
Birds	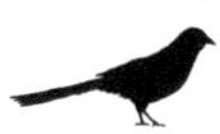	41°C	0.7 hours

Note: The numbers in this table are drawn from Siegel (2022d, Figure 4, p. 942); the correlation coefficient (Pearson's *r*) between temperature and REM time is –.97.

2019, p. 311). However, there is one exception, which already has been noted. Core body temperature and brain temperature differ greatly during REM sleep because, as discussed earlier in the chapter, core body temperature is not regulated during REM sleep. This means that body temperature can fall toward the ambient temperature, even while brain temperature is rising during REM sleep (Siegel, 2022d, p. 943). This disconnect is one of the main reasons why some sleep researchers may be skeptical about the brain-warming function of REM sleep. The emphasis therefore has to be on the fact that the body can withstand colder temperatures, whereas the increasingly complex mammalian brain has to be fully functional at the time of arousal.

In addition, it is useful to highlight the fact that the same pattern of increasing core body temperature holds for birds as well. The most recently evolved birds have much higher brain temperatures than do placental mammals (41°C/105°F), and an even lower amount of REM sleep (0.7 hours) (Siegel, 2022d, p. 942, Figure 4). The usefulness of the findings on the higher brain temperatures of birds has been extended by a study showing that the most recently evolved classification of birds has a higher brain temperature than the most primitive extant species of birds (Gavrilov et al., 2023, p. 12, Figures 4 and 5). If current understandings of the independent origins of mammals and birds continue to hold true in the future, then the relationship between brain temperature and hours of REM sleep in birds provides an impressive example of convergent evolution.

To provide a sense of the range in the amount of REM sleep and the percentage of total sleep time that is spent in REM, Table 6.2 provides an overview of this information for a variety of mammals, with a focus on the variations among placental mammals. The placental mammals used for illustrative purposes in Table 6.2 are either generally known to most people or else are discussed in this or a later section of the chapter. The table includes three atypical placental mammals—the Arabian oryx, a powerfully built species of antelope, the cat-sized hooved mammal called the mouse-deer, and the fur seal. All three of these placental mammals have theoretically important variations in their amount and percentage of REM sleep. The nature of those variations is noted in Table 6.2 and discussed at various points in the remainder of the chapter.

As revealed in Table 6.2, there are unexpected absences of REM sleep in at least some marine mammals. These absences, as shown in the next several paragraphs, provide support for the idea that the adaptive function of REM sleep is to raise brain temperature. The first of two very detailed and useful case studies concerns fur seals, which evolved from land-bound ancestors beginning about 17–24 million years ago. (Naturalistic studies of highly unusual cases are often called "natural experiments" because evolution has created a very extreme case in comparison to what is typically the case (i.e., evolution also has produced the necessary control group).)

TABLE 6.2 Variations in percentage of REM sleep, hours of REM sleep, and total hours of sleep in a wide range of mammals

	Percentage of sleep in REM	*Total REM time (hours)*	*Total sleep time (hours)*
Platypus	57.1%	8.0	14.0
Common opossum	30.5%	5.8	19.0
Eastern American mole	25.0%	2.1	8.4
Big brown bat	19.5%	3.9	20.0
Owl monkey	11.2%	1.9	17.0
Giraffe	11.1%	0.5	4.5
Sheep	8.5%	0.6	5.9
Lesser mouse-deer	3.2%	0.03	11.9
Arabian oryx (summer/winter)	2.1%/4.2%	0.1/0.3	3.8/6.7
Fur seal (in water/on land)	0.0%/18.8%	0.0/1.4	4.0/7.5
Commerson's dolphin	0.0	0.0	0.0

Source: These figures are drawn from four sources: Lyamin et al. (2022, p. 1), Siegel (2022b, p. 97, Figure 10.3; 2022d, p. 941, Figure 2; 2022c, p. 82, Figure 12.6).

Notes: Note that mammals are ordered by the percentage of REM sleep they experience; the Arabian oryx and fur seal are ranked by the lowest of their two REM percentages.

Fur seals forage in the ocean for about seven months a year and live on rocky island beaches for the rest of the year. During their five months on land, they have a typical non-REM/REM cycle over the space of 7.5 hours of sleep and spend about the same amount of time in REM sleep (18.8%) as is found in several land mammals. However, during their months of foraging in the ocean, they have little or no REM sleep, and their non-REM sleep occurs in only one brain hemisphere at a time ("unihemispheric slow-wave sleep").

Fur seals remain in continuous motion during unihemispheric slow-wave sleep, albeit motion at a slower rate than during waking. This continuous motion during unihemispheric sleep occurs because the forelimb contralateral to the activated half of the brain remains active (Lyamin et al., 2018; Siegel, 2022d). At the same time, the environment is monitored for predators with the contralateral eye (Kendall-Bar et al., 2019; Lyamin et al., 2018). The result is about 4 hours of non-REM sleep in each brain hemisphere.

This pattern suggests that the ancestors of fur seals, who share a common terrestrial ancestor with bear-like mammals, gradually lost their REM sleep as they adapted to living in the ocean. They lost their REM sleep, according to the adaptive inactivity theory of sleep, because their brain temperature remains at an adequate level while in the ocean environment. This adequate brain temperature is due to the fact that it is lower in only one hemisphere at a time during non-REM sleep. Nor do fur seals compensate for any seemingly "lost" REM sleep once back on land.

The conclusion that there are no increases in REM sleep after living fully in the water was established experimentally in a study of four fur seals that swam in a large pool for up to two weeks while their unihemispheric electroencephalogram (EEG) sleep patterns were being recorded with implanted electrodes. Then a platform was placed in the pool, which allowed them to be out of the water, at which time they returned to their normal whole-brain, non-REM/REM sleep pattern (Lyamin et al., 2018). This finding suggests that there are no cellular-level adaptive brain processes occurring exclusively during REM sleep in fur seals that are suspended during their time in the ocean.

The sleep pattern found in fur seals when in the water is paralleled by those found in a second natural experiment, the near-absence or complete absence of REM sleep in at least two species of dolphins, which have larger brains than humans and are known for their ability to solve complex cognitive tasks; this loss of REM sleep has been found in harbor porpoises as well (Siegel, 2022b, pp. 96, 100). Dolphins and porpoises, who share a common terrestrial ancestor with pigs, giraffes, and hippos, began their evolutionary journey to living only in oceans and ocean harbors about 47–55 million years ago, which is approximately 30 million years before fur seals became aquatic mammals (Lyamin et al., 2008, 2024; Lyamin & Siegel, 2019).

The apparent absence of REM sleep in dolphins and harbor porpoises, when paired with the similar absence of REM sleep in fur seals while in the ocean, is another example of convergent evolution. It further supports the hypothesis that REM sleep in the earliest known mammals, the monotremes, is an adaptation that periodically increases their brain temperatures so that energy-saving non-REM sleep can be continued. (Whales also share a common ancestor with dolphins and porpoises, but they are too big to study, and it would be unethical to study this endangered species in any case.)

Finally, and importantly, the hypothesis that REM sleep acts as a heating system also receives significant support from a surgical lesion experiment on domestic cats. The relevant REM-generating regions in their brainstems—the lateral pons and the midbrain—were surgically disconnected from the forebrain. Under these conditions, there was little or no REM sleep if their body temperatures were maintained at the normal levels. However, if their body temperature was allowed to fall toward the ambient room temperature, REM sleep in the severed lateral pons and midbrain increased to as much as 70% of the time during which the recordings were being made. The dramatic nature of these findings also can be seen by noting that REM periods never last longer than 5 minutes in intact domestic cats sleeping normally, and that REM sleep typically accounts for about 15.5% of their total sleep time (Jouvet et al., 1990; Siegel, 2022c, pp. 72–73; 2022d, p. 942).

These experimental results address a second reason why some sleep researchers may be skeptical when they encounter the brain-warming hypothesis that is central to the adaptive inactivity theory of sleep. With the exception of the study discussed in the previous paragraph, there is an absence of direct experimental evidence concerning the direction of causality with regard to the higher brain temperatures that are found during REM sleep.

However, when the experimental lesion results in cats are considered in conjunction with the widely differing brain temperatures of monotremes, marsupials, placental mammals, and birds—along with the natural experiments provided by marine mammals—the overall results seem sufficient to suggest that this new theory of sleep should be taken seriously. The suggestion that "REM sleep might be thought of as a thermostatically controlled brain-heating mechanism, which is triggered by the temperature reduction linked to the reduced metabolism and the decrease in energy consumption in Non-REM sleep," now appears in a wider comparative context (Siegel, 2022d, p. 942).

Further, the idea that "REM sleep ends after the amount of REM required to raise brain temperature to close to the waking temperature of the body has occurred" gains plausibility on the basis of the case studies that serve as natural experiments. In addition, this claim about the relevance of case studies of atypical mammals includes additional cases of extreme variations in total sleep time and the percentage of REM sleep. These cases are discussed in a later section of this chapter. The extreme variations in these cases seem to be due to a range of ecological factors (Siegel, 2022d, p. 942).

The REM-Generation Network

The experimental lesion experiment discussed at the end of the previous section, which showed that there are large increases in the amount of REM sleep whenever the relevant REM-generating regions in the brainstem are disconnected from the forebrain, leads to a discussion of the location and nature of the REM-generation network. This network is understood in considerable detail due to a combination of experimental transection studies, lesion studies, and cell-stimulation studies. And once again, each of these methods has different strengths and limitations (Siegel, 2022c, pp. 70–72).

It is therefore reassuring that "transection, lesion, and stimulation studies all point to the same regions of the pons and caudal midbrain as the 'critical region' for the generation of REM sleep" (Siegel, 2022c, p. 76). (The "caudal midbrain" refers to the part of the midbrain that is adjacent to the pons.) In addition, recordings of the activity of single neurons in intact animal models provide "a powerful insight into the precise time course of neuronal discharges," which can be leveraged to study several of the processes that generate the onset and offset of REM sleep (Siegel, 2022c, p. 71).

More specifically, it is likely that "the pons is the crucial region for the generation of REM sleep," but the medulla is necessary to generate the muscular atonia that accompanies REM sleep, and portions of the midbrain are "critical for REM sleep generation" (Siegel, 2022c, p. 73). This REM-generation network then sends its messages, using a complex array of chemically distinct neurotransmitters, to areas in the basal forebrain and the hypothalamus, which in turn propagate these messages to other areas of the brain. Although much is now known about the REM-generation network at the neurophysiological level, further progress at the cellular level may be slow due to the fact that the REM-on and REM-off cells are so closely intertwined that it is "very difficult to identify the sequence in which these cell groups are normally activated…" (Siegel, 2022c, p. 83).

The neuroimaging studies of REM sleep are consistent with the experimentally based REM-generation network discussed in the previous paragraph. They, too, find that the REM-generation network begins in the pons and the midbrain. They further reveal that the pons/midbrain portion of the network propagates its activation signals to the basal forebrain. Unlike during waking, however, these signals are blockaded at the thalamus, which means that the heating of cortical regions during REM sleep relies entirely on the ventral/basal forebrain path. Neuroimaging researchers also discovered that the dorsal/thalamic network that is essential to brain activation during waking is blockaded during N3 sleep as well. As is the case during drowsiness and the sleep-onset process, parts of the posterior cingulate cortex are therefore relatively deactivated during sleep according to these neuroimaging studies (e.g., Braun et al., 1997; Chow et al., 2013; Picchioni et al., 2014).

Based on the overall findings, one team of neuroimaging researchers suggested that the sole reliance on the ventral/basal forebrain pathway to activate cortical regions may be one of the key factors in making REM sleep different from waking (Braun et al., 1997, p. 1185). More generally, a neurophysiological expert on sleep and arousal concludes that the basal forebrain may have a "fundamental role in determining the wake-sleep states" (Jones, 2020, p. 7). To underscore these conclusions, Table 6.3 compares the activation patterns during waking, REM sleep, and N3 sleep.

TABLE 6.3 A comparison of the activation levels in the dorsal/thalamic and ventral/basal forebrain pathways during waking, REM sleep, and N3 sleep

Wake/sleep state	*Dorsal/thalamic pathway activated?*	*Ventral/basal forebrain pathway activated?*
Waking	Yes	Yes
REM sleep	Yes	No
N3 sleep	No	No

Source: This table is based primarily on Braun et al. (1997, p. 1185).

Returning to a full focus on REM sleep, Figure 6.1 provides a schematic graphic of the REM-generation network, which is based on information from one of the earliest neuroimaging studies of REM sleep (Braun et al., 1997, Figure 6). It highlights the way in which the ventral/basal forebrain pathway activates cortical regions in the midbrain at the same time as the dorsolateral and anterior frontal areas that support the FPCN remain relatively deactivated due to a blockade at the thalamus.

According to the neurocognitive theory of dreaming, the blockade of the dorsal/thalamic pathway during REM sleep is of additional relevance in humans. This is because the propagation of activation messages solely through the ventral/basal forebrain has the inadvertent effect of providing high activation levels in medial cortical areas that support the default network. These areas include the hippocampus, parahippocampus, and the

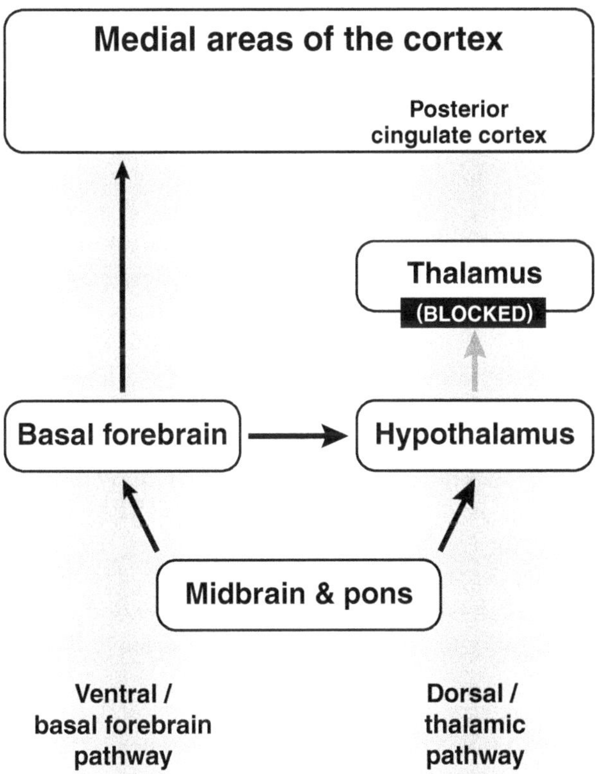

FIGURE 6.1 Schematic diagram of the activated and blockaded subcortical pathways during REM sleep.

Note: The actual locations of the subcortical brain regions in this diagram are shown in Figure 1.3.

medial prefrontal cortex. At the same time, the dorsolateral, ventrolateral, and anterior prefrontal cortex remain relatively deactivated. Thus, the neurocognitive network that gives rise to dreaming can make use of areas that are essential to waking thought because the FPCN is relatively deactivated. Based on this analysis of brain activation patterns during REM, the neurocognitive theory of dreaming suggests that some regions of the brain may experience greater temperature increases than other regions do.

Since the default network only gradually became fully developed in humans in the past 250,000 years, dreaming is therefore an incidental blink of the eye, a by-product, in the 110-million-year history of REM sleep. According to the neurocognitive theory, dreaming is present, at the most, during only the last 0.2% of the history of REM sleep.

Ecological Factors Explain Variations in REM and N3 Sleep Duration

The combination of comparative, lesion, and stimulation studies of REM sleep, along with the single-cell recording of activation patterns, strongly suggests that the adaptive function of REM sleep involves the maintenance of the necessary minimum brain temperatures during sleep. However, variations in the amount of REM sleep do not fully explain the widely varying amounts of sleep in the great majority of the mammals that have been studied to date. This variation in large part involves variations in the amount of time mammals spend in N3 sleep, which is the most important sleep stage in terms of energy conservation. It is therefore likely that the variations in total sleep time are related to a species' ecological niche.

Adding additional complexity to the equation, there are a few mammals that sleep for relatively long periods of time—17 hours or more—while at the same time having very little REM sleep. This seeming anomaly—which provides another set of natural experiments—actually provides further evidence for the hypothesis that the adaptive function of REM sleep is to periodically warm the brain so that energy-saving N3 sleep can continue. Specifically, if a particular ecological niche is very warm day and night, whether in the summer months or year-round, it might be expected that less REM sleep would be necessary to keep the brain warm during energy-saving N3 sleep.

To understand the variations in total sleep time and total REM sleep time among mammals, and especially in the placental mammals that are the primary focus of this subsection, it is necessary to examine a range of cases, including atypical cases. Understanding these variations is not only essential in demonstrating the comprehensive nature of the adaptive inactivity theory of sleep. It is also necessary for comprehending unique features of human sleep that relate to the timing and length of dreaming, which are discussed in Chapter 7.

To begin at the long-sleep end of the spectrum, three very different mammals that sleep from 17 to 20 hours a day illustrate the ways in which different ecological niches can lead to species that spend more time asleep than they do awake. At the same time, these three species have widely varying percentages of REM sleep as part of their total sleep time, as also indicated in Table 6.2.

The common opossum, the marsupial that was earlier mentioned as being distinctive due to its large amount and percentage of REM sleep (5.8 hours, 30.5%), is also one of the mammals that sleep the most—19 hours. With a lifespan of only two to four years, and living in tropical and subtropical highland regions from Mexico to Bolivia, the common opossum is a nocturnal mammal that sleeps in hollow trees and burrows into the ground or crawls under human-made structures and containers. It survives as a species because it is usually only active between 11 p.m. and 3 a.m., can eat anything that is digestible, lives in a variety of habitats, and feigns death and emits an odor resembling that of a decaying corpse when cornered (Allison & Van Twyver, 1970b; Martina, 2014; Siegel, 2022d, p. 941, Figure 2). At the same time, it has the very high REM sleep percentage mentioned above (30.5%), which is higher than in any placental mammal. This is likely because marsupials have a lower brain temperature than do placental mammals, as explained earlier.

The big brown bat, a species of bats that sleeps about 20 hours a day and is widespread throughout both North America and South America, provides an ideal example of how sleep and wakefulness are closely attuned to a placental mammal's ecological niche. The big brown bat feeds on moths and mosquitos that only become active during dusk and returns to its nest as the evening turns into night. Since its food supply is ample and nutritious, and bats are vulnerable to predation by carnivorous birds, it seems likely that selection processes led to their short waking lives.

At the same time, there are variations between daytime and nighttime temperatures in the climate zones that big brown bats live in, so they spend 19.5% of their total sleep time in REM sleep, which is not much different from the REM percent of fur seals when they are on land (18.8%). Moreover, there are seasonal variations in the wake–sleep patterns of big brown bats. They hibernate during the cold winter months, which is a time when insects migrate, go into a dormancy state, or die (Siegel, 2022d, p. 940). Thus, a combination of food availability, predator avoidance, and night–day temperature variations may explain their long sleep periods, their months of hibernation, and their relatively high REM percent when they are not hibernating.

Owl monkeys, which are the only nocturnal species in the anthropoid group—a classification that includes monkeys, apes, and humans—are also unique because they sleep 17 hours a day, a longer time than any other anthropoid (Siegel, 2022b, p. 97, Figure 10.3). At the same time, owl monkeys have only 1.9 hours of REM sleep (11.2%), which is less than bats (19.5%)

and opossums (30.5%). Owl monkeys go to sleep in tree stumps, holes in trees, or in the foliage high in the forest shortly before sunrise and awaken a few minutes after sunset. Their body temperature is protected by their thick fur, they huddle together to sleep on colder days, and they do not face any serious threats from nocturnal predators. They have a nutritious diet based primarily on a variety of fruits, but they also eat flowers, flying insects, nectar, and leaves, and there are no nighttime competitors for these food sources (Savagian & Fernandez-Duque, 2017). It is likely that the combination of an abundant food supply, low risk from predators, and multiple ways to stay warm lead to their long hours of sleep and a lower REM% than big brown bats.

At the other extreme from the several different types of mammals with lengthy sleep periods and varying amounts of REM sleep, the land mammals that sleep the least, the herbivores such as horses and elephants, have to eat large quantities of the low-calorie vegetation from which they acquire energy in order to survive. Consequently, many of them sleep as little as 2.1–4 hours a day (Siegel, 2022b, p. 98; 2022d, p. 940, Figure 1).

The importance of the relationship between time spent in energy acquisition and sleep duration in herbivores is shown by the large negative correlation (–.80) between their body weight and sleep duration, which means that large herbivores sleep even less than smaller herbivores (Siegel, 2022d, p. 940, Figure 1). On the other hand, there is no correlation between sleep duration and body weight for omnivores and carnivores, which have higher-caloric diets that allow them to spend less time on energy acquisition whatever their size. They also tend to sleep longer than do herbivores (Siegel, 2022d, p. 940, Figure 1).

African bush elephants, the largest living land mammal, and also the land mammal with the largest brain, provide an excellent example of an herbivore that sleeps very little. They are also of interest because they have excellent cognitive skills and live in complex social structures. Under normal conditions, African bush elephants sleep less than any other land mammal, 2.1 hours a day, in four or five separate short phases called "polyphasic sleep." Their polyphasic sleep consists of several bouts of sleep that last from 14 to 23 minutes, along with a longer sleep period of an hour or more. Moreover, when bush elephants are grazing over a range of 25–27 miles, they may not sleep at all for a day or two. Even when they go without sleep, they do not need extra sleep after they return to less vigorous routines (Gravett et al., 2017). For African bush elephants, at least, there is no need to make up lost sleep time.

Demonstrating how much an ecological niche can impact total sleep time, African bush elephants sleep about twice as long when they are held in zoos, where they are fed bales of hay and do not need to make any effort to acquire energy supplies (Siegel, 2022d, p. 940). Since captivity also increases total sleep time in several other mammals, including koalas and sloths, these abrupt human-initiated changes in habitats can in effect be viewed as unintended experiments. Such unintended experiments once again demonstrate the importance of knowing about a mammal's ecological niche in understanding its sleep patterns (Ryan et al., 2013; Siegel, 2022b, p. 98).

Just as months of ocean foraging by fur seals provides excellent evidence that REM sleep is related to regulating brain temperatures, so too, their very distant cousins, northern elephant seals, provide evidence that sleep can be reduced to as little as 2 hours a day when foraging in the ocean. Like bush elephants, to whom elephant seals are of course not related, they also can go without sleep for one or two days at a time in order to find sufficient energy supplies (Kendall-Bar et al., 2023).

Dolphins, in addition to having little or no REM sleep, as discussed in an earlier section of this chapter, also provide evidence that very little if any non-REM sleep is necessary for some mammals (Lyamin & Siegel, 2019; Siegel, 2022d, p. 944). For example, one species of dolphins can continuously distinguish between visual stimuli presented every 30 seconds to either their right or left eye for 24 hours a day in three different five-day sessions without showing any signs of fatigue or failure; one of these dolphins was tested over a period of 15 days with similar results (Branstetter et al., 2012, p. 1; Siegel, 2022b, p. 100).

Further, there is also evidence that at least one species of small dolphins, Commerson's dolphin, is in continuous fast motion within groups ("pods"), which usually range in size from 2 to 30 members, although pods can grow much larger on occasion. Swimming within pods, Commerson's dolphins "never float or sink to the bottom and remain still. They move rapidly, and it is evident that they must have accurate sensory and motor performance and associated brain activation to avoid collisions" (Shpak et al., 2009; Siegel, 2022b, p. 100). The Commerson's dolphin thereby provides strong evidence for the conclusion that "Some vertebrates do not ever appear to meet the behavioral criteria for sleep, remaining responsive, or responsive and active, throughout their lifetime" (Siegel, 2022b, p. 94).

In discussing the complex relationship between sleep and ecological niche, it is also highly relevant, especially in terms of the discussion of human sleep in the next chapter, to stress that some mammals experience large seasonal variations in their amount of sleep. This observation is of theoretical importance because these seasonal differences appear to relate to seasonal temperature variations and as a result are also of interest in terms of a better understanding of the adaptive role of REM sleep.

For example, the Arabian oryx, mentioned earlier as a powerfully built species of antelope, sleeps only half as long in the blazing-hot daytime summer months in the Saudi Arabian desert (100°F–130°F) as it does in the comparatively cooler (70–75°F) winter months (3.8 hours of sleep in summer vs. 6.7 hours in winter). Moreover, it has only 4.8 minutes of REM sleep a day in the summer, which is only 2.1% of its total sleep time. Even during the less challenging heat in the winter, when the Arabian oryx sleeps 6.7 hours, mostly at night, it spends only 16 minutes in REM sleep (4.2% of its total sleep time) (Davimes et al., 2018).

The highly atypical sleep patterns and extremely low REM sleep percentages found in the Arabian oryx, especially during the summer months, suggest very directly that less REM sleep may be needed by species that live in very hot climates. This inference is supported by an ideal natural experiment that involves the lesser mouse-deer, a cat-sized, hooved mammal that lives in a tropical area in Southeast Asia. The average daily temperature in this area is around 31°C (88°F) and the humidity is high. Under these conditions, the lesser mouse-deer is most active between 3 a.m. and 6 a.m. and 6 p.m. and 9 p.m. Its brain temperature varies during the waking hours and often goes well beyond 37°C (99°F). It rests numerous times during waking and its frequent panting suggests that it regularly suffers from hyperthermia. Its 12 hours of polyphasic sleep include very little REM sleep (3.2% of total sleep time), and its REM periods last for a mean of 2 minutes (Lyamin et al., 2022). Thus, the higher brain temperatures caused by living in extremely hot year-around climates very likely led to the selection for slightly longer sleep periods than most hooved mammals have, and far less REM sleep.

The large variations in total sleep duration, as well as the variations in the time spent in REM sleep, are consistent with the idea that a complex combination of factors shapes sleep patterns. On the one hand, these variations involve the energy-acquisition and predator-avoidance strategies that are necessary for survival within specific ecological contexts. But the necessity of maintaining adequate brain temperatures during sleep through periods of REM sleep is also essential as well. Ignoring either ecological context or the need to maintain minimum brain temperatures will lead to seemingly anomalous findings and to ad hoc explanations that are likely to be wrong. At the same time, these results further suggest that the cellular-level adaptive processes of removal, restoration, enhancement, pruning, and consolidation, which may occur during sleep in some mammals, instead take place during waking in those mammals that sleep very little or not at all.

These conclusions not only provide evidence that ecological niche is a major factor in determining the total amount of time that any given mammalian species spends in sleep. They also show that temperature variations from ecological niche to ecological niche very likely contribute to, if not greatly determine, the amount of time that a species of placental mammals spends in REM sleep. If ambient temperatures are high, which leads to higher core body and brain temperatures, as in the extreme cases of the lesser mouse-deer and the Arabian oryx, then the amount of REM sleep is very small, as reflected in the lesser mouse-deer's low percentage of REM sleep (3.2%).

The same phenomenon is shown by the even lower percentage of REM sleep found in the Arabian oryx in the even hotter summer months in the Saudi Arabian desert (2.1%). This emphasis on ecological niche in shaping REM percent during sleep is also consistent with the near-absence, if not complete disappearance, of REM sleep in the fur seal when it is in the ocean, and the near-absence or complete absence of REM sleep in dolphins and porpoises.

Finally, the emphasis on ecological niche, the need to maintain minimally necessary brain temperatures, and variations in sleep time in this subsection once again highlight the need for a parsimonious explanation for the variety of brain activation patterns that occur during mammalian sleep. This framework thereby sets the stage for determining the degree to which the various unique aspects of human sleep can be understood within the context of the adaptive inactivity theory of sleep. This determination, which occurs in the next chapter, makes it possible in turn to test the capacity of the adaptive inactivity theory of sleep to strengthen the neurocognitive theory of dreaming by providing an explanation for the activation patterns that underlie dreaming.

Conclusion

The scope of the adaptive inactivity theory of sleep makes it a compelling one to consider. Its breadth, depth, and parsimony are consistent with one of the major goals of all scientific inquiry. That is, the adaptive inactivity theory situates a possible solution to a puzzling phenomenon—in this case, sleep—within a larger theoretical context that is already well established. In terms of the adaptive inactivity theory of sleep, as noted in Chapter 1, the theory first and foremost explains sleep in relation to issues that are essential to all life forms—the acquisition, use, and conservation of energy.

The explanation for REM sleep provided by the theory—the maintenance of a sufficient brain temperature to allow energy-saving non-REM sleep to continue—lies at the heart of this energy-conservation focus. This analysis is compatible with the full range of comparative findings. The emphasis on energy conservation helps to explain the large variations in how long different mammals sleep and links those large variations to the equally large variations in the ecological contexts to which different mammalian species have adapted. And, as stressed in the introductory chapter and throughout this chapter, the theory is compatible with the fact that various cellular-level processes of removal, restoration, enhancement, pruning, and consolidation may occur during sleep in some mammals.

The scope of the adaptive inactivity theory of sleep also makes it a compelling one to consider in the next chapter as a way to understand several unique features of human sleep, including the several factors that lead to the human patterns of brain activation. These activation patterns make dreaming possible not only in REM sleep, but during the sleep-onset process and N2 sleep, especially in the 1.5–2.5 hours of N2 sleep before the spontaneous morning awakening. As explained at a later point in the following chapter, the initial linkage between high brain temperatures and dreaming is made by means of studies of CBF, which is a long-established biomarker of brain activation (e.g., Madsen, Holm, et al., 1991, p. 502).

Specifically, and by way of anticipation of issues that will be discussed in the next chapter, CBF is a useful biomarker because the activated areas of the brain consume more oxygen, leading to increased blood flow into those areas. These increased blood flows can be tracked in a number of ways, all of which eventually led to the discovery of the neurocognitive network that gives rise to dreaming.

7

BRAIN TEMPERATURES, ACTIVATION PATTERNS, AND DREAMING

It is well established that the direct ancestors of the anatomically and cognitively modern humans that appeared about 70,000–250,000 years ago already differed from their anthropoid cousins in terms of living and sleeping on the ground by 3.5–4.2 million years ago at the latest. During this long transitional process, they gradually lost their fur and developed far more sweat glands than other apes have, especially in their scalps, which were very likely selected for in order to deal with hot daytime temperatures and to pursue prey over long distances (Kamberov et al., 2018). Human ancestors also became bipedal about seven million years ago, and probably for many reasons. However, even being a little further above ground level has cooling effects, so the complexities of the evolutionary journey to bipedalism may not be fully understood as yet (e.g., Tuttle, 2024). Moreover, very little was known until recently about the sleep patterns of direct human ancestors or the current-day people who live in habitats and circumstances at least somewhat similar to those of the first *Homo sapiens*.

The Ecology of Human Sleep and Dreaming

Numerous new findings were provided by the first and most detailed longitudinal study of all-night sleep patterns in three of the remaining hunting-gathering and hunting-horticultural societies that have no source of light other than fires (Siegel, 2022d, pp. 937–938; Yetish et al., 2015). The Hadza are a frequently studied hunting and gathering people, who live in the wooded grasslands and hills of Northern Tanzania, about 2° south of the equator. The San are a hunting and gathering group in the Kalahari Desert in Namibia, about 20° south of the equator. Both the Hadza and the San are

DOI: 10.4324/9781003732969-7

among the most genetically diverse people who have been studied, which supports the theory that anatomically and cognitively modern humans first appeared in the southern half of Africa (Henn et al., 2011). The third group, the Tsimané, are a hunting-horticultural society that lives in the lowland Amazonian forests on the eastern slopes of the Andes Mountains in Bolivia, about 15° south of the equator. The Tsimané are distinctive as one of the indigenous societies that has migrated the furthest from the African ancestral home, via southern Siberia and the Bering Land Bridge, and at the same time live about the same distance below the equator as do the San.

In carrying out their investigations, the team of anthropologists and sleep researchers used an ActiWatch, a movement-detection wristband that distinguishes between sleep and waking nearly as well as the electroencephalogram (EEG) (Yetish et al., 2015, Supplementary Experimental Procedures, for full details). In addition, the researchers also "precisely measured ambient temperature at the sleeping sites along with finger temperature and abdominal temperature" for several participants in the San group, which corroborated and augmented the findings with the ActiWatch (Yetish et al., 2015, p. 2865). However, the ActiWatch is not able to distinguish between rapid eye movement (REM) and non-REM sleep, so much still needs to be learned about the timing and duration of REM sleep in indigenous societies without electricity.

Although it is often assumed that humans living a hunter-gatherer lifestyle sleep from dusk to dawn, the Hadza, San, and Tsimané participants in this study slept for a mean of only 5.7–7.1 hours a night (Yetish et al., 2015, p. 2862). In addition, there were few nighttime awakenings, and very few daytime naps. In a subsequent study of sleep in the Hadza, an independent group of investigators, who made use of the MotionWatch 8, found that their participants had a mean of 6.25 hours per night (Samson et al., 2017, p. 576, Table 1). Although this study had its own agenda, this particular finding from it can serve as a conceptual replication of the original study of the Hadza. The 5.7–7.1 hours of sleep in these three societies is 4–5 hours less than the 9.5–15 hours that most other diurnal anthropoids sleep (Nunn & Samson, 2018, p. 603, Figure 1; Yetish et al., 2015, p. 2862).

According to the adaptive inactivity theory of sleep, these notable differences from other diurnal anthropoids are due to the further discovery that the inherited biological rhythms that control human sleep patterns in indigenous societies without electricity are linked to the daily temperature cycle, not the light–dark cycle, as is the case with all other anthropoids. This unexpected finding provides further evidence for the importance of temperature in understanding sleep. This conclusion is first of all supported by the finding that the people in all three of these societies fell asleep on average 3.2 hours after sunset. Moreover, these post-sunset evening hours were filled with social activities and conversation, which suggests considerable alertness: "The time between sunset and sleep onset was filled with conversation, socializing, and cooking over small fires, with a light intensity (i.e., from the fires) generally below levels shown to alter circadian rhythms" (Siegel, 2022d, p. 938).

The fact that members of the three groups did not fall asleep until nightly temperatures actually began to decline significantly provides additional evidence that human sleep patterns are related to the daily temperature cycle. Further revealing the close link between the temperature cycle and human sleep, members of all three groups woke up in the morning at the lowest temperature point in the 24-hour cycle. For members of the Hadza and Tsimané groups, this meant they woke up 30–60 minutes before daybreak in both the winter and summer months. For the San, it meant awakenings 50+ minutes before sunrise in the winter, but an hour after sunrise in the summer months, which is when the ambient temperature reaches its nadir in those warmer months (Yetish et al., 2015, pp. 2864–2866).

Still other new findings from this study concerned changes in core body temperatures throughout the course of the night. As people in the three groups fell asleep, their core body temperatures showed a steady decline in the first half of the sleep period, reaching a low point about 2–3 hours before the morning awakening. (Recall here from Chapter 6 that core body temperature is not regulated during REM sleep, so core body temperature can fall even while REM sleep is raising brain temperature 4–6 times per night). After core body temperature reaches its low point, it begins a continuing rise in the hours before the spontaneous early-morning awakening. This continuing rise in core body temperature is very likely due to evolved circadian rhythms that anticipate spontaneous morning awakenings. They make it possible for humans to be highly functional upon awakening shortly before dawn (Siegel, 2022d, p. 938; Yetish et al., 2015, pp. 2864–2866). These temperature changes are consistent with, and provide ecological validity for, laboratory studies of the human temperature cycle by biologists and sleep researchers (e.g., Benington, 2004; Nielsen, 2004).

The emphasis on the importance of dealing with the increasingly lower ambient temperatures that occur late in the sleep period was examined in more detail by studying vasoconstriction—as manifested in what are commonly known as "goose bumps." In this study, vasoconstriction was measured with a skin-temperature device (the "iButton"), which was worn by 15 San participants over the course of the summer and by 13 of those 15 in the winter months (Tartarini & Schiavon, 2020, for information on the iButton device; Yetish et al., 2015, p. 2866, Figure 4, for the methodological details and findings). The fact that vasoconstriction occurred right around the morning awakening in "both summer and winter" indicates that the participants "were not vasoconstricted prior to awakening" (Yetish et al., 2015, p. 2865). This is further good evidence that awakening occurs when the ambient temperature reaches its nadir.

In addition, there are seasonal differences in the total sleep time of the members of these three indigenous groups. After sleeping only 5.7–6.1 hours in the summer months, when they go to sleep later, the people in these three societies sleep nearly an hour longer (53–56 minutes) in the winter. This extra sleep time during the coldest part of the night in the winter leads to a considerable energy savings because it would be "metabolically costly" for furless humans to rest quietly while awake during cold nights, when much more energy is required to stay warm (Yetish et al., 2015, p. 2867). As in the case of seasonal differences in the amount of sleep experienced by one of the mammals discussed in the previous chapter, the Arabian oryx, temperature differences are therefore very likely the primary factor in the seasonal differences in the amount of sleep time.

Taken together, the findings in the field studies in three indigenous societies suggest that human sleep is as unique in its own ways as is the sleep of other species. People in societies that rely on hunting-gathering, or hunting-horticulture, and with no access to electricity, sleep less than their anthropoid relatives, and their sleep is attuned to the 24-hour temperature cycle rather than the light–dark cycle. Humans also have seasonal variations in their total sleep time. Human sleep is thereby consistent with the tenets of the adaptive inactivity theory of sleep.

And so, too, of course, humans are unique in having several hours of alert and fully active hours during darkness before sleep occurs. Since darkness is not a propitious time for humans to be hunting or gathering, it is during this time that lengthy discussions can take place, at least on occasion, as well as dancing, merriment, and healing ceremonies. But such activities are not as frequent as sometimes thought. Most nights are not spent carrying out various ceremonies.

Perhaps the most relevant and comprehensive account of the various nighttime activities of indigenous peoples—chatting about the day's events, playing music, engaging in healing ceremonies, and discussing dreams—can be found in studies of a hunting and horticultural society in the highlands of Malaysia, the Temiar, who were able to retain their traditional culture until fairly recently (Benjamin, 2014, for the most detailed account of all these issues). There is also an anthropological field study of this same indigenous society that focuses on music, with a primary interest in the role of music in the context of healing ceremonies, in which dreams also sometimes play a part (Roseman, 1991).

From Woodland Grasses and Cold Outdoor Sleeping to the Sleep-Dream Lab

One of the key findings in the study of sleep in the three indigenous societies discussed in the previous section concerned the decline in core body temperature from sleep onset until a low point between 3–4 a.m., and a slow rise thereafter. This rise in body temperature very likely contributes to the increasing amount of N2 sleep in the approximately 1.5–2.5 hours before the spontaneous morning awakening. When these findings are combined with the periodic REM periods, these findings conceptually replicate and provide ecological validity for the laboratory findings that body temperature and non-REM sleep increase toward morning. This laboratory finding, in turn, led to a "dual-rhythm" model of activation to explain more frequent dreaming toward morning (Antrobus et al., 1995; Reinsel et al., 1985; Wamsley et al., 2007; Wollman & Antrobus, 1987). According to this model, both circadian rhythms and REM periods contribute to rising brain temperature—and a gradual increase in dreaming—in the 1.5–2.5 hours before awakening.

Drawing on the dual-rhythm model and the findings developed within the context of the adaptive inactivity theory of sleep, the neurocognitive theory of dreaming suggests that there should be sufficient activation to support dreaming during N2 sleep in the 1.5–2.5 hours before the spontaneous morning awakening. Conversely, the neurocognitive theory of dreaming expects that there is little or no dreaming during N3 slow-wave sleep, which is characterized by high-amplitude brain waves, called "delta" waves. Delta waves are also called "slow waves" because they have a cycle of only 1–3 Hz. They are displayed in Table 7.1 in a comparison with theta and alpha waves.

TABLE 7.1 Delta waves—which are a characteristic of N3 sleep—have a much lower frequency than alpha or theta waves

Name of pattern	*Frequency*	*Description*	*Illustration*
Alpha	8–13 Hz	Alpha waves are often present in drifting waking thought. They are also found in the sleep-onset process and sometimes in REM.	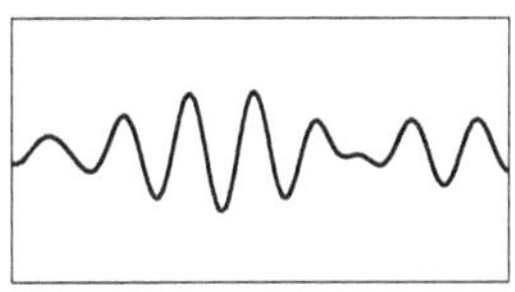
Theta	4–8 Hz	Theta waves are sometimes present in drifting waking thought, are present in the latter half of the sleep-onset process, and are prominent in REM sleep.	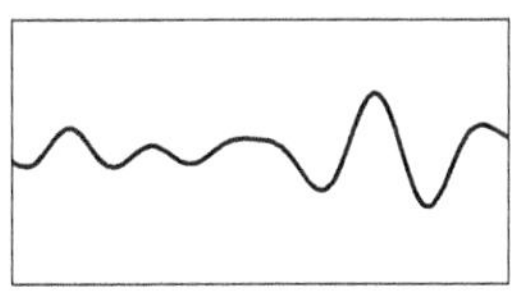
Delta	0.1–4 Hz	Delta waves are slow, rhythmic high-amplitude waves; they appear briefly in N2 sleep, but are the electrophysiological signature of slow-wave sleep (SWS).	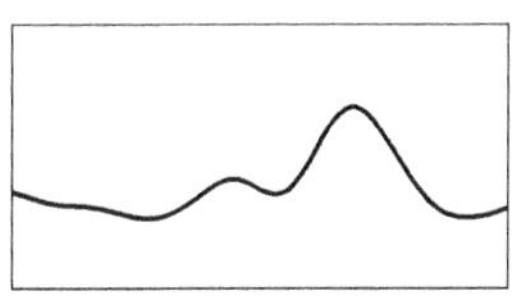

In developing a step-by-step analysis that assesses the expectations concerning the presence or absence of dreaming, which is based on the sleep findings discussed above, the remainder of this chapter makes use of three different sets of studies—(1) laboratory studies of cerebral blood flow (hereafter CBF) during waking, REM sleep, N2 sleep, and N3 sleep; (2) neuroimaging studies of waking, REM sleep, N2 sleep, and N3 sleep; and (3) sleep-dream laboratory studies that included awakenings from N2 sleep or from both N2 and N3 sleep. The final section of the chapter suggests new ways in which the adequacy of this analysis could be tested in lab or non-lab settings using a new portable and wearable neuroimaging technology.

All that said, it is important to emphasize that this analysis can only be considered suggestive in terms of its claims about dreaming in the 1.5–2.5 hours before the morning awakening. First, neuroimaging studies would be needed to demonstrate the presence of functional connectivity between anterior and posterior regions of the default network in N2 sleep late in the sleep period, which is necessary for dreaming to occur. Second, it would be necessary to carry out Hall/Van de Castle content analyses of post-awakening reports in order to distinguish dream reports from the mind-wandering reports that often occur in N2 sleep, as shown shortly.

To begin, the findings on core body temperature changes in the three indigenous societies are paralleled by laboratory studies in which the levels of regional CBF in the brain were assessed during the resting state and three sleep stages: REM sleep, N2 sleep, and N3 sleep. As discussed below, these parallels support the earlier assertion that wake-like brain temperatures are necessary to produce the activation levels needed for dreaming. This conclusion provides the initial evidence for the possibility of dreaming during N2 sleep within the framework of the neurocognitive theory of dreaming.

The first relevant study of human CBF, which involved 11 participants, found that CBF increased by 4% in secondary visual areas during REM, as compared to waking. On the other hand, CBF declined by 9% in frontal areas, which are now thought to provide the neural substrates for the frontoparietal control network (FPCN) (Madsen, Holm, et al., 1991, pp. 503–504). Using a slightly different and more precise measure of regional CBF, these results were later conceptually replicated and extended in the PET-scan studies by Braun et al. (1997, pp. 1183–1184, 1189). It unexpectedly found that CBF *in REM-activated* brain regions is in general slightly higher than it is during waking, not simply higher in secondary visual areas. Since PET scans are no longer used very often, if at all, in neuroimaging studies, it is therefore reassuring to know that PET-scan studies nonetheless still set "the gold standard" when it comes to studying CBF (Al-Shama et al., 2024, p. 4).

In addition, it is also reassuring that the wake-like levels of CBF found in the REM-activated regions are supported in a systematic overview of more recent neuroimaging studies that compared CBF levels in waking and the various stages of sleep (Al-Shama et al., 2024). In the case of REM sleep, the review found ten studies of varying quality in which participants had not been sleep deprived or else had been sleep deprived for less than 24 hours. Seven of these ten studies found CBF in REM-activated areas and waking to be the same. Two found that REM-activated areas had higher CBF than during waking, and one found that CBF in waking was higher than during REM (Al-Shama et al., 2024, pp. 1, 7). It therefore can be concluded with considerable confidence that CBF in REM-activated areas is equal to or higher than during waking.

This surprising conclusion fits well with the expectations of the adaptive inactivity theory of sleep and supports the neurocognitive theory of dreaming in claiming that wake-like activation levels are necessary for dreaming to occur. At the same time, the neural substrates that support goal-directed waking thought—basically, what is now meant by the FPCN—do not show any increases in CBF during any stage of sleep (Braun et al., 1998, pp. 93–94). Thus, the results from studies of CBF are consistent with a conclusion stated in Chapter 2. Dreaming occurs when portions of the default network, the secondary visual cortex, and the secondary sensorimotor cortex are activated at the same time as the areas supporting the FPCN and the two attention networks are relatively deactivated (Uitermarkt et al., 2020, pp. 5–6).

The results from the CBF studies of REM sleep also provide a baseline and starting point for considering the possibility that brain activation levels may be high enough to support dreaming during N2 sleep. The information needed to assess this possibility was first provided by a second phase of the first study of regional CBFs discussed above (Madsen, Holm, et al., 1991). This second phase was based on 8 of the 11 participants who were involved in the first phase. It concluded that there were no statistically significant differences in regional CBF between waking and N2 sleep (Madsen, Schmidt, et al., 1991, p. 219). Once again, that is, the activation levels during N2 sleep appear to be sufficient to support dreaming. On the other hand, the results from the eight participants in the second CBF study further revealed that CBF declined by fully 25% during N3 slow-wave sleep, as compared to N2 (Madsen, Schmidt, et al., 1991, p. 219).

The high levels of CBF in N2, and the considerably lower values during N3 sleep, are supported in a systematic review of a large number of studies (Al-Shama et al., 2024). These replication studies are essential in rendering the claims made by the neurocognitive theory of dreaming more plausible for all three sleep states—REM, N2, and N3.

In addition, the overall CBF findings are supported at the behavioral level by studies of auditory waking thresholds, which are determined by the intensity of the tone that is necessary to arouse a sleeping participant. Two separate studies with large sample sizes found that this threshold is the same for REM and N2 sleep, but higher for N3 (Rechtschaffen et al.,

1966; Zimmerman, 1970). Two other studies with smaller sample sizes also found that the auditory waking thresholds for REM and N2 sleep are similar (Cartwright & Ratzel, 1968; Watson & Rechtschaffen, 1969).

Sleep Activation Patterns and the Neural Substrates that Support Dreaming

The findings on wake-like CBF during the resting state, REM sleep, and N2 sleep provide a neurophysiological rationale for assuming that the neural substrates that subserve the neurocognitive network for dreaming are sufficiently activated during N2 to support dreaming. On the other hand, the diminished levels of CBF during N3 sleep suggest that these lower levels of brain activation rarely or never provide sufficient activation to support the functional connectivity of the neurocognitive network that engenders dreaming.

To explore these possibilities by means of sleep/dream lab studies, the neuroimaging findings on brain activation patterns during the sleep-onset process and REM sleep can be used as a starting point. This is because it is certain that portions of the default network are functionally connected during these two states, as discussed in Chapters 2 and 4.

Dreaming during Early N2 Sleep

As discussed in Chapter 5, which focused on the sleep-onset process, several neuroimaging studies show that the neural substrates that support dreaming remain functionally connected and gradually become ascendant in relation to the FPCN as the sleep-onset process unfolds (e.g., Horovitz et al., 2009; Kaufmann et al., 2006; Picchioni et al., 2008; Sämann et al., 2011; Tagliazucchi et al., 2013; Tarun et al., 2021). Thus, it is only necessary to recall that there is ample evidence from sleep-dream laboratory studies that awakenings during sleep onset often lead to dream reports (e.g., Foulkes & Schmidt, 1983; Foulkes et al., 1966; Foulkes & Vogel, 1965; Hayashi et al., 1999; Hori et al., 1994; Tanaka et al., 1996). These findings concerning the sleep-onset process therefore provide a non-REM starting point for determining the degree to which dreaming can occur during N2 and N3 sleep.

Moreover, this baseline starting point can be immediately put to use, thanks to the fact that several of the functional Magnetic Resonance Imaging (fMRI) studies of the sleep-onset process also extended into the relatively few minutes that are spent in N2 sleep before the beginning of a long period of N3 sleep, which is then followed by a REM period of about 5–10 minutes and a rapid return to N3 sleep (Dement & Kleitman, 1957). These fMRI studies reveal that the relevant portions of the default network remain functionally connected during N2 sleep (Horovitz et al., 2009; Sämann et al.,

2011; Stevner et al., 2019; Tagliazucchi et al., 2013; Tarun et al., 2021). Thus, awakenings from N2 sleep should lead to dream reports according to the neurocognitive theory of dreaming.

Unfortunately, and unlike in the case of the sleep-onset process, the available data for examining the possibility of N2 dreaming in the first hour or two of sleep in any detail are not ideal. First, the exact time at which the awakenings were initiated is not usually specified. Second, the studies do not often mention whether the awakening came from N2 sleep or N3 sleep. Third, these studies did not include at least one adaptation night, so higher activation levels due to sleeping in a new place, as discussed in Chapter 3, may be a confounding factor by inflating the number of post-awakening reports that are designated as dreams (Tamaki et al., 2016; Wick et al., 2020).

Fourth, and finally, most of the studies of dream reports obtained from N2 awakenings only used rating scales that provide one overall number to assess the degree to which the report had dreamlike qualities (e.g., Pivik & Foulkes, 1968). Such rating scales lack the capability of making fine-grained distinctions between dreaming and mind-wandering, both of which are known to occur during N2 sleep. Still another study of early N2 sleep used the total word count in the post-awakening reports as its single indicator of cognitive activity, but this measure cannot distinguish between reports of mind-wandering and dreaming (Antrobus, 1983).

For all these reasons, the main focus of this chapter will be on N2 sleep in the 1.5–2.5 hours before the spontaneous morning awakening, for which there are relevant data and analyses. In addition, the findings from N2 later in the sleep period are better suited for comparisons with the N3 findings from the middle of the night, when activation levels appear to be well below what is likely needed for dreaming to occur.

Fortunately, there is somewhat better information available on N3 sleep and dreaming. First, several of the sleep-onset neuroimaging studies that continued into N2 sleep also extended into the early minutes of N3 sleep. These extended studies discovered that the anterior and posterior portions of the default network lose functional connectivity during the early phases of N3 sleep (e.g., Horovitz et al., 2009; Sämann et al., 2011; Tarun et al., 2021). According to the neurocognitive theory of dreaming, it therefore would be expected that dreaming would not be reported after awakenings from N3 sleep.

With these various problems and limitations in mind, there is first of all a large-scale descriptive empirical study of dream reports following awakenings from both non-REM sleep and REM sleep throughout the night. It provides a good general indication of the degree to which dreaming occurs during non-REM sleep in general (Rechtschaffen et al., 1963). In addition, the reports from REM awakenings in this same study provide an excellent baseline for a comparison with the non-REM findings. The study also contains very useful observations concerning the mind-wandering that most likely occurs during N2 sleep.

This general non-REM/REM study is based on 186 awakenings of 17 male participants over the course of three non-consecutive nights, with the lack of one or two adaptation nights perhaps elevating the activation levels and increasing the number of post-awakening reports. Moreover, the study does not provide any information on the time of awakenings, so any differences in post-awakening N2 reports from early and late in the sleep period cannot be assessed.

After being awakened, the participants were asked to verbally respond to a series of questions, which appeared on a lighted screen at the foot of the bed. (The responses were tape-recorded.) The participants reported "some specific content of mental experiences" after 86% of REM awakenings and after 23% of non-REM awakenings. In addition, the participants themselves characterized 87% of their REM reports as dreams, compared to only 41% of their many fewer non-REM reports (Rechtschaffen et al., 1963, pp. 409–410). Basic arithmetic tells us that these percentages mean that 74.8% of the REM reports are dream reports, but only 9.4% of the non-REM reports are dream reports according to the participants who made the reports. At the least, this large difference testifies to the salience of REM sleep as the primary platform for sustained dreaming.

The process of examining the contents of the non-REM reports that were considered to be thoughts by the participants, not dreams, led to a new discovery that was not sufficiently appreciated in the pre-neuroimaging era. The non-REM cognitive activity that is not characterized as dreaming often "resembles that large portion of our waking thought which wanders in seemingly disorganized, drifting, non-directed fashion whenever we are not attending to external stimuli or actively working out a problem or a daydream" (Rechtschaffen et al., 1963, p. 411). The researchers came to this conclusion because the participants rated the non-REM reports that they did not classify as dreams as being less visual, more under their own control, more plausible, and more concerned with their current lives (Rechtschaffen et al., 1963, p. 411).

These several different ratings add up to a very plausible distinction between dreaming and mind-wandering. Similarly, an overview of N2 studies between the early 1960s and early 1980s concludes that 20% of all non-REM awakenings involve thinking and that this thinking often involves "some aspect of their workaday world" (Foulkes, 1985, p. 58). These overall findings and observations therefore suggest that awakenings from N2 sleep might lead to either mind-wandering or dreaming reports, which is also the case during the sleep-onset process.

It is therefore likely that these researchers documented mind-wandering during N2 sleep in numerous instances. In retrospect, this finding is an important discovery from the perspective of a neurocognitive theory of dreaming. This is because it is now known from neuroimaging studies that the same two subsystems of the default network, the dorsomedial prefrontal cortex subsystem and the medial temporal cortex subsystem, are the primary basis for both mind-wandering and dreaming. This finding therefore supports the hypothesis that dreaming is a form of mind-wandering and daydreaming (Domhoff, 2011; Domhoff & Fox, 2015; Fox et al., 2013).

Thus, future studies that carry out detailed Hall/Van de Castle quantitative content analyses of both N2 post-awakening reports and waking-state mind-wandering reports could assess the hypothesis that mind-wandering is the bridge between directed waking thought and nighttime dreaming. This might be especially the case if such studies were carried out using portable and wearable neuroimaging technologies, such as those discussed later in this chapter. Such a bridge finding would provide significant support for the neurocognitive theory of dreaming.

Dreaming during N2 Sleep in the 1.5–2.5 Hours Before Morning Awakening

As already mentioned earlier in this chapter, many studies in the pre-neuroimaging era were not as precise concerning the time at which non-REM awakenings were made as would be needed for the purposes of this book. Nor did they regularly distinguish between N2 and N3 awakenings or make detailed assessments of the contents of the post-awakening reports. As a result, the most useful evidence concerning the occurrence of dreaming during N2 sleep comes primarily from awakenings during this sleep stage in the last 1.5–2.5 hours before the morning awakening. For example, one pioneer dream researcher, who carried out several studies of non-REM sleep in laboratory settings over the space of 35 years, later concluded that non-REM dreams "are more likely to occur in the later hours of sleep, when, by physiological critcria, non-REM sleep shows greater cerebral activation" (Foulkes, 1985, p. 61).

The initial findings concerning the nature of dream reports from N2 awakenings later in the sleep period are supported by a secondary analysis of a database from an earlier study that included both REM and non-REM awakenings (Foulkes & Rechtschaffen, 1964, for the source of the database). Drawing on several categories in the Hall/Van de Castle coding system, the secondary analysis found that the N2 reports from late in the sleep period, after there have been three REM periods, were different from early N2 reports, and also more like REM reports. For example, 54% of the early N2 reports had codeable elements, but later reports had 70%. More exactly, the number of elements in one of seven frequently used coding categories for social interactions and events—aggression, friendliness, misfortune, good fortune, success, and failure—went from 7% in early N2 reports to 14% in later reports. The latter figure is higher than the 10% for such elements in the third REM period of the night in the same study (Domhoff & Schneider, 1999, pp. 149–150, for a summary of these previously unpublished results, which are based on codings in the late 1960s by one of the co-creators of the Hall/Van de Castle system, Calvin S. Hall).

Using dream reports collected by means of a small portable awakening device that can detect eyelid and head movements by means of movement sensors, dream reports were collected over a two-week period from 15 college students, 7 women, and 8 men, living in their dormitory rooms or apartments. Although there was no distinction between N2 and N3 awakenings, the non-REM dream reports were examined to determine if there were any changes over the course of the night. The researchers found that "directed thinking [which likely included instances of mind-wandering] decreased by 56% and hallucinations [their term for dream imagery] increased by 62% from the second segment to the last segment of the night" (Fosse et al., 2004, p. 301). They concluded that "as the night progresses, non-REM approaches the neurocognitive characteristics of REM" (Fosse et al., 2004, p. 302). Information on the awakening device and the general findings in this field study are reported in an earlier study by these researchers (Stickgold et al., 2001).

The likelihood that dream reports explicitly from N2 sleep toward morning increasingly resemble REM dream reports is supported by still another study, this one by proponents of the dual-rhythm model. The study examined changing levels of activation during N2 periods in the second half of the sleep period. Based on a good sample size of 20 participants (15 women, 5 men), the researchers found that there were more dream reports from N2 awakenings toward morning. They also reported that both N2 and REM reports became longer and more dreamlike toward morning when compared to reports from the likely low point for brain activation in the middle of the sleep period (Wamsley et al., 2007, pp. 352–353).

The increasing length and substantive content in N2 dream reports as the night progressed in the three studies discussed above suggest that most, if not all, of the N2 dream reports that were used in the most detailed study comparing REM and N2 dreams came from late in the sleep period (McNamara et al., 2007). Drawing on the same sample collected in the two-week dormitory study discussed above, a team of independent investigators drew combined female–male samples of 100 REM dream reports and 100 non-REM dream reports, which were of roughly equivalent lengths. Using numerous Hall/Van de Castle content indicators, they found there were no differences in terms of (1) any character category; (2) settings (indoor vs. outdoor, familiar vs. unfamiliar); or (3) in the percentage of dream reports with at least one friendliness, misfortune, success, or failure (McNamara et al., 2007, p. 122, Table 3).

However, there were differences on aggression indicators. Specifically, the at-least-one-aggression percent was 24% in REM and 12% in the N2 reports, and the A/F% and the Aggressor Percent were higher in REM as well. On the other hand, there was a higher Befriender Percent in the N2 dream reports (McNamara et al., 2007, p. 122, Table 3). In addition, the results with aggression indicators replicated similar findings in an earlier study carried out by the same lead investigator and his colleagues (McNamara et al., 2005, p. 134, Tables 2 and 3). The researchers note that the findings on aggressions in their two studies are consistent with the differences on aggression that are found in cross-cultural, gender, age, and lab/non-lab comparisons (McNamara et al., 2007, p. 124).

Finally, the possibility that N2 dream reports become increasingly similar to REM reports in the morning hours is further supported in a sleep-dream laboratory study of the cognitive activity reported after spontaneous morning awakenings. The study first of all discovered that the 20 female and 16 male participants awoke from non-REM sleep 73% of the time and from REM sleep in the other 27%, which is similar to the percentage of spontaneous awakenings from REM and non-REM sleep in three earlier studies that did not focus on dream content (Cicogna et al., 1998, p. 463, Table 1).

The study further revealed that there were very similar percentages of dream recall after awakening from either sleep state: 90.7% from the non-REM awakenings and 95.0% from the REM awakenings. Moreover, based on the 54 non-REM dream reports and 24 REM dream reports that were collected, there was only one small difference in the content of the dream reports, a conclusion drawn from findings using a variety of rating scales (Cicogna et al., 1998, pp. 446–447). The conclusion that the reports from the REM and non-REM awakenings are very similar is supported by a later analysis of a subset of the same dream reports, which made use of a narrative analysis of temporal sequence (Montangero & Cavallero, 2015).

The dream reports from this study also were translated into English and coded with several categories in the Hall/Van de Castle coding system. Focusing here on the more frequent reports from women, the character density per 50 words was almost identical in the REM and non-REM dream reports, and both the REM and non-REM reports were similar to the Hall/Van de Castle norm sample for women in terms of the Male/Female Percent and the Familiarity Percent. However, the percentage of non-REM dream reports with at least one aggression was slightly lower compared to REM reports ($h = -.19$). The Physical Aggression Percent (calculated by dividing all physical aggressions by the total number of aggressions, physical and non-physical) was much lower in non-REM reports than in REM reports ($h = -.57$),

TABLE 7.2 Italian women's REM dreams compared to their NREM dreams

	NREM (n = 31)	*REM (n = 11)*	*Female Norms*
Male/Female Percent	52%	45%	48%
Familiarity Percent	51%	54%	58%
Aggression/Friendliness Percent	41%	46%	51%
Physical Aggression Percent	28%	56%	34%
At Least One Aggression	45%	55%	44%
At Least One Friendliness	45%	45%	42%

Notes: The sample sizes in the Italian study are too small for detecting significance levels. The findings show that the Italian women's dream reports, whether from NREM or REM, are mostly similar to the American women's normative sample discussed in Chapter 3, except on the aggression indicators in the 11 REM dreams from the Italian women.

which is consistent with the two studies discussed above (McNamara et al., 2005, 2007). However, the trends for these two aggression indicators did not come close to statistical significance in this study due to the small frequencies involved. The overall results with women are presented in Table 7.2. (The dream reports from this study can be found under "Italian REM and non-REM dreams," in both Italian and English, on the DreamBank.)

On the basis of the overall results from these several different studies, it seems highly plausible that the increasing brain temperatures in the last 1.5–2.5 hours of sleep can support the functional connectivity of the neural substrates that produce dreaming during N2. This conclusion is also supported by the ecologically valid findings on rising core body temperatures in the hours before morning in the hunting-gathering and hunting-horticultural groups that were studied in connection with the adaptive inactivity theory of sleep (Yetish et al., 2015). To provide further perspective on the importance of brain activation levels to dreaming, it is also useful to contrast these findings from N2 awakenings to reports after awakenings from N3 sleep, when brain temperature is known to be at its lowest.

Dreaming during N3 Sleep?

The finding in several fMRI neuroimaging studies that the anterior and posterior parts of the default network become disconnected during N3 sleep, along with the lower brain temperatures during this stage of sleep, leads to the expectation that there should be little or no dreaming reported after N3 awakenings (Horovitz et al., 2009, p. 11378, Figure 2; Sämann et al., 2011; Tagliazucchi et al., 2013; Tarun et al., 2021, for the neuroimaging studies detecting the disconnection of the default network during N3 sleep). This expectation is supported in a systematic overview and analysis of the results of 21 studies based on awakenings from both REM and non-REM sleep.

These studies were carried out between 1962 and the mid-1990s in a variety of sleep-dream laboratories (Nielsen, 2000, p. 855, Table 1).

This synthesizing analysis first of all found that 84.1% of REM sleep awakenings in these 21 studies led to reports of dreaming, compared to only 12%–25% of non-REM reports (Nielsen, 2000, pp. 854–855). The overall figure for REM recall of 84.1% is consistent with the general conclusion from many studies that 80%–85% of REM awakenings lead to dream reports. Moreover, the overall findings based on 21 previous studies are only slightly higher than those in the earlier-mentioned study in which the 17 male participants were awakened 186 times over the space of three non-consecutive nights. In that study, as may be recalled, 74.8% of the REM reports were dream reports and 9.4% of the non-REM reports were dream reports (Rechtschaffen et al., 1963, pp. 409–410). The similarity of these results increases the possibility that both sets of results are solid.

More directly relevant to the inference concerning the absence or near-absence of dreaming in N3 sleep, many participants never recalled any cognitive activity in the relatively few studies in which awakenings from N3 sleep were specified (Nielsen, 2000, p. 854). For example, in the largest study focused primarily or strictly on awakenings during N3 sleep, which began with 60 participants, 10 of the participants were excluded from the data analysis "because they failed, over repeated attempts, to produce a content report in the slow-wave condition" (Cavallero et al., 1992, p. 564).

Further, of the remaining 50 participants, 27 of them "required some additional nights to remember a dream," which means that as many as five more nights were spent in the sleep-dream lab for the 20 participants who did not recall a dream from N3 sleep (Cavallero et al., 1992, p. 564). In addition, the request to sleep in the lab for one or more extra nights also might have generated very strong demand characteristics to report dreams (Corneille & Lush, 2023, for the continuing problems related to experimenter effects on studies, which are thought to contribute to the difficulties in replicating many psychological studies).

Overall, the results from past studies of post-awakening reports from N2 sleep and N3 sleep support the hypothesis that dreaming increases during N2 sleep toward morning and occurs rarely if at all during N3 sleep. However, these conclusions are not firmly established. They therefore await further study using portable and wearable neuroimaging technologies, along with Large Language Model (LLM)-based Hall/Van de Castle codings of post-awakening reports from both of these sleep states (Bongalon, 2025).

New Possibilities for Studying N2 Dreaming

Due to the difficulties of studying sleep throughout the night using the noisy and uncomfortable fMRI neuroimaging technologies currently available, there are as yet no neuroimaging studies that focus on the 1.5–2.5 hours of sleep before the morning awakening. The conclusions drawn in this chapter therefore invite further testing through the use of a new portable and wearable neuroimaging technology that makes such studies feasible in non-laboratory settings, and in home settings, too. This relatively inexpensive ($50,000–$100,000) neuroimaging technology is based on high-density diffuse optical tomography (HD-DOT) (e.g., Vidal-Rosas et al., 2023, for a general overview). In technical terms, it measures changes in the concentrations of the oxygenated and deoxygenated forms of the red blood cells (hemoglobin) that carry oxygen throughout the body. However, for most purposes "oxygenation" provides a good proxy term for what is being measured.

By tracking changes in blood oxygenation levels, researchers can then generate 3-D images of the brain. This technology therefore has "the potential to open new fields of real-world neuroscience by enabling functional neuroimaging of the human cortex at a resolution comparable to fMRI *in almost any environment and population*" (Vidal-Rosas et al., 2023, p. 1, italics added).

The HD-DOT technology already has been used to study the waking brain during the resting state in one participant: Robert J. Cooper, a brain research scientist, who helped lead the development of the wearable HD-DOT. He studied himself in 14 separate sessions of 12 minutes each over the course of three weeks. (Each session was also videotaped, which made it possible for colleagues to determine the degree to which the sessions were similar.) The study reliably detected canonical neurocognitive networks. Moreover, in keeping with several studies cited earlier, this self-study found that the default network was negatively correlated with the FPCN and negatively correlated with the salience portions of the salience/ventral network (Uchitel et al., 2022, Figure 4). Figure 7.1 shows multiple views of the HD-DOT headcap.

As noted earlier in the chapter, this new technology also may make it feasible to carefully compare mind-wandering and dreaming reports from N2 sleep. Such comparisons in turn might make it possible to examine the hypothesis that mind-wandering is the bridge between directed thought and dreaming.

The only necessary addition to future studies of this kind would be to ask the participants to keep their eyes closed, which most closely approximates the conditions during sleep and changes the functional connectivity patterns within the waking brain. This is especially the case with regard to the relationships among the primary visual cortex, the salience network, and the default network (Costumero et al., 2020; Ingram et al., 2024). Such studies also could make use of high-frequency dream recallers to maximize the possibility of detecting functional connectivity with a small handful of participants, an innovative approach that has been used successfully in past

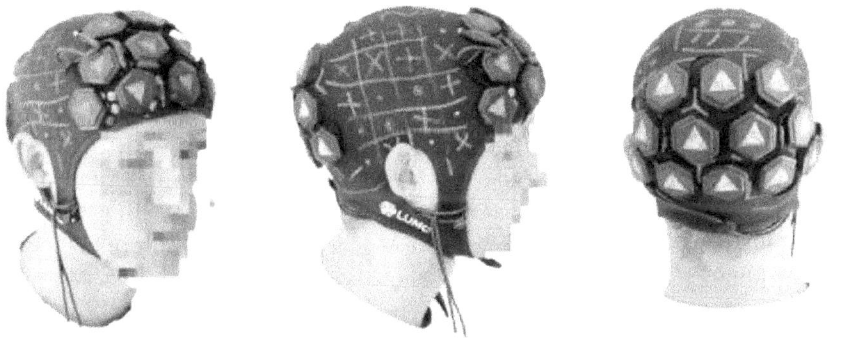

FIGURE 7.1 The wearable HD-DOT system that makes it possible to carry out imaging studies of the neurocognitive networks in the brain.

Note: The wearer's face has been pixelated for privacy's sake.

Source: Adapted from Uchitel et al. (2022), under CC BY license.

neuroimaging studies of the default network related to dreaming (Eichenlaub et al., 2014; Vallat et al., 2018, 2020).

Conclusion and Transition

As noted in the conclusion to the previous chapter, the breadth and depth of the adaptive inactivity theory of sleep make it a compelling one to consider in order to understand the variations in the length of sleep, and in the frequency and length of the REM periods within sleep, throughout the mammalian kingdom. In this chapter it has been shown that the explanatory power of the adaptive inactivity theory extends to the unique features of human sleep, which include the linkage of the human sleep cycle to the daily temperature cycle, not the light–dark cycle. The theory also can explain the seasonal variations in the length of human sleep in indigenous societies in terms of energy conservation.

Then, too, the adaptive inactivity theory of sleep can explain the gradual rise in brain temperature in the hours before a spontaneous morning awakening in terms of rising body and brain temperatures entrained by circadian rhythms. This higher brain activation level leads to the N2 sleep that makes dreaming increasingly possible toward morning. By relying on the adaptive inactivity theory, the neurocognitive theory of dreaming does not have to call upon one or more of the cellular-level theories to explain why there is sufficient activation for dreaming to occur during the sleep-onset process and REM sleep, as well as during N2 sleep in at least the 1.5–2.5 hours before the spontaneous morning awakening.

At the same time, and as noted in earlier chapters, the adaptive inactivity theory of sleep is compatible with the fact that various cellular-level processes of removal, restoration, enhancement, pruning, and consolidation may occur during human sleep. However, it is not readily apparent as to how any of the cellular-level theories could explain the differing times—during the sleep-onset process, REM sleep, and N2 sleep—when there are high activation levels that make dreaming possible. Further, most memory consolidation during sleep appears to happen in NREM sleep, so activation during REM sleep is not explained by the memory consolidation theory (Chen & Wilson, 2017; Cordi & Rasch, 2021a). (This theory is among the adaptive theories of dreaming that are discussed in more detail in Chapter 10.)

It is also important that the adaptive inactivity theory can explain the absence or near-absence of dreaming during N3 sleep on the basis of its low brain activation levels. The functional connectivity of the default network is lost during N3 sleep—due to the low activation levels in the service of the greater energy conservation that occurs in this sleep stage. This lack of functional connectivity within the default network also explains why there are very few thoughts reported after awakenings from N3, and why the relatively few reports that are made consist of static imagery or isolated thoughts (e.g., Foulkes, 1985, pp. 58–59; Kamiya, 1961, pp. 168–170; Nielsen, 2000, pp. 854–855).

The findings presented in this chapter bring the adaptive inactivity theory of sleep to its explanatory endpoint at the moment of awakening. It now becomes necessary to call upon another set of studies to understand how the processes of arousal, self-awareness, and alertness bring people back into the waking state. In addition, and of relevance for the purposes of this book, this is the time during which dream recall is most frequent for a majority of people.

8

THE AWAKENING BRAIN

From Dreaming to Consciousness

This chapter begins with a focus on how processes of arousal, self-awareness, and alertness return people to the waking state in a matter of seconds. It does so in order to provide a solid neurophysiological and neurocognitive basis for understanding dream recall and the verbal reports that sometimes eventuate from this recall. As noted earlier, verbal reports are still the only way in which the contents of dreaming can be known, a situation that is likely to continue for the foreseeable future.

The three-phase process of arousal, self-awareness, and alertness can also be thought of as a somewhat unusual state in that self-aware autonoetic consciousness returns very quickly, but alertness returns more gradually. Unless the salience/ventral network sends urgent messages to the frontoparietal control network, this groggy level of alertness often leads to mind-wandering, which sometimes includes the recall of a dream, and then perhaps to reflections about the dream itself.

Although self-aware consciousness usually returns very quickly, the nature of the network that supports autonoetic consciousness is not discussed in detail until the next chapter. Instead, this chapter prepares the ground for an understanding of the consciousness network by showing how a subcortical neurophysiological network activates the neurocognitive network that reaches into areas in the frontoparietal control network through several pathways, which are now known to go through the default network. Thus, the emphasis in this chapter is on the default network, even though it is only part of the intermediate level of the multistate hierarchical network that supports autonoetic consciousness. This analysis of the steps that lead to the full activation of the networks that support autonoetic consciousness also includes findings on lesions in the default network, which can lead to one or

DOI: 10.4324/9781003732969-8

another of the slightly differing "disorders of consciousness" (DoC). DoC are defined by an inability to achieve normal waking consciousness (e.g., Colombo et al., 2023).

The Neurophysiological Arousal Network

Arousal from sleep requires the activation of a subcortical network that is located in the pons/midbrain portion of the brainstem, the basal forebrain, the hypothalamus, and the thalamus (Jones, 2020, pp. 6–8). The same neurophysiological researcher who was cited at the end of the previous sentence further concluded that "Arousal circuits comprise multiple, diverse, partially redundant systems which promote behavioral arousal that is accompanied by cortical activation" (Jones, 2020, p. 6). If this brief two-sentence overview has a familiar ring to it, that is because the arousal process is similar to the sleep-onset process discussed in Chapter 5. Even further, the arousal-suppression network that leads to sleep, and the arousal networks that lead to consciousness, may eventually be found to be one and the same network—which discharges its neurotransmitters in different ways and to different degrees at sleep onset than it does during the arousal process.

Perhaps the best summary of current understandings of the relationship between the sleep-onset and arousal processes at the neurophysiological level is that "the early idea that sleep and waking centers were present in the brain is too simplistic" (Jones, 2018, p. 17). Further details related to this point are then added in a more comprehensive account of arousal and sleep circuits (Jones, 2020, pp. 9–10). Adding to the complexities that remain to be sorted out in the future, it should be emphasized that "no one neuromodulatory system is essential for waking or sleep nor would any one by itself be sufficient" (Jones, 2018, p. 17). Redundant subcortical arousal systems make evolutionary sense in that they enhance survival, but they make unraveling these complex processes even more difficult for sleep researchers.

The Neurocognitive Network That Supports the Return to Autonoetic Consciousness

The findings on arousal networks are consistent with and support detailed research at the neurocognitive level. This new research at the neurocognitive level is reported in a pair of studies that add many new insights and details not available in the past (Edlow et al., 2024; Li et al., 2021). In the first study, the researchers examined what they called the subcortical "candidate regions" that support the nearly immediate activation of the posterior cingulate cortex, a region in the default network, which quickly propagates the activation message to other regions in the default network as well. Based on resting-state functional magnetic resonance imaging (fMRI) studies of 168 participants whose scans are included in the Human Connectome Project, the research team found that the ventral tegmental area of the midbrain and the intralaminar nuclei located in the thalamus provide the main connections to several areas in the default network: the "posterior cingulate, precuneus, medial prefrontal cortex, and inferior parietal cortex." These areas appear to be the "primary contributors to the neural correlates of consciousness" (J. Li et al., 2021, p. 2).

The same large team of researchers then compared 84 resting-state scans from the Human Connectome Project with the results of even more detailed studies of three neurologically normal *ex vivo* human brains. The study of the *ex vivo* brains used "deterministic tractography," a more refined form of "diffusion tractology." By diffusing water through *ex vivo* brains, it is possible to obtain more detailed and higher-quality information for tracing the connections among different brain regions. Perhaps most importantly, the study confirmed that "All midbrain candidate nodes connected with the intralaminar nuclei of the thalamus," but it also added many new details and discoveries as well. The new findings that are most relevant to the neurocognitive theory of dreaming are brought together in the schematic diagram in Figure 8.1—which builds upon the very similar schematics of Figure 5.1 (the sleep-onset network) and Figure 6.1 (the REM-generation network).

As the emphasis on the dorsal/thalamic pathway to consciousness in these studies shows, autonoetic consciousness has a broader activation basis than does rapid eye movement (REM) sleep. As readers may recall from Chapter 6, activation for REM sleep follows a ventral/basal-forebrain pathway because the dorsal/thalamic pathway is blockaded during sleep. Arousal from sleep is therefore different from the activation during REM sleep because it activates both the posterior cingulate cortex via the thalamus and the basal forebrain (e.g., Braun et al., 1997; Chow et al., 2013; Picchioni et al., 2014).

The neuroimaging findings on *in vivo* and *ex vivo* brains, which highlight the role of the default network in generating consciousness, and the importance of the intermediate level of the multistate hierarchical model of consciousness more generally, are further supported by studies of neurological patients who lose consciousness due to lesions caused by accidents or illnesses. As the title of one study puts it, "Default network connectivity reflects the level of consciousness in non-communicative brain-damaged patients"; this conclusion is based on a study of 14 "non-communicative brain-damaged patients and 14 healthy controls" (Vanhaudenhuyse et al., 2010, p. 161). In addition, this research group found that patients with DoC have "significant impairments" in the networks that connect "the posterior cingulate cortex/precuneus with the thalamus" (Fernández-Espejo et al., 2012, p. 335).

Then, too, when the sedative Propofol was used to induce either mild sedation or unconsciousness, the same core group of researchers who studied DoC found

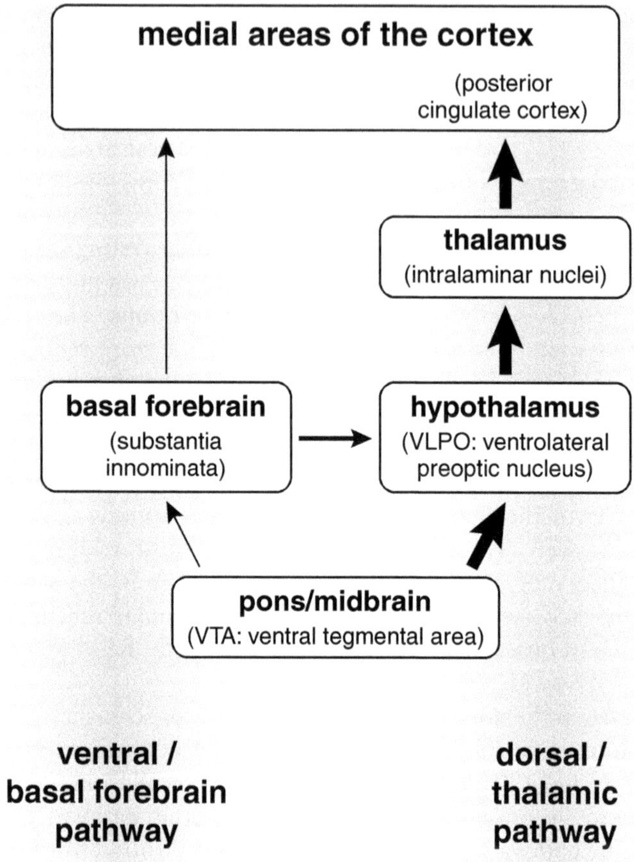

FIGURE 8.1 A schematic diagram of the pathways in the subcortical areas of the brain that lead to arousal and autonoetic consciousness.

Note: The phrases that appear in parentheses denote the specific locations within these regions that are responsible for the rapid brain arousal that makes consciousness possible (Edlow et al., 2024).

that the salience network "disintegrated" and that the thalamus decreased its connectivity with the default network as consciousness was lost (Guldenmund et al., 2013, p. 273). The findings in this and the previous paragraph once again highlight the importance of the nexus of the salience/ventral network, the posterior cingulate cortex, and the anterior thalamus in relation to drowsiness, the sleep-onset process, and REM sleep (Braun et al., 1997; Chang et al., 2013; Chow et al., 2013; Horovitz et al., 2009; Picchioni et al., 2014).

The Gradual Return to Alertness May Aid in Dream Recall

Although the return to consciousness is almost immediate as sleep ends, there is a more gradual return to alertness in normal circumstances. This lack of full alertness within the context of waking consciousness leads to slower reaction times, a feeling of fogginess or grogginess, and a period of mind-wandering and drifting waking thought. This interlude of "sleep inertia," as this gradual return to alertness is sometimes called by sleep researchers, is highly relevant from the perspective of the neurocognitive theory of dreaming. This is because the great majority of dream recall occurs during this time period, as do any initial reflections based on the dream itself, a point that was foreshadowed earlier in the chapter.

This distinction between consciousness and alertness is clearly shown in an early PET-scan study of the arousal process. It drew upon findings from the same 27 healthy adult participants, ages 21–32, who were also studied with regard to the differences between waking, REM sleep, and N3 sleep (Balkin et al., 2002, for the full results of the arousal study; Braun et al., 1997, for the details on the participants and methodologies involved in tracing CBF using PET scans). The study outlined the same direct pathway from the pons, midbrain, hypothalamus, and thalamus to areas in the default network that is more fully delineated in the later studies by Edlow et al. (2024; J. Li et al., 2021).

The PET-scan study also found that several areas in the lateral prefrontal cortex are not fully activated in the first 10–20 minutes after arousal if the participants are allowed to lie quietly (Balkin et al., 2002, p. 2318). These findings suggest that mind-wandering is indeed frequent during the gradual return to full alertness unless people are forced by circumstances to drag themselves out of bed shortly after they awaken.

Studying Dream Recall during the Night, Morning, and Daytime

As stated at various points in this book, it is likely that most people have at least four to six dreams each night. Furthermore, people are often dreaming just before they awaken, as demonstrated in the study of spontaneous awakenings in a sleep-dream laboratory (Cicogna et al., 1998). Nevertheless, people remember very few of their dreams, although it turns out to be surprisingly difficult to determine the frequency of dream recall with a high degree of certainty. This is because participants often tend to overestimate or underestimate their dream recall when responding to questionnaires. This finding is based on studies in which participants who made initial estimates of their dream recall on a questionnaire also kept daily logs of their dream recall (Beaulieu-Prévost & Zadra, 2005a, 2005b, 2007).

With these cautions about the difficulties of assessing the frequency of dream recall in mind, one analysis based on several survey studies concluded that "mean dream recall is once per week" outside of laboratory settings (Schredl et al., 2022, p. 113). Roughly speaking, then, if it is conservatively assumed that people dream at least four to six times per night, then most people remember only 2%–4% of their dreams—or more likely, fragments of their dreams in most cases. In addition, according to studies that will be cited below, as much as 65%–75% of dream recall occurs during the morning awakening. These studies suggest that much is riding on the understanding of the reasons for high morning recall.

Systematic Studies of Dream Recall in a Laboratory Setting

The effort to understand the low levels of everyday dream recall begins with laboratory-based evidence. This evidence "consistently" demonstrates that "dreams are difficult if not *impossible* to recall unless the sleeper awakens during or shortly after the dream experience itself" (Goodenough, 1991, p. 144, italics added). In striking contrast, 80%–85% of REM sleep awakenings lead to what are often lengthy and detailed dreams reports. However, and this is where the mystery of low everyday dream recall may start to unravel, even a gradual awakening from REM sleep, as compared to an abrupt one, reduces dream recall "substantially" (Goodenough, 1991, p. 144). Specifically, if people do not encode dreams into memory shortly after having them, they may not remember them at all.

As a result, the mystery may be closer to a resolution when it is added that the "percentage of recall drops dramatically if the awakening is delayed for even a few minutes after the end of REM sleep" (Goodenough, 1991, p. 144). This finding supports the hypothesis that it may not be possible to recall a dream if the attempt to recall it for encoding occurs after it has ended. The possibility that a majority of dreams are not encoded in the first place does not fit into any conventional definition of "forgetting" because there is nothing in any memory system to be forgotten. These findings support the first systematic study of all-night EEG sleep recordings that focused on REM and non-REM sleep:

> It is apparent that most of the dream experience in normal sleep is never recalled. That which is recalled can probably be accounted for by the fortuitous interruption of dreaming, as for instance when the alarm clock goes off in the morning.
>
> *(Dement & Kleitman, 1957, p. 685)*

These findings become of greater interest when it is noted once again that 65%–75% of dream recall tends to occur during the morning awakening (Elce et al., 2025; Meier et al., 1968). This 65%–75% morning recall figure, which fits well with the necessity of an immediate post-dream awakening to make recall possible, leaves only 25%–35% of everyday dream recall to be explained by factors other than the encoding and recall of the ongoing dream when people awaken in the morning.

These conclusions on the importance of post-dream awakenings and encodings are supported and given a neurocognitive basis in a study showing that people who remember dreams frequently also tend to have more frequent arousals during sleep. This finding suggests that these arousal periods may provide the opportunity to encode dreams into long-term memory. The researchers who carried out this study further "propose that the minimum necessary duration of an awakening during sleep for a successful encoding of dreams into long-term memory is approximately 2 minutes" (Vallat et al., 2017, p. 1). They further explain that "these intra-sleep awakenings would finally give more opportunities to the brain to restore memory-encoding abilities and therefore to encode the dream in long-term memory" (Vallat et al., 2017, p. 10).

The possibility that spontaneous night awakenings might allow for the encoding of dreams into memory, and therefore for their morning recall, is supported by one of the unexpected findings in the Miami laboratory study discussed in Chapter 3. As readers may recall, the 11 participants had a total of 57 spontaneous awakenings, after which they voice-recorded their dreams. Moreover, when these 57 dream reports were compared to their dream reports after REM sleep awakenings, the spontaneous reports were very similar in their content to the other lab dreams (Hall, 1966a, p. 26). Since it was already established in Chapter 3 that dreams reported after systematic REM awakenings provide a representative sample of dream content, these further results suggest that dreams that are encoded after spontaneous awakenings, if they are remembered in the morning, also provide a normative sample of dream reports.

The importance of morning recall as the primary factor in everyday dream recall is supported in a neuroimaging study of the functional connectivity of the default network shortly after awakening. The study was carried out by the same team of neuroimaging researchers who studied spontaneous awakenings during the night (Vallat et al., 2020). They discovered that participants who have higher levels of dream recall also have greater functional connectivity within their default networks shortly after awakening. In addition, high recallers also have greater default network connectivity to the "regions involved in memory processes" (Vallat et al., 2020, pp. 1, 6). This finding is also consistent with the emphasis on the default network in neuroimaging studies concerning the rapid return to consciousness after awakening, which were discussed in the previous section (Edlow et al., 2024; J. Li et al., 2021). More generally, these findings are consistent with current understandings on the relationship between short-term and long-term memory (Norris, 2017).

The Morning Recall of Dreams Reported After REM Awakenings

The likelihood that spontaneously recalled dreams after arousals during the night can be remembered in the morning is supported by four separate lab studies that included a total of 35 participants. In each study the participants were awakened one or more times during or at the end of REM periods to recall dreams. They were then asked to recall those dreams in the morning. Overall, they spontaneously recalled 56.5%–95% of those earlier-recalled dream reports in the morning (Cipolli et al., 1981, 1984; Meier et al., 1968; Strauch & Meier, 1996, pp. 66–67). These high rates of recall suggest that the dreams were indeed encoded into memory when they were reported after night awakenings from REM periods.

The first of these studies involved 198 awakenings from every REM period that occurred over the space of 50 nights. However, there was only one participant, a "middle-aged" male pharmaceutical executive in Zurich, who had a Ph.D. in physical chemistry. Previous to his 50 non-consecutive nights in the sleep-dream lab, he had kept a dream journal for 1.5 years during a Jungian analysis. He recalled 105 dreams in a period of 560 nights, which is a recall rate of 1 dream every 5 or 6 nights (Meier et al., 1968, p. 552). This modest rate of everyday recall provides a baseline for considering his recall in the sleep lab.

Within the laboratory setting, the participant recalled 138 dreams after 198 REM awakenings (83.8%), which is within the 80%–85% range that is found in most studies of REM dream recall. Most importantly for the purposes of this chapter, he spontaneously recalled 56.5% of his earlier REM dream reports when asked what dreams he still remembered in the morning. Since he often remembered three or more dreams in the morning during his nights in the lab, the sample size was large enough to determine the relative importance of several classic waking memory variables in understanding which REM dreams were recalled.

First, the dream reports from the more recent REM awakenings were spontaneously recalled more frequently in the morning (83.3%) than those from earlier REM awakenings, so the "recency" of an encoded dream is an important factor in recall. Second, the longer REM dream reports were recalled more frequently, which suggests that "length" is also a factor in everyday dream recall. Third, the more "intense" or "salient" REM dream reports, a concept that includes dimensions such as "novelty" and "dramatic impact," were recalled more frequently than low-intensity dreams (Meier et al., 1968, Table 1). These three factors—recency, length, and intensity/salience—are three of the main factors that are found to be important in waking studies of the recall of newly learned material.

On the other hand, two other classic memory variables are not useful in understanding everyday dream recall. "Primacy," which refers to the first piece of information in a list of items that has to be memorized, proved to be an insignificant factor statistically and with regard to its relative importance. On the other hand, "serial interference," which was operationalized by comparing nights in which one to four dreams were recalled with nights in which five to ten dreams were recalled, is not useful because it would be a rare night in which people sleeping at home would awaken after five or more dreams.

The ample sample size in this study also made it possible to examine the interaction effects among recency, length, intensity/salience, and intraserial interference in a further attempt to understand the relative importance of four of the main factors involved in waking memory recall. The analysis first of all found that recency can compensate for both the shortness of a dream report and for low intensity/salience. Further, longer dream reports can compensate for low intensity/salience. Finally, the researchers found that "intraserial interference is independent of the other three factors" (Meier et al., 1968, p. 555). The fact that intraserial interference is independent of the other factors reinforces the earlier point that intraserial effects are not likely to be important in explaining everyday dream recall.

The overall results of the interaction portion of the study not only demonstrate how important recency is in and of itself. The fact that recency compensates for short length and low intensity/salience, and that length can compensate for low intensity/salience, is important in understanding why many dreams that have a low intensity/salience level are part of morning recall. These findings thereby support a conclusion that was reached in Chapter 3 based on the comparison of the four Hall/Van de Castle studies—everyday dream recall can provide a normative sample of dream reports in well-controlled studies with adequate sample sizes. Put another way, the issue of dream intensity and salience does not seem to bias samples of everyday dream recall, as was sometimes claimed in the past. Then, too, further evidence disputing the over-emphasis on salience was presented in a later study of dream recall (Schredl, 2000).

In the first well-controlled follow-up study on the findings with the single participant, the ten young adult participants were awakened from only one REM period a night over the space of two nights. Nineteen of the 20 awakenings led to a dream report, and all 19 of those dream reports were remembered in the morning (95%), which is far higher than the pharmaceutical executive's recall rate either at night or in the morning (Cipolli et al., 1981, p. 397). This study was then replicated by the same lead investigator and his colleagues with a different set of ten young male participants. In this study the participants were awakened from four REM periods on each of four nights (Cipolli et al., 1984).

The participants in this second study reported dreams from 92.5% or more of the awakenings from each of the four REM awakenings. However, they varied in their spontaneous morning recall of their earlier REM reports: from 70% at the earliest REM awakening to 85% of the REM reports at the third and fourth awakenings (Cipolli et al., 1984, p. 439). The details of these findings are presented in Table 8.1.

TABLE 8.1 A comparison of the percent of REM recall after night awakenings, the morning recall percent for the dreams that were recalled at night, and the morning recall percent after being given a retrieval cue

REM period	*Recall from REM*	*Spontaneous morning recall*	*Additional morning recall based on cues*	*Combined morning recall*
1	97.5%	70.0%	20.0%	90.0%
2	95.0%	77.5%	10.0%	87.5%
3	100.0%	85.0%	12.5%	97.5%
4	92.5%	85.0%	10.0%	95.0%

Source: From Cipolli et al. (1984).

Notes: There were 160 REM awakenings overall. It is notable that the overall recall rates from REM awakenings by these ten participants are higher than the usual 80%–85% recall in most studies. It therefore is possible that the combined morning recall rate for less-frequent dream recallers would be somewhat lower.

The Cipolli et al. (1984) study added an important new experimental variable. The participants were provided with a "retrieval cue," which in this case consisted of a relevant phrase or sentence from each REM dream that they could not spontaneously recall in the morning. The use of retrieval cues was an especially useful idea because they are known to be important in recalling newly learned material in waking memory tasks (Schacter, 1999; Storm, 2018; Tulving, 1974; Wheeler & Gabbert, 2017).

As can be seen in the third column of Table 8.1, the retrieval cues added from 10 to 20 percentage points to the spontaneous recall figures. Most impressively, the retrieval cues increased the percentage of dreams recalled in the morning from the first REM awakening from 70% to 90%, an improvement of 20 percentage points. Even in the case of the third and fourth REM periods, the retrieval cues raised the total percentage of the dreams that were recalled by 10–12.5 percentage points. The researchers rightly conclude that their findings on the importance of retrieval cues are the "main result" of their study, which reveals that "entire episodes of mental experiences are still present in memory" if a report is made after a REM awakening and thereby encoded into memory (Cipolli et al., 1984, p. 444).

The importance of retrieval cues in increasing the percentage of REM dream reports that are remembered again in the morning was replicated in a lab study that used key words and short phrases from the nighttime REM dream report to trigger recall. Although the authors do not state the percentage of REM awakenings that led to recall, they do report that 67% of the 114 REM-awakening dreams were spontaneously recalled in the morning, and that another 20% were recalled on the basis of the retrieval cues (Strauch & Meier, 1996, pp. 66–67).

In addition to demonstrating the importance of nighttime memory consolidation and the high frequency of morning dream recall, which are consistent with the neuroimaging studies of frequent dream recallers (Vallat et al., 2017, 2020), two of the studies provide sophisticated, extremely detailed psycholinguistic comparisons of the night-recall, spontaneous morning recall, and cued-recall morning reports. These studies revealed that the three types of reports are very similar in their content and structure (Cipolli et al., 1981, 1984). They conclude that "the morning reports reflect the consolidation of the contents in memory" and more specifically, that "the percentage of contents common to night and morning reports was similar for both spontaneous and probed morning reports, as was the stability of the serial position of those contents" (Cipolli et al., 1981, p. 391).

Still another carefully designed and highly focused study, which also included an innovative control condition, offers a further perspective on the degree of detail that may be possible in recalling fully encoded dreams from night awakenings (Montangero et al., 2003). In this study, 20 participants, 12 women, and 8 men, mostly biology and medical students, were awakened after the second REM period of the night on two different nights one week apart. In a counterbalanced design, the participants either took several minutes to recall a dream and then write it down in as much detail as possible, or else they watched a 4-minute video that was made especially for the study. They then wrote down an account of what they had just seen in the video in as much detail as possible.

In the morning, after a shower and breakfast, they were asked to read what they had written the night before and to make any additions or corrections. As part of this morning task, one of the experimenters probed for more detail on any additions they made that were not fully articulated. In both conditions, the participants added many further details. When the additions to the recall of the video were compared to the actual video, they proved to be overwhelmingly accurate, although a few incorrect additions were made (Montangero et al., 2003).

If this inventive control condition—watching and recalling a brief video—is considered plausible, then fully encoded dreams after night awakenings may lead to greater daytime recall than had been thought possible in the past. If that turns out to be the case, this study provides a basis for understanding why highly motivated participants can recall very detailed dream reports in the morning, which were consolidated into memory after awakenings from REM sleep.

In addition, this study also provides evidence as to why people who keep dream journals out of their own personal interest are very likely documenting accurate recall. They clearly have a great interest in dreams, and they take the time to think about a dream when they recall it. Under these conditions, they may recall more details when they begin to write down or tape-record a dream report.

The possibility that a high percentage of encoded dreams are forgotten, but could be recalled if there is an intention to do so, is consistent with findings in waking memory studies. These studies suggest that the forgetting of unimportant information makes the retrieval of valuable information more efficient (e.g., Schacter, 1999, p. 186; Storm, 2011, 2018). That is, it is useful to forget unnecessary memories. Placing dream recall within this more general context developed by memory researchers, it may be adaptive for most people to forget the dreams that are encoded into memory.

According to this perspective, retrieving *relevant* information is what makes memory adaptive for humans in general and useful for individuals. Moreover, experimental studies during waking demonstrate that the retrieval of information depends on rehearsing it and relying on many different kinds of retrieval cues, including thoughts and the context the person is in at any given moment (Storm, 2018, for a detailed overview). This perspective supports an earlier claim that consolidated memories of dreams are often not recalled because of the lack of relevant retrieval cues after a night awakening (Cipolli et al., 1984, pp. 445–446). This insight may be yet another factor in why dreams are generally more difficult to remember than waking events.

In the next section, several of the ideas and experimental findings discussed in the previous few paragraphs are examined in the context of a field study of dream recall. The study is suggestive in that it provides some evidence that retrieval cues may be important in explaining dream recall in the late morning, afternoon, and evening.

A Field Study of Everyday Dream Recall Provides Ecological Validity for These Laboratory Findings

Several of the laboratory-based findings reported in the previous subsection are consistent with, and become more closely linked to everyday life by, the findings in a small two-week field study of everyday recall in the 1960s. The sample consisted of the first 12 college students who responded to an ad in the student employment office at a large American university. The ad simply asked for volunteers who would be paid to take part in a two-week study of dream recall, with no details provided. Thus, the participants were not screened for frequency of dream recall, attitude toward dreams, or any other factor. They were, for all intents and purposes, self-selected. For one week they reported any dreams they recalled by using their telephone—a land line in those days—to call in their dream report as soon as it was feasible. They did so by calling an "Ansaphone," a now-outdated tape-recording answering machine that first became publicly available in 1960. During the second week, they wrote down the relevant information as soon as possible on the written form that was provided (Domhoff, 1969, pp. 208–211).

Using a counterbalanced design, half of the participants began with a week of phone-recording, and the other half began by writing down the requested information on the open-ended report form. Prior to providing their dream reports, the participants reported the time, the location, and the number of people they were with, if any, at the time the dream was recalled, along with any cues, thoughts, or moods that may have triggered their recall. (As it turned out, there were no differences on any factor between the telephone reports and the written reports.)

Two participants dropped out after reporting dreams in the first week. Consistent with many other studies to be discussed in the next section, there were individual differences in dream recall for the remaining ten participants. Two participants reported, somewhat apologetically, that they had recalled no dreams over the two-week period, and two others recalled only one dream each. Thus, the remaining six participants provided 23 of the 25 telephone reports that were received, along with all 27 written reports. Overall, then, these six participants averaged 8.3 dreams each, which is a recall rate of about 4.2 dreams per week. However, none of the participants provided more than 10–12 of the dream reports, so it turned out that no one in the sample remembered one or more of their dreams each day, which is in recent decades one usual definition for frequent dream recall.

As might be expected from the laboratory studies cited in the previous subsection, 36 of the 52 dream reports (69.2%) came during morning awakenings. Another two came from night awakenings, both from the same participant. There were no mentions of any cues being involved in the recall of either the morning dreams or the night-awakening dreams. (Although only one of the six participants recalled dreams from spontaneous night awakenings, this finding is consistent with the findings in one of the neuroimaging studies cited above. It found that an as-yet-unknown percentage of people do awaken *and* recall dreams during the night (Vallat et al., 2017).)

On the other hand, the 14 reports from late morning, afternoon, and evening often occurred after hearing, seeing, or even feeling an incidental retrieval cue. This finding is consistent with the effect of retrieval cues on recall in the aforementioned laboratory studies, in which the participants recalled dreams in the morning that they had encoded into long-term memory after REM sleep awakenings. It is also consistent with the importance of cued recall in waking memory studies (Storm, 2018; Tulving, 1974; Tulving & Thomson, 1973).

For example, a male participant was talking to a friend about his car, and at that point he suddenly remembered a dream in which the paint was peeling off of his car. A woman participant recalled a detailed dream when she was walking into her chemistry class and saw one of her friends who was also in the class. The dream she then recalled concerned the fact that still another student in the class had for some reason or another received a failing grade (Domhoff, 1969, pp. 209–210). These findings lend ecological validity to the laboratory findings mentioned earlier, in which small retrieval cues from the researchers could trigger morning recall of seemingly forgotten dreams that were reported earlier during a REM awakening (Cipolli et al., 1984; Strauch & Meier, 1996, pp. 59–60).

Dreams were also recalled in the two-week field study when participants were alone and in a "relaxed mood," which since the turn of the 21st century has been called "drifting waking thought" or "mind-wandering." A woman participant provides a prototypical example of the way in which retrieval cues, mind-wandering, and being alone can combine to produce the recall of a dream in the early afternoon:

> It's 1:15 Sunday afternoon and I was doing my homework; I've been sitting in the sunshine, but the sun is moving and so it's getting to be half sun and half shade in my chair, and I was starting to get cold, and when I got cold I started thinking about the trip I'm going on in two weeks with the Photo Club, and while I was thinking about the trip I happened to remember the dream I had last night.
>
> *(Domhoff, 1969, p. 210)*

This example suggests that a combination of an external retrieval cue (starting to feel cold) and an internally generated retrieval cue (thinking about an upcoming trip) led to dream recall.

Similarly, the interaction of retrieval cues, mind-wandering, and being alone are exemplified in an early-evening recall of a dream, which was the only dream reported by this male participant:

> "I'd come home and I was relaxing and sitting around. I lit a cigarette and all of a sudden, I remembered that this is what I'd dreamed about." (Specifically, he dreamed he burned his fingers lighting a cigarette, then the cigarette burned down and burned his fingers again). "I wasn't thinking about anything in particular at the time," he continued. "I was kind of relaxed and sitting alone...I was relaxed I think for the first time today."
>
> *(Domhoff, 1969, p. 210)*

As both this small field study and the laboratory studies suggest, it seems very likely that dream recall in the morning, along with daytime recall due to retrieval cues, are the most important factors in explaining the small amount of dream recall that most people experience. However, there are also individual differences that need to be explained.

Studies of Individual Differences in Dream Recall in Non-Lab Settings

Despite the methodological difficulties in studying the frequency of dream recall, which were mentioned earlier in this chapter, such studies provide a starting point for understanding why there are individual differences in the frequency with which people recall their dreams. The studies reviewed in the remainder of this section boil down to the conclusion that an "interest" in dreams, which is sometimes discussed in terms of a "favorable attitude toward dreams," is the major factor in explaining individual differences (Cohen, 1974, 1979, Chapter 6; Elce et al., 2025; Horton, 2009).

The possibility that people with little or no interest in dreams are less likely to recall their dreams is consistent with the finding by waking memory researchers mentioned in the previous subsection. Forgetting things that are not important to a person is useful in terms of making the retrieval of relevant information more efficient, and perhaps more creative in terms of problem-solving (e.g., Ditta & Storm, 2018; Storm, 2011). However, that conclusion leaves the origins of an interest in dreams unexplained. For example, an interest in dreams could be due to cultural factors or personal factors. It is also plausible that people who have a proclivity to more frequent dream recall, whatever the reason may be, would be more likely to develop an interest in dreams (A. Zadra, personal communication, December 17, 2024). For example, such a proclivity might be due to more frequent nighttime arousals, or to greater functional connectivity of the default network immediately after the morning arousal (Vallat et al., 2017, 2020).

On the other hand, personality variables do not seem to be among those various reasons. They have low correlations with dream recall. In a study of 87 participants that used a battery of personality and attitude tests, it was found that the personality tests only had correlations with a person's estimated recall frequency that were between .01 and .08. On the other hand, the degree to which a person had a favorable attitude toward dreams correlated far higher with the frequency of dream recall ($r = .56$) (Tonay, 1993, p. 6, Table 1). The finding that most personality variables do not seem to be a major factor in dream recall is further supported in a detailed critical analysis of a large body of literature (Blagrove, 2007). These negative assessments are consistent with earlier findings on the relative unimportance of personality factors in dream recall (e.g., Blagrove & Akehurst, 2000; Cohen, 1979; Cohen & Wolfe, 1973; Levin et al., 2003).

There is one interesting exception: A fantasy-proneness scale, which arguably might be a cognitive variable, not a personality variable, showed a relatively high correlation with dream recall ($r = .29$) (Tonay, 1993, p. 6, Table 1). This finding was later supported in a study that found a correlation between dream recall and "openness" to new experiences, which is one of the dimensions on the Five-Factor Personality Inventory (Horton, 2015). Both fantasy proneness and openness are thought to involve imaginative thinking, and in one study openness mediated the relationship between fantasy proneness and creative thinking (Bunce & Boerger, 2022).

Still another study then found a relationship between openness and dream recall, although a later review of the literature on dream recall, within the context of a new study using the Five-Factor Personality Inventory, concludes that the relationship with openness is "small" in terms of the effect size (see Schredl & Göritz, 2017; Schredl et al., 2022, p. 113, for the finding on the small effect size). These several studies suggest that fantasy-proneness and openness may be two of the several avenues that can lead to a personal interest in dreams, and then to an intention to recall, and then perhaps to a higher frequency of dream recall.

Interviews with people who provide autobiographical accounts of how they became interested in dreams support the conclusion that an interest in dreaming can develop for a variety of reasons. To take an example that might not come readily to mind, some people report that they developed an interest in dreams because of one or more allegedly parapsychological experiences (e.g., Krippner, 2011, a pioneer dream researcher, who began his career in the 1960s on the basis of seemingly parapsychological occurrences he had experienced when he was younger). The importance of a seemingly parapsychological dream—such as a dream about an unexpected illness of a loved one, who turns out be ill—may be impactful enough to create an interest in remembering dreams. This possibility is suggested by studies asking people if they have ever had a psychic experience. Perhaps to the surprise of the parapsychological researchers who carried out these studies, "spontaneous case collections have shown that ESP is most likely to occur during dreaming, followed closely by daydream-like states" (Broughton, 2015, p. 415). Then, too, the reasons why people keep a dream journal for months or years at a time are very diverse, as recounted at the end of Chapter 3.

New Ways to Study Dream Recall More Thoroughly

Thanks to the fact that an estimated 86% of the world's population own a cell phone, which includes 42% of American children by age 10, and over 90% of American teenagers by age 14, it is now possible to carry out larger and better-controlled field studies of the frequency of morning and daytime dream recall. Then, too, the factors that lead some people to recall more dreams than do other people could be studied. In the process, it would be possible to collect a large sample of representative dream reports to compare with the Hall/Van de Castle normative samples for women and men.

These assertions are based not only on systematic lab and non-lab studies, as well as the two-week field study of dream recall, all of which reveal the primary importance of memory factors, not personality factors, in dream recall (e.g., Goodenough, 1991; Vallat et al., 2017, 2020). They are even more importantly based on the fact that research-oriented psychologists have been successful in using cell phones in field studies on a variety of topics in waking life (Harari et al., 2016; Mehl et al., 2024, for an edited volume of chapters on the use of cell phones in psychological research).

Although any representative sample of available participants would be suitable for such a study, college students provide an excellent starting point for systematic studies because many of them have two important qualities that are a function of their age and situation. Many are open to sharing their inner experiences due to their own desire for knowledge, and some are eager to contribute to the development of knowledge. As part of such studies, asking the participants to fill out the Five-Factor Personality Inventory, which takes about 10–15 minutes, would make it possible to replicate earlier studies concerning the role of openness in explaining individual differences in dream recall.

For studies with smaller sample sizes, such as pilot studies, it might be helpful to use women as the participants. Whatever the reasons may be, women in Western industrialized societies tend to have more interest in dreams than men. This generalization is supported by the fact that there are more women participants in most published dream studies, who generally provide more and longer dream reports (Domhoff, 2022, Chapter 7, for evidence on this point in daytime studies of dream reports from children in middle school to young adults). This generalization is also true for longitudinal laboratory studies from early childhood to ages 15–16 (Foulkes, 1982; Strauch, 2005).

In addition to examining anew the factors involved in everyday dream recall, field studies of this kind would make it possible to identify a large pool of both frequent dream recallers and infrequent dream recallers. Those participants who expressed a willingness to continue to be involved in the study could be asked to serve in laboratory-based replications of studies that concerned spontaneous night-arousals after REM periods, or in further studies of the functional connectivity of the default network after spontaneous morning awakenings (e.g., Eichenlaub et al., 2014; Ruby et al., 2021; Vallat et al., 2017, 2020).

As also noted at the outset of this brief subsection, such a study would provide a very large sample of dream reports that could be used to compare present-day dream reports with the Hall/Van de Castle norms. Such a study would provide a more rigorous examination of the extent to which the dream life of humans is ahistorical, as defined by the degree to which it can be shown that a large majority of dreams continue to revolve around family, friends, waking personal concerns, and current personal avocational interests. However, such a study would be very labor-intensive and require a large employment budget. This study therefore might need to make use of an

AI-based tool like DreamCoder for automated coding of Hall/Van de Castle content categories (Bongalon, 2025).

Implications, Conclusions, and Transition

The findings on the neurophysiological arousal system and the rapid reestablishment of the neurocognitive foundations of consciousness after the morning awakening, which were presented at the outset of this chapter, provide a solid foundation for a more detailed discussion of consciousness in the next chapter. They also show that the drifting waking thought that often occurs during the gradual return to alertness provides a favorable occasion for the recall of the dreams that were encoded during relatively brief post-dream arousals during the night, or during the morning awakening.

In addition, the dreams that are encoded into memory after post-dream arousals of 2 or more minutes during the night, or after the morning awakening, may be recalled during the day due to incidental external or internal retrieval cues. Further, it may be that such incidental retrieval cues are more likely to lead to the recall of a dream if the person has slipped into a few moments of drifting waking thought.

Taking this hypothetical causal chain one step further, the substantial individual differences in dream recall may be due to the fact that incidental cues are more likely to lead to dream recall for people who have an interest in dreams. Such people may therefore have a mindset to pay attention to the incidental retrieval cues that occur in the course of the day, or during drifting waking thought. New studies of this topic are clearly needed.

Although many different factors can lead to an interest in dreams, two of the more promising factors for further study are fantasy proneness and an openness to new experience (one of the five personality factors included in the Five-Factor Theory). Most interesting of all, perhaps, it seems plausible that at least a small subset of frequent dream recallers develop an interest in dreams because they tend to recall more dreams.

All that said, the realization that a majority of dreams are very likely not encoded into memory is one of the most unexpected conclusions that was reached in the process of an examination of the research literature on memory encoding. This conclusion is also based on lab findings on how difficult it is to remember a REM dream if the experimenter waits for even a short time after the REM period ends to initiate an arousal. It is also grounded in the fact that the necessity of memory encoding during waking life has been firmly established in waking studies. Within that context, the problem of understanding dream recall begins with whether a dream is encoded in memory or not. When dreams are encoded into memory, then retrieval cues and an interest in dreams become the most relevant factors in dream recall.

The possibility that a large majority of dreams are not encoded into memory creates further problems for the several adaptive theories of dreaming which assume dreams that are not recalled nonetheless can have an impact on waking cognitive functioning. If, however, a majority of dreams are not encoded into memory, then it may be difficult for most researchers to accept the assumption that a fleeting dream experience nonetheless could have an impact on cognitive processes that are operative during the waking state. These doubts about the impact of dreams that are not encoded into memory are paralleled by the doubts about dreams having any impact on task-oriented cognitive networks that in fact are relatively deactivated throughout sleep. These problems for several adaptive theories are discussed in more detail in the concluding chapter.

Then, too, both the overall low levels of nighttime memory consolidation and of dream recall after the morning awakening raise strong doubts about the problem-solving theory of dreams. This is because the theory implies that the insights purportedly found within adult dreams should lead to higher dream recall than is the case (e.g., Barrett, 2007, Chapter 6; Cohen, 1979, Chapter 10). Instead, as stated in one early study of 71 nights of sleep in 33 participants, "most of the dream experience in normal sleep is never recalled," and the small amount of recall is likely due to "the fortuitous interruption of dreaming" (Dement & Kleitman, 1957, p. 685). The problem-solving theory will be analyzed in more detail in the concluding chapter.

By the time that most people have recalled a dream, or thought of a new way to tackle a project during their early-morning mind-wandering, they are nearing a state of full alertness. They are planning for the day that will soon unfold, or perhaps dreading a task they are not fully prepared to undertake. The world of sleep and dreams is once again behind them for another 14–17 hours. They are at this early point in their day mostly involved in task-oriented thinking, and they are fully consciousness.

From a dream researcher's point of view, they are now back in the hands of the many thousands of psychological scientists and cognitive neuroscientists across the world who study every conceivable form of waking thought and behavior. It is therefore time to examine the neurocognitive networks that give rise to the human capacity for self-knowing (autonoetic) consciousness. It is then possible to show how the neural substrates that support the neurocognitive process of dreaming fit into this larger network.

9

DREAMING AND WAKING CONSCIOUSNESS

The previous chapter demonstrated how rapidly the neurophysiological arousal networks that arise from the pons and midbrain are able to propagate their arousal signals—primarily through the dorsal/thalamic pathway—to the posterior cingulate cortex and most of the anterior regions in the prefrontal cortex. These millisecond-level messages activate the neurocognitive networks that make it possible for people to quickly return to waking self-awareness. But what is the full nature of the neurocognitive networks that are necessary for consciousness to be experienced?

And how do the neurocognitive networks that produce autonoetic consciousness on the one hand, and noetic (fact-knowing) dreaming on the other, relate to each other? By comparing the neurocognitive network that creates autonoetic consciousness with the neurocognitive network that gives rise to dreaming, it also becomes possible to determine the degree to which noetic dreaming has the cognitive capacity to make use of episodic memories, figurative thinking, and five of the most frequent emotions that are experienced during waking—fear/apprehension, disgust, anger, sadness, and happiness/joy.

The Multistate Hierarchical Model of Consciousness

As noted in Chapter 1, the multistate hierarchical model of consciousness, when placed within the seven-network framework for analyzing perception and cognition, provides an excellent start point for analyzing self-knowing (autonoetic) consciousness. The lower-order sensory and sensorimotor networks receive and then send forward any new sensory information that arrives from either the external world or the body. Then the intermediate-level

DOI: 10.4324/9781003732969-9

networks, which importantly include the default network, process and assimilate this new sensory information to update existing memory schemas and cognitive concepts. These areas are "thus sources of complex cognitive representations that can, like perceptual, mnemonic, and conceptual representations, be used in the assembly of conscious experiences by the higher-order network" (LeDoux, 2019, p. 360). These schemas and concepts also can be described as "complex collections of memories about specific things, such as situations, one's self, and also about emotions" (LeDoux, 2021b, p. R828). Put in still another way, the intermediate areas have an important role in creating the conceptual systems that are the basis for both thinking and dreaming.

Thirdly, the intermediate areas then "re-represent" the newly updated and revised schemas and concepts, which can be used by the higher-order network that is part of the frontoparietal control network (FPCN). To recall discussions in Chapters 1 and 2, the FPCN is based on neural substrates in the dorsolateral and ventrolateral prefrontal cortices, and the lateral frontal pole, as well as parietal areas that have greater functional connectivity to frontal area in humans than they do in other anthropoids (Garin et al., 2022). Moreover, the parietal lobe is larger in humans and has distinctive areas within it that contribute to higher-order processing (Verendeev & Sherwood, 2017, pp. 42, 44, Figure 2).

And, as shown in Figure 9.1, the lateral frontal pole is the only brain region that is unique to the cognitively modern humans that emerged 70,000–250,000 years ago (LeDoux, 2020a, 2021b, Figure 3). Its importance is revealed by the fact that it is necessary for highly abstract conceptual thinking and is fully involved in future planning and problem-solving (Hartogsveld et al., 2018; Mansouri et al., 2017; Miyamoto et al., 2023; Rolls et al., 2024). Further, the lateral frontal pole interacts with the dorsolateral and ventrolateral prefrontal cortices in exerting control over areas in both the intermediate and lower-order levels according to the multistate hierarchical model of consciousness. Finally, the FPCN's near-instantaneous analyses of the re-representations provided to it by the intermediate areas are among the final steps that makes autonoetic, self-reflective consciousness possible (e.g., LeDoux, 2019).

The complexity of the human brain, and the resulting complexity of the multistate hierarchical model, can be seen in LeDoux's succinct summary of the entire model, which begins with the processing of the inputs received by the various levels of the three overall networks:

> Within the lateral frontal areas, a gradient of processing from the posterior to anterior end exists, with processing becoming less stimulus-specific and more abstract in progressively more anterior areas. The gradient is defined

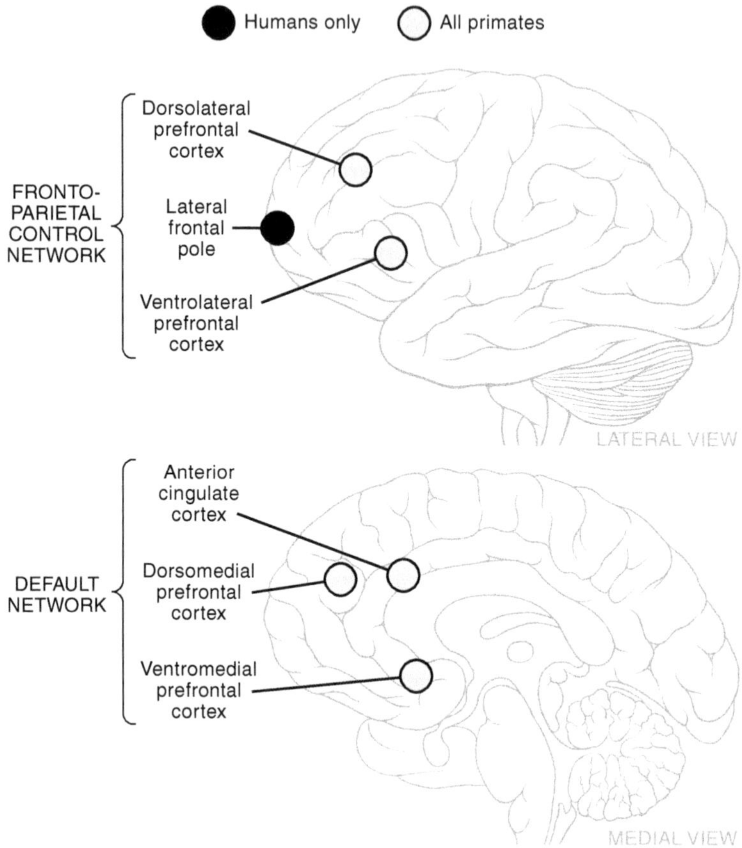

FIGURE 9.1 How human brains are unique compared to other primates' brains.

Notes: As noted in the text of this chapter, the human brain has enlarged areas in the parietal lobe as well as the enhanced prefrontal areas, which leads to much greater functional connectivity between the prefrontal cortex and the parietal cortex.

Source: Adapted with permission from LeDoux (2021b).

> by the bottom-up inputs to the prefrontal cortex. The more posterior areas of the prefrontal cortex primarily receive inputs from unimodal secondary sensory areas. Intermediate regions, like the dorsal lateral and ventral lateral prefrontal cortex, receive a combination of unimodal and multimodal inputs; these areas exert top-down control over their posterior inputs.
>
> *(LeDoux, 2019, p. 252)*

Having established the highest levels of processing and the top-down control over posterior inputs, LeDoux goes on to explain how abstract thinking occurs and how it relates to executive control of the overall multistate hierarchical model:

> The most anterior region, the frontal pole, only receives inputs from multimodal convergence zones, and creates the most abstract conceptual representations in the brain; it allows maintenance of long-term goals for future planning, and contributes to reasoning and problem solving. It interacts with the dorsal and ventral lateral prefrontal regions, and these together allow executive control over both unimodal (sensory) and multimodal (conceptual) processing in posterior areas, as well as control of deliberative behavior by way of connections to the motor cortex.
>
> *(LeDoux, 2019, pp. 252–253)*

These complex processes are shown in Figure 9.2—which is more complete than Figure 1.2, the schematic that was presented in Chapter 1. It includes several of the neural substrates that support the default network, which is an important part of the multimodal intermediate areas.

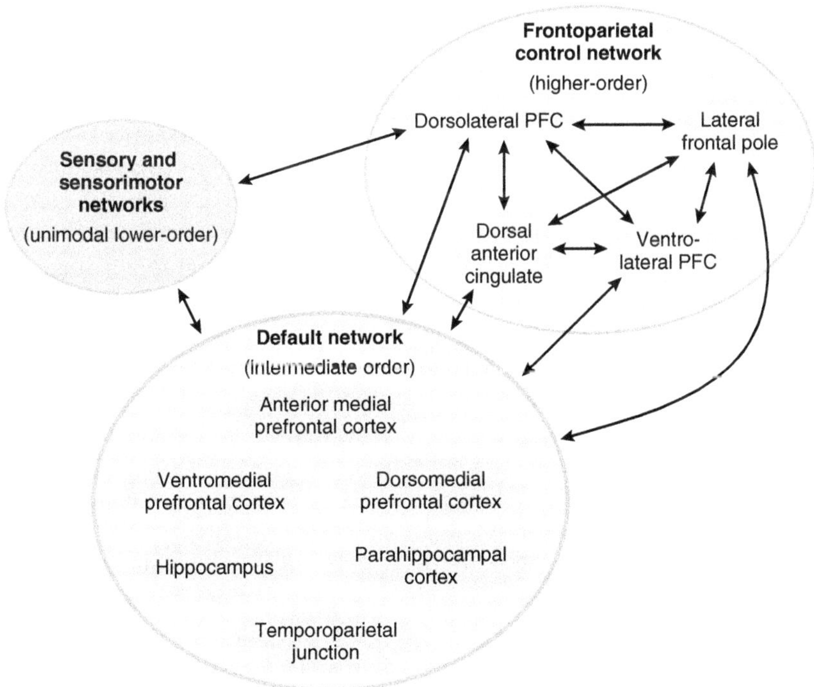

FIGURE 9.2 The main neural substrates that support autonoetic consciousness.

Source: Adapted with permission from LeDoux (2020a).

Based on this analysis, it can be suggested that consciousness is a property of this overall multistate hierarchical network. If one or more of the key network areas are damaged in some way, then consciousness can disappear, as seen in the discussion in Chapter 8 of disorders of consciousness that are due to injuries in the default network (Fernández-Espejo et al., 2012; Laureys et al., 2005; Vanhaudenhuyse et al., 2011; Vogt & Laureys, 2005). In a similar fashion, lesions in still other areas can lead to defects in consciousness. In particular, lesions in the areas of the prefrontal cortex that support the higher-order network may lead to more subtle defects—including attention deficits and deficiencies in planning—thanks to the ability of the highly complex cells in the anterior regions of the prefrontal cortex to compensate for lesions in nearby cells (e.g., LeDoux et al., 2020, pp. 255–258; Odegaard, 2019; Odegaard et al., 2017).

The autonoetic consciousness that is produced by this complex hierarchical network is not a mere by-product that accompanies the abstract conceptual representations and problem-solving that are carried out within the higher-order network. Autonoesis has evolutionarily adaptive value in and of itself by going beyond "simply detecting risk and avoiding it"; autonoesis makes it possible to "personalize risk" by asking, "How dangerous is it to *me*?" (LeDoux, 2019, p. 375, italics in the original). Further, this personalization of risk "is how autonoesis made emotions possible" because "emotion is the experience that something of value is happening to you"; if there is "no self, [there is] no fear—nor other emotions" (LeDoux, 2019, p. 375).

This analysis of the emergence of emotions as a crucial aspect of human consciousness is supported by a series of studies of "affective meaning," which is defined as "the attitude or emotion elicited by a stimulus" (APA, 2024). These studies, which were carried out in 21 different languages in 30 different cultures, found that people in all of these geographical regions and countries assess the personal meaning of the new information they receive primarily in terms of three basic dimensions. There is first of all an "evaluative" dimension, which concerns the degree to which the new information is "good" or "bad" from a personal perspective. The second dimension concerns the "potency" of the person, animal, plant, or object that is being assessed, which is best defined in terms of powerfulness vs. powerlessness. The third dimension, the "activity" dimension, is defined by a fast-slow—or liveliness-quietness—dimension (Heise, 2014, p. 1).

In terms of the personalization of risk made possible by autonoetic consciousness, the importance of the three dimensions of affective meaning discussed in the previous paragraph lies in their "survival significance in the evolutionary sense" (Osgood, 1971, p. 88). That is, they are important because it is essential to distinguish things "which are good from those which are bad, those which are strong from those which are weak, and those which are active from those which are passive" (Osgood, 1971, p. 89). In LeDoux's

(2021a) terms, one of the initial and foremost concerns of all living organisms is to detect and deal with danger.

For example, a person or animal that is judged to be very bad, very powerful, and very active clearly represents a great personal risk. At the other extreme, a person or animal that is judged as very good, without power, and only somewhat active might be viewed as a potential helper or ally. At the least, this would not be a person or animal to fear. Similar judgments are made about plants, which can be prickly and dangerous or laden with fruit, and about objects, whether they be boulders sitting precariously on a mountain side, or shiny pebbles that glisten in a smoothly flowing creek bed.

This three-dimensional evaluative framework is assessed by having people rate any person, animal, color, object, or situation on a series of seven-point rating scales that contain adjectival opposites (e.g., good/bad, fast/slow, strong/weak, warm/cold, bitter/sweet, beautiful/ugly, and many more). The overall set of scales is called the "semantic differential" (Heise, 2010; Kervyn et al., 2013; Osgood et al., 1959, 1975). Within the context of the multistate hierarchical model of consciousness, the three dimensions of the semantic differential—evaluative, potency, and activity—provide a pathway to studies of how humans perceive and judge the dangers and opportunities that exist within the highly varied ecological and social settings in which they live (e.g., Mukherjee & Heise, 2017, for an analysis of how well the 250 million people in Bangladesh and parts of India who speak Bengali fit within this framework).

Placing the Multistate Hierarchical Model within the Seven-Network Framework for Analyzing Perception and Cognition

The placement of the multistate hierarchical model of consciousness within the seven-network framework for analyzing perception and cognition makes it possible to incorporate a wide range of ongoing research that focuses on hierarchical reasoning, directed thought, and top-down commands. The use of the seven-network framework also can help in delineating the relationship between consciousness and dreaming more fully.

First, the sensory and sensorimotor networks that comprise the lower-order network are well established within the seven-network framework. This differentiation between sensory and sensorimotor networks is useful in terms of the emphasis on mental imagery and the sense of movement in the neurocognitive theory of dreaming. Second, the intermediate-level areas are in large part located in the default network. This point highlights just how readily the neurocognitive theory of dreaming can be incorporated into the multistate hierarchical model of consciousness—especially for those cognitive neuroscientists who work within the seven-network framework. Finally, placing the higher-order network within the FPCN makes it clear that consciousness is related to directed thought, working memory, hierarchical reasoning, and top-down commands (e.g., Levy, 2024, as discussed in Chapter 1).

This emphasis on the FPCN as the basis for the higher-order network is in good part due to a series of studies by the neurocognitive psychologists who found that a specific subnetwork of areas in the anterior prefrontal cortex focuses attention internally or externally. As might be expected on the basis of the lateral frontal pole's recent evolutionary development and importance, it is included in this subnetwork. This inclusion makes it possible for this augmented subnetwork to produce both higher-order thinking and consciousness (e.g., Burgess et al., 2007; Christoff, 2014; Christoff & Gabrieli, 2000; Christoff et al., 2003; Henseler et al., 2011; LeDoux, 2019, pp. 256–257). In particular, a study showing that there are two subsystems within the FPCN provides a further specification of how top-down commands operate. One of these subsystems regulates the dorsal attention network during attention and action. The other subnetwork interacts with the default network when the focus is on personal thoughts (Dixon et al., 2018).

The subsystem of the FPCN that interacts with the default network when there is a focus on personal thoughts leads to the concept of "metacognition." Metacognition is a mental state that involves reflecting on one's own current mental state. It serves as a bridge to autonoetic consciousness in that metacognition includes mental states in which people are thinking about the fact that they are thinking about themselves (Dixon et al., 2018). Two other studies support the likelihood that the internally oriented portion of the FPCN plays a role in this type of metacognitive self-reflectiveness. First, a study of the lateral frontal pole found that participants could use immediate feedback about electrical signals in this region to increase or decrease its activity, which provides tentative indirect evidence that people can gain control of their thoughts (McCaig et al., 2011). A second study found that this same internally oriented region within the FPCN interacts with regions in the default network that are concerned with self-referential information and also contribute to metacognition (Dixon et al., 2022).

Then, too, situating the higher-order network within the FPCN makes it possible to draw upon work concerning "cognitive control networks" (e.g., Christoff & Gabrieli, 2000; Christoff et al., 2001, 2016; Dixon et al., 2014a, 2014b). As their definition of cognitive control in the next sentence makes clear, this concept has close parallels with the idea of top-down commands. For these neurocognitive researchers, cognitive control is "the process by which PFC [i.e., prefrontal cortex] selectively biases currently relevant representations in other parts of the brain, thereby helping focus attention on currently relevant stimuli while diminishing attention toward other competing stimuli" (Christoff, 2014, p. 319).

In addition, a large part of the success of the higher-order network in carrying out sophisticated hierarchical reasoning and top-down directed thought is due to the fact that the human brain has a far greater capacity to hold several pieces of information in its working-memory subsystem than is the case for our closest cousins, chimpanzees. Chimpanzees have at most a working memory that can work with two separate pieces of information at the same time (WM = 2±1) (Read et al., 2022, pp. 1, 23). This figure is not even close to the working memory of 7±2 in humans. As additional evidence for this point, the gradual evolution of human working memory has been delineated in detail through careful studies of the "archeological evidence for qualitative changes marking different stages in the design and technological complexity of tool manufacture" (Read et al., 2022, p. 23 for this quotation, and pages 22–23, including Figure 12 and Table 6, for this elegant and mathematically informed analysis). More generally, humans have the "metacognitive ability" to develop strategies that "vastly" exceed the computational power of non-human primates (Read et al., 2022, p. 25).

In terms of the seven-network parcellation of the human brain, the FPCN and the default network are the primary basis for the unique human abilities, including a large working memory, that make possible problem-solving, hierarchical reasoning, and imaginative constructions. However, it is the constant change in activity and connectivity patterns across the five association networks that creates the kaleidoscope of networks that underlie the constantly changing thought patterns that occur during waking. For example, these thought patterns can shift from focused thinking to mind-wandering and back again to focused thinking in a matter of seconds.

The Contrasts between Waking Thought and Dreaming

Within the context of the seven-network framework and the multistate hierarchical model consciousness, the differences between waking thought and dreaming can be stated very clearly. First, due to the blockade of sensory stimuli at the thalamus during sleep, as stressed in Chapters 2 and 6, dreaming lacks the perceptual inputs that represent the demands and opportunities presented by the waking world. During waking, external and internal stimuli are received by the lower-order sensory and sensorimotor areas and then sent to relevant intermediate areas for recognition, memory storage, and incorporation into schemas and concepts.

The lack of these perceptual constraints leaves the neurocognitive network that produces dreaming with little or no sensory input, and therefore without any external guidance. This is a very large contrast with the waking state, in which sensory information is a near constant. Even during contemplative states, or drifting waking thought, sudden and highly amplified sensory information can put the brain on full alert.

At the same time, the capacity to redirect thought through top-down commands is also lost during dreaming, due to the relative deactivation of the FPCN. The imagination network therefore can roam through the memories and concepts that are stored in the expansive semantic network located in the intermediate-level networks within the multistate hierarchical model of consciousness (Binder & Desai, 2011; Duff et al., 2020; Sridhar et al., 2023, for analyses of the semantic network). As part of this process, the neurocognitive network that produces dreaming can draw upon semantic memories and the self-system to create dream scenarios that range from highly realistic dramatizations of ongoing personal concerns to adventurous dreams that do not appear to be related to personal concerns, as discussed in Chapters 3 and 4. The only constraints are the limits of imagination. That is, if a person can imagine something, then that person has the capacity to create a dream about it.

However, no matter how realistic, frightening, or inspiring dreams may be, the fact remains that dreaming is based on portions of the intermediate areas that are functioning on their own. Dreaming occurs without inputs from either the lower-order network on the one side, or the higher-order network on the other. Table 9.1 provides an overview of the analysis that is presented in this subsection.

In comparison to waking thought, dreaming suffers from "cognitive deficiencies." These cognitive deficiencies are primarily due to the deactivation of the FPCN and the two attention networks during dreaming, but the concept

TABLE 9.1 A comparison of the main neural substrates that support autonoetic consciousness and noetic dreaming

	Consciousness network	*Dreaming network*
Lateral frontal pole	Activated	Relatively deactivated
Dorsolateral PFC	Activated	Relatively deactivated
Ventrolateral PFC	Activated	Relatively deactivated
Ventromedial PFC	Activated	Activated
Dorsomedial PFC	Activated	Activated
Hippocampus	Activated	Activated
Parahippocampal cortex	Activated	Activated
Episodic memory network	Activated	Relatively deactivated
Semantic memory network	Activated	Activated
Lingual gyrus (visual processing)	Activated	Activated
Secondary visual areas	Activated	Activated
Primary visual cortex	Activated	Relatively deactivated

Note: This table is based on the discussions and graphics in Domhoff (2022, Chapter 2) and LeDoux (2019, Chapter 57).

of cognitive deficiencies also is used to understand the deficiencies in dreaming during childhood, such as the lack of complexity and the relative absence of the self in young children's dreams. Within this context, cognitive deficiencies provide the final and perhaps most compelling evidence that dreaming has no evolutionarily adaptive value. Unlike the waking default network, which is in constant dialogue with the FPCN, the portions of the default network that are active at various times during sleep are not interacting with the FPCN. This point is demonstrated in detail in the next section.

Cognitive Deficiencies during Dreaming

The fact that dreaming is supported by only portions of the intermediate areas in the multistate hierarchical model of consciousness, with no help from lower-order sensory inputs or higher-order hierarchical reasoning, suggests that there are cognitive deficiencies in dreaming. For example, as noted briefly in Chapter 1, there appears to be a relative absence of episodic memories during dreaming according to two studies with large sample sizes.

In a study of 299 spontaneously recalled dreams that were documented in14-day daily logs by 29 participants, it was found that no more than 1%–2% involved any form of episodic replay, even though as many as 65% of the reports seemed to relate to one or more waking experiences during the day. The researchers therefore suggest there is a "functional dissociation" between dreams and episodic memory (Fosse et al., 2003, p. 1). In a similar study, 32 participants kept daily records of their dreams and any related waking experiences, which led to only one dream with an episodic memory out of 186 dream reports (Malinowski & Horton, 2014, p. 444). These findings are consistent with the fact that several of the areas that support episodic memory during waking are relatively deactivated during dreaming, including the anterior prefrontal cortices, the dorsolateral prefrontal cortex, and the ventrolateral prefrontal cortex, which are also among the most essential neural substrates that support the FPCN (Cooper & Simons, 2019; Simons et al., 2022, pp. 174–175; Yoo et al., 2021, for neurocognitive analyses of the episodic memory network during waking).

Following a similar line of reasoning, it can be suggested that there is little or no symbolism in dreams (see Domhoff, 2022, Chapter 5, for a detailed presentation of the various findings that lead to this conclusion). This is because the FPCN works closely with areas in the default network on both the production and understanding of figurative thought during waking (Beaty & Silvia, 2013; Beaty et al., 2017; Benedek et al., 2014; Holyoak & Stamenkovic, 2018; Rapp et al., 2012; Vartanian, 2012, for the neurocognitive networks that support figurative thought during waking). However, the FPCN is relatively deactivated during all stages of sleep, as shown in Chapter 2, which very likely limits figurative thinking during dreaming.

In terms of the networks that are most active during metaphor production, which seems to be the type of figurative thought that is most akin to what is meant by symbolism in dreaming, they show "increased cooperation among brain regions involved in mental simulation, executive control, and semantic integration" (Beaty et al., 2017, p. 170). As already stated above, the network that involves executive control is relatively deactivated during dreaming, which is one strong reason why there may be little or no metaphoric thinking during dreaming. On the other hand, the pervasiveness of metaphoric thinking during waking may be the main reason why metaphoric interpretations are often made of dreams. That is, metaphoric interpretations are a good example of a wake-state bias, in which it is assumed that thinking and dreaming are very similar because of some of the parallels in content, and also because dreams often have a "realistic" feeling to them.

These conclusions are also consistent with a meta-analysis of studies focused on metaphor comprehension. It found that the comprehension of metaphoric thinking is supported by the inferior frontal gyrus and "sometimes the dorsolateral prefrontal cortex," as well as by "broad regions of the temporal cortex" (Holyoak & Stamenkovic, 2018, p. 653). Since the inferior frontal gyrus and the dorsolateral prefrontal cortex are relatively deactivated during REM sleep, this finding reinforces the inference that there is little or no complex metaphorical thinking during dreaming. Recalling the neuroimaging studies of REM sleep that were discussed in Chapter 2, the neurocognitive network that supports dreaming does not include any parts of the FPCN. It is therefore unlikely that the portions of the default network that are active during dreaming receive enough support from regions in the FPCN to generate metaphors.

This conclusion, in turn, is consistent with the several unsuccessful attempts to use content analysis to study symbolism as a form of metaphoric thinking in dream reports (Domhoff, 2022, Chapter 5, for a detailed summary of past studies, starting with Freud's claims based on psychotherapy sessions and other sources). Several of these efforts were developed on the basis of the field of cognitive linguistics, which has shown how pervasive metaphoric thinking actually is in all forms of waking thought, including philosophy (Gibbs, 1994, 2014; Lakoff, 1987; Lakoff & Johnson, 1999). This work revived early hopes that studies of symbolism in dream content might move beyond clinical case studies and anecdotal examples (Domhoff, 1996, p. 210, for a summary of the possibilities that seemed to exist in the 1990s; Hall, 1953, for a cognitive theory of dream symbols based on metaphoric thinking during waking; Lakoff, 1997, for an application of cognitive linguistics to dreams). However, the systematic studies of symbolism based on large representative samples of REM dream reports and of the dream reports in personal dream journals have not been successful in moving beyond the conclusion that symbolism is very likely rare at best in dreams.

The next subsection focuses on a likely cognitive deficiency during dreaming that concerns what is perhaps the most controversial issue in the study of dreaming and dream content. To what degree do emotions appear in dreams?

Are Emotions as Frequent during Dreaming as They Are Claimed to Be?

According to many characterizations of dreaming, dreams are noteworthy for their frequent and strong emotions. However, waking neuroimaging studies of the neurocognitive networks that give rise to five important emotions (fear, disgust, anger, sadness, and happiness), when combined with numerous studies of dream content that are based on the four Hall/Van de Castle coding categories for emotions, suggest that emotions are far less frequent in dreams than is generally suggested (Domhoff, 2022, Chapter 8, for full background information and a more detailed analysis).

The waking neuroimaging findings presented in this section may be surprising for at least two reasons. They first of all call into question the idea that all animals experience emotions in any human sense of the term, which became accepted knowledge in the sciences because Charles Darwin presented strong observational and behavioral evidence for this idea in *The Expression of the Emotions in Man and Animals* (1872/1998). Secondly, the new neurocognitive findings refute the idea that each emotion is based on a dedicated area in the brain that was created throughout innumerable generations of mammals due to natural selection.

These issues were first discussed at length in a larger historical context by a long-time researcher on emotions, who later turned his attention to the development of the multistate hierarchical model of consciousness. He concluded on the basis of existing scientific evidence that mammals other than humans lack the prefrontal neural substrates that make human emotions possible (LeDoux, 2015, 2020b; LeDoux & Brown, 2017).

Building on the cognitively oriented approach to emotions that first appeared in psychology in the early 1960s, the relatively recent neurocognitive analyses of emotions that provide the basis for this subsection are rooted in a series of four meta-analyses of neuroimaging studies of emotions by the same team of researchers. These meta-analyses began at the neurophysiological level, which concluded that different emotions do not have separate neural substrates within the autonomic nervous system, based on 202 studies of induced emotions in representative samples of adults. It further concluded that most of the autonomic nervous system variables are generally involved in all five of the emotion states, although there was some variation in their roles for each of the emotions (Siegel et al., 2018).

The second meta-analysis, based on 397 neuroimaging studies, found no evidence of a neural substrate underlying a positive–negative dimension, which is generally characterized as the "hedonic tone." The existence of such a dimension was assumed in the past on the basis of "hundreds of studies of semantics, self-reports of experience, and emotions perceptions in faces and vocal acoustics…" (Lindquist et al., 2016; Polner-Clark et al., 2016, p. 147, for a summary statement of these findings). Nor was there any evidence for the idea that positivity and negativity are independent dimensions. Instead, several brain regions are involved in shaping hedonic tone, including two neural substrates that are frequently mentioned in this book, the dorsomedial prefrontal cortex, and the ventromedial prefrontal cortex, both of which are part of the default network.

The third meta-analytic study provided important new evidence on another longstanding issue. Does each emotion category have a "specific, dedicated neural circuitry in the brain?" (Polner-Clark et al., 2016, p. 152). Contrary to textbook expectations, the researchers found that a variety of brain regions, primarily in the prefrontal cortex, but also in regions in the amygdala, are involved in supporting all five of the emotions, and that these same brain regions are frequently involved in supporting non-emotional cognitive processes as well (Lindquist et al., 2012).

The fourth and final meta-analysis focused on the degree to which all five of the emotions that were studied make use of one of more of the five association networks that are essential to waking thought. The surprising result is that each of the five association networks is involved to varying degrees in creating all five of these emotions (e.g., L. F. Barrett, 2017; Barrett et al., 2025; Polner-Clark et al., 2016). For example, both the default network and the salience/ventral network are involved in the construction of all five emotions, but the degree of their involvement varies with each emotion (Raz et al., 2016, p. 721; Touroutoglou et al., 2015, pp. 1257, 1261–1262).

Fear and anger, to take another example, involve greater activation in the default network, the dorsal attention network, and the FPCN, along with secondary visual areas. But those same areas are less activated when sadness, disgust, or happiness was experienced. In a result that may seem paradoxical on the basis of many past perspectives, both sadness and happiness share greater activation of the salience/ventral and sensorimotor networks (Polner-Clark et al., 2016, pp. 155–156). Put another way, the overall results of these studies demonstrate that emotions can be "distinguished by their profiles of relative activation across networks," which includes the limbic network mentioned briefly in Chapter 1 (Polner-Clark et al., 2016, p. 155).

Based on waking-state findings on the importance of the five association networks in the creation of emotions, the neurocognitive theory of dreaming would expect that emotions are more limited during dreaming than during waking. Although portions of the default network, which are involved in all five of the emotions that were studied, are relatively activated during dreaming, the FPCN, the two attention networks, and the limbic network are relatively deactivated. It therefore seems unlikely that the portions of the default network that are relatively activated during dreaming are sufficient to produce the range and frequency of emotions that can occur during waking.

This expectation first of all can be studied by making use of studies of dream content that relied on the categories for studying emotions that are included in the Hall/Van de Castle coding system. As readers may recall, the measurement and statistical issues related to this coding system were discussed in detail in Chapter 3 (Hall & Van de Castle, 1966, Chapter 5). By coincidence, this coding system includes coding categories for the same emotions that are the focus of the series of neuroimaging studies discussed above. They are labeled fear/apprehension, anger, sadness, and joy/happiness in the Hall/Van de Castle coding system.

Further, the emotion of disgust, which is very infrequent in dream reports, is part of the fear/apprehension category, which means that there is a complete overlap with the five emotions examined in the neuroimaging studies that were cited above. The inclusion of disgust in the fear/apprehension category is consistent with analyses suggesting that disgust seems to have its origins in a fear of contamination by bodily excretions and specific types of food, along with a similar fear of specific immoral actions, often related to sex (e.g., Gifuni et al., 2017, p. 1171, for recent evidence concerning this point).

In addition, the fear/apprehension category also includes guilt, shame, and embarrassment, which are also rarely expressed in dreams according to Hall/Van de Castle studies of emotions in dream reports. Guilt, shame, and embarrassment are included in the fear/apprehension category because they are due to the fears people have about being caught in a lie, being socially ridiculed for something they said or did, or facing social rejection by family members and friends.

The content analyses of emotions in the rest of this subsection begin with findings based on the dream reports collected in the Miami laboratory/non-laboratory study (Domhoff & Schneider, 1999, p. 144). The emotion results for the normative samples of women and men are also included in this analysis. The overall results are expressed by a "No-Emotions Percent," which is simply the inverse of the percentage of dream reports that include at least one emotion.

The No-Emotions Percent is useful here because it immediately makes clear that in all but one of the samples that will be discussed in this subsection, a majority of dream reports had no emotions in them. For example, two-thirds or more of the dreams in the three samples from men in Table 9.2 have no emotions, according to studies using the Hall/Van de Castle coding

TABLE 9.2 Percentage of dreams that contain no emotions, from Hall and Van de Castle's studies

	n	*Dream reports with no emotions*
Miami lab (men)	167	76.0%
Miami non-lab (men)	106	67.0%
Male norms	500	66.8%
Female norms	491	49.7%
Combined male and female norms	991	58.3%

Notes: The codings for the Miami lab and non-lab dreams were carried out by coders who were blind to the provenance of the dream reports. They were hired by G. William Domhoff and trained by Adam Schneider. The new codings were necessary because Hall and Van de Castle did not code the Miami dream reports for emotions. Note also that the women's sample size was 491 and the combined sample size was 991 because nine of the women's dreams and coding cards were lost when Hall and Van de Castle were mailing materials back and forth between California and Virginia after they both left Miami in 1966 (Domhoff, 2022, pp. 211–212).

system. For the sample of women in Table 9.2, 49.7% of their dreams have no emotions. The findings for the combined normative findings for women and men are also included in this table to make it possible to compare Hall/Van de Castle findings with later studies that analyzed combined samples of women and men.

The no-emotions findings in the Miami lab/non-lab study and the Hall/Van de Castle normative dreams were conceptually replicated in a study that was based on the researcher's own independently developed coding categories for emotions (Snyder, 1970). The 635 REM dream reports were collected in sleep-dream laboratories at the National Institute of Mental Health in Bethesda, Maryland, and the Downstate Medical Center in Brooklyn, New York, over the space of "250 subject nights." Although the exact number of participants is not stated, 30% of the participants were women and 70% were men. In the analysis of the combined sample of women and men, 65% of the dream reports contained no emotions, which is close to the Hall/Van de Castle combined norms (58.3%) (Snyder, 1970, p. 141).

Similarly, a study of 104 REM dream reports collected from 20 college-age men, which made use of new coding categories created by the researchers, found that a minimum of 62% of the dream reports contained no emotions (McCarley & Hoffman, 1981, pp. 908, 912). (If "surprise" is removed from their emotions scale because it is not unambiguously an emotion, then the percentage of dream reports with no emotions is 66.8% (Domhoff, 2022, pp. 82–87 and pp. 209–210 for a discussion of why the cognitive appraisals called "surprise" and "confusion" are no longer considered to be emotions within the context of the Hall/Van de Castle coding system).

Using a German translation of the Hall/Van de Castle coding system, the Hall/Van de Castle normative findings were directly replicated for a third time based on a combined sample of 180 women and men's non-lab dream reports collected by researchers associated with the Central Institute of Mental Health in Mannheim. Fully 60.6% of the dream reports in this combined sample had no emotions, which is almost identical with the 58.3% of dream reports with no emotions in the combined American normative sample of women and men (Domhoff, 2022, p. 215; Schredl & Doll, 1998, p. 640, Table 1).

The Hall/Van de Castle normative findings were conceptually replicated again in a series of three studies by researchers at the University of Turku in Finland, who developed their own coding system for emotions. Their coding system included ten categories for positive emotions and ten categories for negative emotions. The first study focused on 115 REM dream reports provided by 17 participants—10 women and 7 men (Sikka et al., 2014, pp. 54–55). Based on a combined sample of the women and men, the coders found that 61.3% of the dream reports had no emotions, which is similar to the 58.3% found in the combined American normative results (Sikka et al., 2014, pp. 56–57). The second study was based on 552 non-lab dream reports provided by 44 participants, 28 women, and 16 men. The two coders found that 52% of the dream reports in a combined sample of women and men did not include any emotions, which is slightly lower than the American normative figure for a combined sample (58.3%) (Sikka et al., 2017, p. 367).

In their final study in this series, the University of Turku researchers compared 120 REM laboratory dream reports with 151 non-lab reports. The two coders, once again working independently and then meeting to resolve any differences, concluded that more than half of the dreams reported in both the laboratory setting and the non-laboratory setting contained no emotions: 54.6% in the non-lab dreams and 70.7% in the lab dreams (Sikka et al., 2018, p. 210, Table 2). The no-emotions percentage for non-lab dreams is, again, very similar to the Hall/Van de Castle normative results (58.3%). (There is no comparable Hall/Van de Castle combined sample for lab dream reports collected from REM awakenings because only men were used in their lab study.)

The results from all ten of the studies discussed above are summarized in Table 9.3. It shows that the No Emotions% Percent is over 50% in every case except for the Hall/Van de Castle American female norms.

Although the three studies by Sikka et al. at the University of Turku in the 2010s and the Hall/Van de Castle studies in Miami in the 1960s were carried out 50 years apart in two different countries and used different categorical-level coding systems, they are in many ways very similar. They both had large samples based on everyday recall and smaller samples of lab and non-lab dream reports from the same participants. In addition, their results are

TABLE 9.3 Percentage of dream reports that contained no emotions in ten different samples

	Gender	*n*	*Dreams with no emotions (Non-lab/ home)*	*Dreams with no emotions (Lab/REM)*
H/VdC norms (1947–1950)	Female	491	49.7%	
H/VdC norms (1947–1950)	Male	500	66.8%	
H/VdC norms (1947–1950)	Combined	991	58.3%	
Miami lab (1966)	Male	167		76.0%
Miami non-lab (1966)	Male	106	67.0%	
Snyder (1970)	Combined	635		65.0%
McCarley and Hoffman (1981)	Male	104		66.8%
Schredl/Doll (1998)	Combined	180	60.6%	
Sikka et al. (2014)	Combined	115		71.3%
Sikka et al. (2017)	Combined	552	52.2%	
Sikka et al. lab (2018)	Combined	120		70.7%
Sikka et al. non-lab (2018)	Combined	151	54.6%	

remarkably similar. In conjunction with the three previously mentioned studies carried out by three different investigative teams, the three studies from the University of Turku provide a strong case that the frequency of emotions in dreams is much lower than is generally believed.

There is one dissenting voice, however. The study from the Central Institute of Mental Health, which reported very similar results to the Hall/Van de Castle normative findings using a German translation of the coding system, also included a rating scale. The rating scale was used by the 263 participants to rate their own dream reports, for a total of 964 self-ratings. The-self-raters concluded that only 7.3% of their dream reports were without emotions.

Next, an independent rater was asked to rate the subset of the 180 reports that had been coded using the Hall/Van de Castle coding system, as discussed earlier in this chapter. The independent rater found that only 14.4% of the dream reports did not include an emotion, which is a very large difference from the 60.6% of the dream reports that had no emotions according to the Hall/Van de Castle codings (Schredl & Doll, 1998, p. 640, Table 1, in which their no-emotions findings are summarized). This large discrepancy led them to claim that this "inconsistency" is "best explained by the *underestimation* of emotions by external raters in general, but particularly by the strong *underestimation* of positive emotions and the low rate of explicitly mentioned positive emotions in a dream report" (Schredl & Doll, 1998, pp. 642–643, italics added). From a neurocognitive point of view, this claim of underestimation does not fit with the relative deactivation during sleep of four of the five associative networks that are necessary for waking emotions to occur (e.g., L. F. Barrett, 2017; Polner-Clark et al., 2016; Touroutoglou et al., 2015).

This dissenting conclusion was then amplified in a further study 19 years later by the same lead researcher and a new co-worker. The 413 participants documented 1207 dreams over a two-week period. The self-ratings were again clear in stating that only 4.7% of the dream reports did not contain an emotion (Röver & Schredl, 2017, pp. 66–68). Contrary to their results and conclusions, it seems more likely that the rating results greatly underestimated the absence of emotions for several methodological reasons, including the fact that the dreamers were instructed to include any "implicit" emotions and "moods" in their self-ratings (Schredl & Doll, 1998, p. 638). Thus, it is very likely that they are claiming there is far more emotion in dreams than is found in other studies because of the rating systems and instructions used in the dissenting studies. Due to the detailed methodological arguments that are involved in resolving this issue, it is therefore discussed in greater depth in Appendix A.

The no-emotions findings in the ten studies of women and men's dream reports reported in Table 9.2 are supported by the even higher percentages of dream reports that contain no emotions in the longitudinal laboratory studies of children's dream reports. These findings with children cannot be doubted as easily as the adult results were by the researchers associated with the Central Institute of Mental Health because they are consistent with the paucity of other types of adult-like dream content in children's dream reports (Domhoff, 2022, pp. 225–226, for a summary). In the longitudinal study of 14 children at ages 3–5, 5–7, and 7–9, 92% of the dream reports at ages 3–5 contained no "feelings," the term used for discussing fear/apprehension, anger, sadness, and happiness, as well as feelings of hunger and fatigue. Further, most of these feelings concerned hunger or fatigue (Foulkes, 1982, p. 331, Table B.1). This lack of emotions was also present at ages 5–7 and 7–9 (Foulkes, 1982, pp. 50, 86).

In the second longitudinal study by this researcher, which involved children at ages 9–11, 11–13, and 13–15, the girls had a No-Emotions Percent of 50% or above at all three ages: 50% at ages 9–11, 58% at ages 11–13, and 60% at ages 13–15 (Domhoff, 2022, p. 226 for a summary; Foulkes, 1982, Tables B.2 and B.3).

Even higher no-emotions percentages were reported in the REM dream reports from lab awakenings in the Swiss replication and extension longitudinal study of 12 girls and 12 boys at ages 9–11, 11–13, and 13–15. Using the Hall/Van de Castle codings for Fear/Apprehension, Anger, Sadness, and Joy/Happiness, 91.2% of the girls' dream reports in the first year of the study contained no emotions, compared to 88.4% for the boys. After that first year in the lab, the girls had lower no-emotions percentages than did the boys: 85.0% vs. 89.3% at 11–13 and 78.7% vs. 85.9% at 13–15 (Strauch, 2005, p. 161, Table 4).

The complex neurocognitive basis necessary for emotions to occur in waking life, and the relative deactivation during sleep of all but portions of the default network, explains why emotions are relatively infrequent in dream reports from adults. Further, the gradual maturation of the default network until ages 9–11 explains why there are even fewer emotions in dream reports of children and young adolescents. Looked at from a neurocognitive perspective, the quantitative findings on the lack of emotions in dreams are consistent with the idea that there are cognitive deficiencies in dreams due to the limited cognitive capacities available to the neurocognitive network that supports dreaming (Domhoff, 2022, Chapter 8 and pp. 268–273).

But Why Are Emotions Thought to Be Very Frequent in Dreams?

If the quantitative findings on the infrequency of emotions in dreams are correct, then why do so many people think otherwise? This subsection suggests there is a neurocognitive explanation for this widely shared belief. As a starting point, it is very likely that this belief is in good part based on nightmares. Neuroimaging studies of people who suffer from frequent nightmares suggest that the neurocognitive network that produces dreaming has been enlarged due to extreme stress. In particular, this expanded neurocognitive network very often includes at least portions of the usually deactivated salience/ventral network in neuroimaging studies of post-traumatic stress disorder (PTSD) victims, waking or sleeping (Abdallah et al., 2019; Ebdlahad et al., 2013; Germain, 2013; Germain et al., 2013; Mysliwiec et al., 2014; Simor et al., 2013).

As highly personal accounts of what it is like to experience PTSD nightmares make painfully clear, these very frightening nightmares are impossible to forget, and they create a dread of going to sleep, which further compounds the problem (Paulson & Krippner, 2010). A video-taped set of frank and startling interviews with four Vietnam veterans at the Palo Alto VA Medical Center, who describe the circumstances that triggered their PTSD, demonstrates how much their nightmares impact their lives—and sleep—in totally negative ways (Shapiro & Notowitz, 1988/2016, for a 25-minute video available on YouTube).

Moreover, there are other frightening states that occur during sleep, which also may contribute to the beliefs about high emotionality in dreams. “Disorders of arousal,” which most frequently occur in preschool children during N3 sleep relatively early in the night, are sudden awakenings that include screaming and yelling. However, they are also experienced by 2%–3% of adults as well. These disturbing episodes cannot be ended by the verbal reassurances, holding, or the gentle patting that is provided by concerned parents, or partners in the case of adults (Avidan, 2017; Broughton, 1968; Fisher et al., 1973). Most of the time, those who suffer from disorders of arousal cannot remember any of their seeming terror during the sudden arousal, but these frightening events are not forgotten by the parents of young children, who often talk with relatives and friends about these upsetting experiences.

There is also a more common and generally non-pathological experience that occurs during awakenings from sleep, especially in the morning, and can be very frightening. During this experience, called "sleep paralysis," people sometimes have "complete awareness of their surroundings" or else feel "partially asleep with awareness." And yet, they are "unable to move even the fingers or to vocalize" (Vaughn & D'Cruz, 2017, p. 582). Although sleep paralysis is often very frightening, it can include feelings of warmth, with a sensual tinge, along with the sense that there is some human, animal, or alien in the room (Clancy, 2005; McNally & Clancy, 2005). More generally, it is conjectured by clinically oriented sleep researchers that sleep paralysis is one basis for the widespread cultural belief that demons and other spirits attack people during sleep (Cheyne & Pennycook, 2013).

These and other harrowing states during the course of a night's sleep ("parasomnias," in the parlance of sleep medicine) are conveyed to family members, friends, and neighbors by word of mouth, and eventually appear in published accounts, which are sometimes written by those who experienced such events. Nightmares, disorders of arousal, and sleep paralysis then become prototypes for artists and science fiction writers, who strive to portray the strong emotionality and terror that sometimes occur during the night.

The Developmental Relationship between Consciousness and Dreaming

Turning now to developmental issues with regard to both dreaming and consciousness, it seems likely on the basis of the research that will be discussed in this section that autonoetic consciousness and noetic dreaming are closely intertwined developmentally. This possibility is first of all consistent with the fact that neither of them is very often present, if they are present at all, during the first five years of a person's life. It therefore follows that there should be a close relationship in their parallel developmental patterns in both neuroimaging studies and developmental studies of children's waking cognitive capacities (Foulkes, 2017, for argument and evidence to this effect).

If, for example, the FPCN is an essential foundation for consciousness, and if the default network is the main foundation for dreaming, then their relative immaturity and the nature of their relationship should be visible in developmental neuroimaging studies. More specifically, as noted in

Chapter 2, and also earlier in this chapter, both dreaming and consciousness are dependent upon the development of an intact semantic memory network during the preschool years, which is located in good part in the brain regions that support the intermediate multimodal areas in the multistate hierarchical model of consciousness (Vargha-Khadem et al., 1997, for a remarkable study of two participants who suffered brain lesions before age 5 that left them unable to develop an episodic memory network, but who nonetheless developed a normal semantic memory network).

As a starting point, the cross-sectional neuroimaging study of the development of the default network from ages 7–9 to 19–31, a topic that was discussed with regard to dreaming in Chapter 2, also discovered that the FPCN is more functionally connected than the default network throughout middle childhood and adolescence (Fair et al., 2009). At age 8 years, 6 months, for example, the FPCN is more integrated than the default network (Fair et al., 2008, 2009). By way of contrast, the medial prefrontal cortex, one of the default network's most central areas in adults, and an area that is involved in dreaming, is on the periphery of the default network at ages 7–9 and only indirectly connected to the network's parietal areas (Fair et al., 2009, pp. 6–7, 11). However, by ages 9–11, the FPCN is becoming very similar to that of adults. The differences in the degree of integration within, and segregation between, the FPCN, and the default network at ages 8, 12, 15, and 24 are displayed in Figure 9.3.

Over time, the FPCN and the default network become increasingly segregated, which makes it possible for the FPCN to more readily modulate and control the default network. This finding is supported by the findings in the longitudinal neuroimaging study of children at ages 10 and 13, which was discussed in Chapter 2. The FPCN is very similar to that of adults by age 10, but the segregation between the default network and the FPCN is a work in progress between 10 and 13 (Sherman et al., 2014, pp. 151, 155). The details of how this increased segregation occurs throughout preadolescence are found in several studies (Campbell et al., 2012; Fair et al., 2007; Gordon et al., 2011; Supekar et al., 2010; Uddin et al., 2011). Most of these studies are summarized in Domhoff (2022, pp. 166–168).

Within the context of these neuroimaging findings, it is useful to turn to developmental studies of memory and other cognitive abilities, on the one hand, and observational studies of mother–child interactions on the other. In terms of understanding the development of autonoetic consciousness, it is first of all relevant to note that preschool children "don't understand that your thoughts can be internally generated," or that "thoughts can simply follow the logic of your internal experiences instead of being triggered from the outside," until the ages of 5–6 (Gopnik, 2009, p. 152).

Similarly, preschool children do not understand that their dreams are internally generated, and they sometimes think dreams are a shared

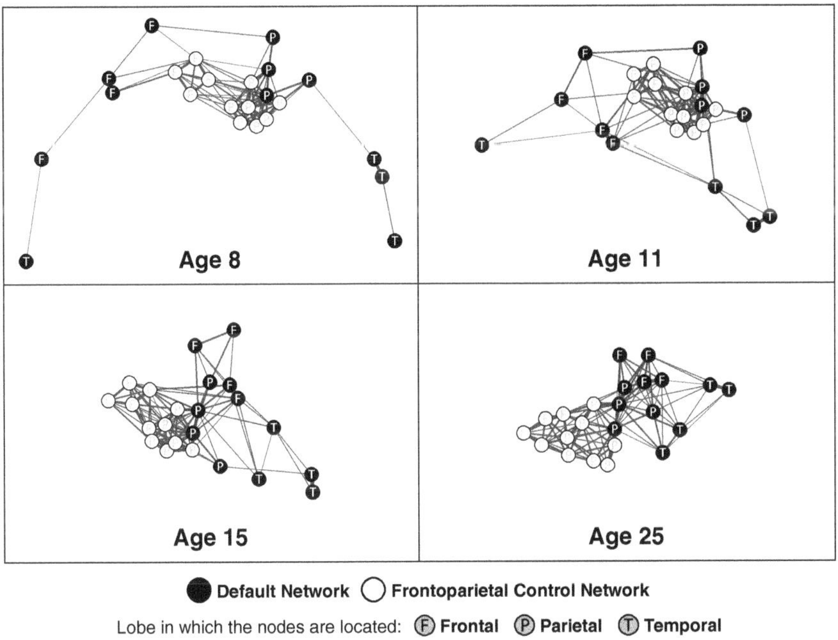

FIGURE 9.3 Maturation of connectivity in the default network and frontoparietal control network.

Notes: Note that the frontoparietal control network is more functionally connected than the default network between ages 8 and 15. As in the two similar graphics in Chapters 1 and 2, the nodes are depicted as spatially closer if they are functionally closer.

Source: Adapted from Fair et al. (2009), under CC BY license.

experience. This lack of understanding of where dreams come from may be due to the fact that preschool children do not dream very often, if at all, as discussed in Chapter 2. They therefore may rely on what their parents and children's books tell them about dreaming (Meyer & Shore, 2001; Woolley & Boerger, 2002; Woolley & Wellman, 1992).

In addition, preschool children "don't experience their lives as a single timeline stretching back into the past and forward into the future"; nor do they "feel immersed in a constant stream of changing thoughts and feelings" (Gopnik, 2009, p. 153). Furthermore, if preschool children are asked during an idle moment what they were just thinking, they usually say "nothing," which actually may be the case if they are not proficient at simulating and imagining.

Based on these various findings, it seems likely that children need to have an autobiographical self—a self-memory system—in order to experience autonoetic consciousness (Conway et al., 2019; Gopnik, 2009, p. 153; Ross et al., 2024). However, before age 5 children do not have "the basics of autobiographical memory" and only develop "a roughly adult understanding of consciousness" around the age of 6 (Gopnik, 2009, p. 156). This conclusion has been enriched by numerous studies of the ways in which discussions between mothers and their children aid in the development of an autobiographical self (e.g., Fivush, 2020; Nelson, 2005; Nelson & Fivush, 2020).

These various studies also lead to the conclusion that children need to have an episodic memory, which they lack until about age 5, for an autobiographical self to develop (Tulving, 2005). More recently, it has become clear that in addition children must have a memory for the "source" of their memories, a specific type of episodic memory that also develops during this same age period. These capabilities are closely intertwined in the development of the self-memory system (Ross et al., 2024, for historical background in the context of a new study showing the close relationships among episodic memory, source memory, and the development of the self-memory system).

The emphasis on the importance of autobiographical memory suggests that the development of autonoetic consciousness has a developmental trajectory similar to that of noetic dreaming between ages 5 and 8, but with dreaming developing a little more slowly. For example, the five-year longitudinal study of dreaming discussed in Chapter 2 discovered that the few and brief accounts of dreams after REM sleep awakenings by preschool children rarely include the dreamer herself or himself until ages 5–6. Even then, the dreamer was primarily an observer until ages 9–11 (Foulkes, 1999, p. 75, Table 3, for a summary of these revealing findings).

These findings are also consistent with studies of the development of mind-wandering, which is not present—or at least recognizable to the children—until the 5–7 age period, during which the autobiographical/self-memory system develops. In a developmental study of children's familiarity with mind-wandering, only 44% of children in the first grade (ages 6–7) understood what mind-wandering is, compared to 65% of third-graders (ages 8–9), 86% of sixth grades (ages 10–11), and 100% of college students (Eisbach, 2013, Table 2).

Taking the development of the FPCN and consciousness to age 10, which is also about when adult-like dreaming develops, a longitudinal experimental study of 135 children found that the FPCN continued to be more integrated than the default network. This conclusion is based on tests of working memory, the ability to inhibit irrelevant thoughts, and attention-shifting between the mean ages of 8 years, 3 months and 10 years, 3 months (Brydges et al., 2014, pp. 34, 40). The results of this study support the idea that the integration of the executive network leads to better working memory, more planning for the future, more sophisticated inferences about other people's mental states, and improved inhibitory control of irrelevant responses.

The neurocognitive developments that occur between the ages of 5 and 10 were long ago detected at the behavioral level in the indigenous societies that it has been possible to study, as well as in Western history. For example, a large-scale study that included several indigenous cultures concluded that children are first given more responsibilities between the ages of 5 and 7, and gradually even more thereafter (Rogoff, 1993; Rogoff et al., 1975; White, 1965, for the classic analysis of the various changes during ages 5–7). Then, too, the age of 7 is considered the "age of reason" in Western traditions, both in English law and the Catholic Church (Sameroff & Haith, 1996).

Based on both the neuroimaging and developmental psychology findings, it seems likely that the FPCN and, by inference, waking consciousness, develop sooner than does dreaming. At the same time, both waking consciousness and dreaming seem to become increasingly sophisticated during early adolescence due to greater integration within both networks, greater segregation between the two networks, and a closer working relationship between them.

The overall findings in this section, and perhaps especially the finding that both dreaming and consciousness first appear between ages 5 and 7 for most children, provide strong support for the conclusion that noetic dreaming and autonoetic consciousness have a close relationship. However, they do not have quite the same properties. Moreover, consciousness appears earlier than dreaming.

In the next section, the relationship between noetic dreaming and autonoetic consciousness is explored from a very different angle. There are dreamlike cognitive experiences during sleep in adults in which there is also an awareness that the person is dreaming.

Self-Awareness during Dreaming in a Hybrid Sleep State

As one team of neurocognitive researchers notes, "humans typically lack awareness that they are dreaming while dreaming" and "most individuals experience lucid dreams rarely" (Baird et al., 2018, p. 1). The lucid dreaming that is referred to in the previous sentence is the name that those who report awareness during dreaming have used since it was coined in 1913 by a Dutch physician-utopian thinker with an interest in parapsychology. He did so in a lengthy article that appeared in the proceedings of a parapsychology meeting in which he described his experiences in great detail (van Eeden, 1913).

Building on van Eeden, the topic of lucid dreaming was revived by a parapsychologist in the ferment of the 1960s (Green, 1968). An anthology on "altered states of consciousness," which reprinted van Eeden's article, brought lucid dreaming to the attention of dream researchers as well as the general public (Tart, 1969, Chapter 8). Lucid dreaming is now one important part of a more recent paradigm among dream researchers, which focuses on efforts at "dream engineering" (Carr et al., 2020; Mallett et al., 2024).

Although lucid dreaming is rare, it is relevant within the context of the neurocognitive theory of dreaming. This is because it may be a hybrid state of sleep and wakefulness that can be understood on the basis of the neurocognitive theory of dreaming and the multistate hierarchical model of consciousness. Specifically, it is likely that lucid dreaming is based on the relative activation of the internally oriented portions of the anterior prefrontal cortex that support metacognitive self-reflectiveness, which were discussed in a previous subsection (e.g., Dixon et al., 2018, 2022; Domhoff, 2023, pp. 8–10, for an earlier discussion of lucid dreaming as a hybrid state of sleep). Two sleep-lab studies support this supposition.

The first study, which used high-density electroencephalogram (EEG), involved six highly motivated college students, who reported that they remembered three or more lucid dreams each night at home. The participants each spent up to five nights in the sleep lab; three of the six were able to signal one instance each of self-awareness during dreaming, which is a surprisingly small number based on their estimated frequencies of lucid dreaming at home (Voss et al., 2009, p. 1191).

During these three instances, brain patterns were characterized by "wake-like inter-scalp networking, including high-frequency bands," which were "most pronounced in frontal and frontolateral coherences"; the authors concluded that self-awareness during dreaming may occur during a "hybrid state" that has features of waking as well as REM sleep (Voss et al., 2009, p. 1196). These findings are consistent with the emphasis on portions of the default network as the basis for imagination and dreaming in the neurocognitive theory of dreaming and with the emphasis on the dorsal lateral prefrontal cortex and the ventral lateral prefrontal cortex as part of the network that supports self-reflective consciousness in the multistate hierarchical model of consciousness.

The second study of this hybrid state involved 15 nights of functional magnetic resonance imaging (fMRI) studies with four adult male participants between the ages of 27 and 31. All of them had been actively working to have greater self-awareness during dreaming for several years or more for their own reasons. Assuming there were four REM periods for each of the 15 nights, the four participants had an estimated 60 REM periods. However, only two of the four participants were able to provide eye movement signals in one instance each, which were corroborated by their post-awakening reports. These results reinforce the finding that lucid dreaming is usually rare, even for some of the people who strive to experience it. However, the two occurrences seemed clear enough to report "a reactivation of several areas normally deactivated during REM sleep," and especially the dorsal lateral prefrontal cortex, ventral lateral prefrontal cortex, and lateral frontopolar cortex (Dresler et al., 2012, p. 1020). These areas are part of the higher-order network in the multistate hierarchical model of consciousness.

The correlation between activation in prefrontal areas and lucid dreaming also has been supported in an experimental study in which transcranial direct current stimulation was applied to frontal areas of the brain using 19 participants, who spent three consecutive nights in a sleep laboratory. They received the direct current stimulation, or else sham stimulation, during REM periods on the second and third nights. Self-ratings by the participants suggested that the causal effects were "not strong and found only in frequent lucid dreamers" (Stumbrys et al., 2013, p. 1214). The researchers noted that further research on activation patterns during lucid dreaming is necessary, but it is striking that there have been no further nighttime neuroimaging or direct current stimulation studies by researchers interested in lucidity since 2012–2013.

There is, however, one recent neuroimaging study, which was carried out during the waking state. It suggests that there may be individual differences between the many people who do not experience self-awareness during dreaming and the few people who do. This study compared 14 participants, who reported they had three or more instances of lucid dreaming per week, with a control group of the same size, whose members reported they had one or fewer self-awareness dreams per year. The researchers concluded that the awareness of dreaming while dreaming may be "associated with increased functional connectivity between aPFC [i.e., the anterior prefrontal cortex] and temporoparietal association areas, *regions normally deactivated during sleep*" (Baird et al., 2018, p. 1, italics added). This finding is consistent with the findings in the three studies discussed above.

Rather unexpectedly, the idea of a "hybrid state" has been rejected by three lucidity researchers on the basis of a re-analysis of EEG data collected by one of the article's three co-authors in the early 1980s. However, their re-analysis does agree with earlier findings that "lucid dreams are associated with higher-than-average levels of physiological activation during REM sleep, including measures of both subcortical and cortical activation" (Baird et al., 2022, p. 1). This re-analysis of EEG findings also is consistent with the EEG-based findings by earlier dream researchers, who were neutral with regard to the reality of lucid dreams. They reported that the few instances they found of lucid dreaming occurred when the percentage of alpha waves in the EEG records was higher than usual (Ogilvie et al., 1982; Tyson et al., 1984).

Here it also can be noted that the database for the re-analysis consists in good part of the EEG records of one of the three co-authors of the article, Stephen LaBerge, who served as both a researcher and participant in the original published study that made use of this database (LaBerge et al., 1981, p. 728, Table 1, which shows that 14 of the 20 verified lucid-dream signals came from LaBerge as a participant). Then, too, in his dissertation study, LaBerge was responsible for 14 of the 17 verified signals, with the other three participants having 1 verified signal each (Domhoff, 2018, p. 292, for details on the original results; LaBerge, 1980, p. 82 for the fact that he was the participant who provided 82.4% of the successful signals in his dissertation work). It is therefore possible that the re-analysis of 1980 data is based on one highly interested participant who is also a co-author. This possibility suggests that detailed neuroimaging studies of prolific lucid dreamers would be an excellent avenue to understanding lucid dreaming.

Contrary to the re-analysis of the 1980 database, the findings on lucid dreaming provided by several other researchers, which were discussed above, provide a solid case that the neurocognitive network that supports lucid dream overlaps with, but is larger than, the neurocognitive network that supports dreaming. These results therefore strongly suggest that lucid dreaming cannot be used to talk about dreaming in general.

This conclusion is also supported by the fact that the experiences reported by participants in most recent lucid-dream studies do not have a high degree of resemblance to everyday dream content, which most often includes people, social interactions, and activities of various kinds, as explained in Chapter 3. Instead, the reports after the various stimuli that are involved in dream engineering—such as flashing lights and/or beeping sounds in the pre-sleep period, and/or gentle vibrations during sleep—often have an otherworldly quality, with an emphasis on colorful scenic imagery, flying, and highly unusual content (e.g., Carr, 2025, pp. 50–51).

However, the question still remains as to why a small percentage of individuals become lucid dreamers. The need is for further neuroimaging studies of frequent lucid dreamers, who also would provide detailed autobiographical accounts in order to help understand how lucid dreaming develops, whether it be due to genetic predispositions, atypical developmental factors, and/or atypical adult experiences. For now, there are indications in the few autobiographical accounts provided by lucid dreamers that they do have different developmental or adult experiences from the overwhelming majority who do not experience such dreams. For example, one avenue to experiencing lucid dreaming may involve the relatively rare frightening dreams that occur during preadolescence.

According to two of the four lucid dreamers who discussed their experiences decades ago on a panel sponsored by a lucidity conference, frightening dreams during preadolescence, or perhaps somewhat earlier, led them to attempts to avoid such dreams. They also developed a fear of going to sleep, which in turn caused them to sleep more lightly, and perhaps to experience lucid dreams (Lucidity Newsletter, 1986, pp. 75–77). A well-known lucid dreamer of the past, who often spoke and wrote about the topic, also reported similar issues during childhood (Worsley, 1988). This set of circumstances is now called "somnophobia," and recent studies suggest it often develops during childhood (Pacheco & Peters, 2024). Those who suffer from it have difficulties falling asleep and experience frequent awakenings.

As discussed in Chapter 8, frequent awakenings during sleep may lead to higher levels of dream recall.

As noted in an earlier section of the chapter, sleep paralysis, which leads to vivid and often upsetting mental imagery, can also lead to atypical dreaming. As also noted earlier, sleep paralysis usually occurs when the sleepers have an awareness of their surroundings and are in a wake-like state but are not able to move or speak because REM atonia continues for them (Vaughn & D'Cruz, 2017, p. 582). One frequent lucid dreamer told an interviewer that she suffered from nightmares during episodes of sleep paralysis when she was younger. Based on her self-report of her earliest lucid dream, sleep paralysis may be another factor that leads to lucid dreaming (St-Cyr-Leroux, 2024).

Prolonged insomnia, which is now known to involve atypical brain activation patterns, may be yet another pathway into lucid dreaming (e.g., Aquino et al., 2024; Bressera et al., 2025; Kay et al., 2016, for three useful sources on brain activation patterns in those who suffer from insomnia). For example, one of the participants in the 1986 lucidity conference reported that he began experiencing lucid dreaming after a "long period of insomnia." His lucid dreaming occurred in the context of sleeping from shortly before midnight to 4 a.m., when he awakened to drink coffee and read. He then returned to sleep around 6 a.m., at which time he would feel he was awake during dreaming (Lucidity Newsletter, 1986, pp. 93–94). The combination of the increase in general brain activation during the early morning, along with the caffeine in his coffee, may have led to an expansion of the neurocognitive network that produces dreaming in this individual.

Then, too, past use of recreational drugs may provide another way in which people come to experience the fact that they are aware they are dreaming. The fourth participant in the long-ago lucidity conference, a prominent spokesperson in relation to lucid dreaming at the time, reported that she developed her awareness that she was dreaming after ending her use of peyote and LSD when she became pregnant. Her lucid dreaming first occurred late in her pregnancy, a time during which she frequently awakened late at night and often took daytime naps (Lucidity Newsletter, 1986, pp. 84–85). This possible relationship between the past use of psychedelic drugs and lucid dreaming can also be seen in interviews with another prolific lucid dreamer (Libman, 1988; Rolston, 2013).

Many more case studies would need to be carried out to determine the prevalence of lucid dreaming in those who have used recreational drugs in the past. But by now there is much evidence that the sustained use of either psychedelic drugs or alcohol can lead to many sleep disturbances, including "difficulty in maintaining sleep," which leads to frequent awakenings (Roehrs & Roth, 2015, p. 793). Frequent awakenings, in turn, may lead to more frequent recall of cognitive activity that occurs during more wake-like sleep states.

This overview of research on lucid dreaming shows that the extent to which lucid dreaming is similar to typical dreaming or autonoetic consciousness has yet to be fully examined. There is, as noted above, a need for studies with large samples of lucid dreamers. Such studies would include neurocognitive assessments of the participants during sleep, as well as detailed case studies that included autobiographical accounts of when and how the participants first experienced lucid dreaming. However, by now enough is known to be confident that the neurocognitive theory of dreaming and the multistate hierarchical model of consciousness are able to explain this rare hybrid wake-sleep state in terms of atypical brain activation patterns during sleep.

Dreaming during Relaxed Waking Thought?

There is good evidence that daydreaming can become very long and intense for some people, which suggests that the default network may be under less control by the FPCN and the two attention networks at these times (Klinger, 1971, 2009; Singer, 1975). These waking-state findings raise a final question concerning dreaming. Is dreaming possible during waking? According to the neurocognitive theory of dreaming, dreaming during waking is possible in theory. But it can only occur if the neurocognitive network that generates dreaming becomes ascendant, however briefly, in comparison to the FPCN, a situation that may occur on occasion when people are reclining in a quiet solitary setting in which external stimuli are absent.

The statement of these possibilities is based on replicated evidence from the pre-neuroimaging era, which suggests that such dreaming may occur during waking (Foulkes, 1985, pp. 70–77, for an overview). This evidence was first discovered serendipitously in the mid-1970s by unsuspecting dream researchers (Foulkes & Scott, 1973). Now, 50+ years later, based on the technological advances since then, the original study and the two direct replications of it that followed could be more rigorously replicated and extended on the basis of systematic information collected in neuroimaging studies. Such studies would require about a dozen observational-and-report sessions with each of five to ten participants. Each of the observational-and-report sessions could last for perhaps as little as 30–35 minutes.

The unexpected discovery of what seemed to be dreaming during waking occurred in daytime practice sessions for a nighttime study in a sleep-dream laboratory in 1973. During these practice sessions, 16 new women participants were learning how to focus on the last thing that was going through their minds just before their names were called. To make the daytime practice sessions as similar to the upcoming sleep-dream study as possible, each participant spent 10 or more minutes reclining alone in a dimly lighted room. To further simulate the forthcoming night sessions, electrodes were attached and their EEG records were being monitored.

The participants were then instructed to relax but stay awake, and their wakefulness was monitored by the EEG recordings. They then responded to random verbal requests from the experimenters to report "the very last thing going through your mind just before I called you" (Foulkes, 1985, p. 71). To the researchers' surprise, they learned that 24% of sampled waking thoughts reported by the 16 women were described as visual and dramatic and experienced by them as dreams (Foulkes & Scott, 1973, for the details of the study).

Then, in a direct replication study that included ten women and ten men, who were asked to report their thoughts at 12 random times in sessions of 45–60 minutes, the research team found a very similar figure for dreaming episodes: 19% (Foulkes & Fleisher, 1975). To provide an indication of what these dream reports are like, one participant reported she was watching a judicial sentencing by a judge, who was wearing an old-fashioned powdered wig. Another woman said she was pressing down on a vein in an effort to stop it from bleeding. A third woman first reported she had been sitting in her dormitory room, watching her boyfriend drink beer, and thinking she was very upset about it. When contacted again later in the session, she dreamed she was in her dormitory room and smoking a cigarette. After a final contact, she was watching a man leaning out of a window and taking pictures of clouds (Foulkes, 1985).

Another 20% of the responses in this replication study also contained "what might be called *mind-wandering* (the subject is not controlling his thoughts, but he is aware he is in the laboratory...)." Yet another 22% of the responses indicated a state of "what might be called '*lost in thought*' (the subject may or may not be controlling his thoughts, but he is not aware he is in the laboratory...)" (Foulkes & Fleisher, 1975, pp. 68–69, italics in the original). In addition, 38% of the probes revealed that the participants were in full reality contact; they were completely aware of where they were and what they were doing. Making clear that the participants were awake, "only 3 of the 120 probes showed anything other than a clearly waking polygraph tracing," a conclusion based on both brain-wave and eye movement patterns. Then, too, no "instances of self-described sleep were observed" (Foulkes & Fleisher, 1975, p. 70). The main findings are presented graphically in a pie chart in Figure 9.4.

Finally, these findings were replicated once again as a preliminary part of a study that also included probes during the sleep-onset process, REM sleep, and Non-REM sleep, but the waking-state results were not formally published (Foulkes, 1985, pp. 70–77, for a summary of all three studies that concerned dreaming during relaxed waking). Added together, half of the 52 participants (42 women, 10 men) in one of the three separate studies sometimes reported brief episodes of dreaming after they were asked to report what they were experiencing when they were contacted by the experimenter (Foulkes, 1985,

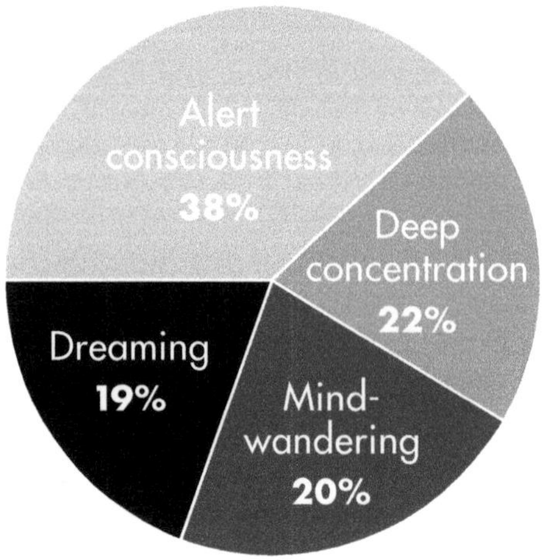

FIGURE 9.4 The four types of cognition reported by participants when asked about the last thing going through their mind when queried by the researchers.

Source: Data from Foulkes and Fleisher (1975).

pp. 89n39–90n49). Starting with the 26 participants who did not experience any dreaming, their non-dreaming sessions make clear that brief episodes of dreaming clearly do not happen for everyone during relaxed moments when they are alone. On the other hand, the fact that 50% of the participants did experience moments of dreaming suggests that further studies based on the technological advances in the past 50 years might prove to be very fruitful.

The findings in these three EEG-based studies are given some neurocognitive credence by one of the EEG/fMRI studies mentioned in the analysis of the default network and its relationship with the FPCN in Chapter 2 (Chang et al., 2013). This study showed that the anterior regions of the default network, which are the portions of the default network that are relatively activated and more functionally connected during dreaming, also become more connected to each other as the posterior regions in the default network begin to decouple from the dorsal attention network during moments of drowsiness. As also discussed in Chapter 2, there was an increase in alpha in anterior regions of the brain as this decoupling occurred, and evidence of theta rhythms as well (Chang et al., 2013, p. 230). In addition, recall that several studies suggest that theta increases when portions of the default network become more activated during the sleep-onset process and REM sleep.

Studying Dreaming and Consciousness at the Same Time?

The three sleep-dream laboratory studies of dreaming during waking lead to the possibility that their findings could now be re-examined and extended in apartment-like laboratory settings or home settings. Such studies would be possible by making use of the wearable and portable HD-DOT technology, which was discussed in the final section of Chapter 7 (Uchitel et al., 2022). As also noted at that earlier point, the HD-DOT technology already has been used to study the waking brain during the resting state in one participant, a brain research scientist who studied himself at home in 14 separate sessions of 12 minutes over a three-week period. Here it also can be recalled that the HD-DOT cap reliably detected the default network and its negative correlation with the FPCN, and with the salience portions of the salience/ventral network as well (Uchitel et al., 2022, p. 6, especially Figure 4).

Although it was cautioned in that earlier context that this new technology still may not be comfortable enough to be worn for very long periods during sleep, there is no question that it would be ideal for relatively short sessions during waking, as shown by the success of the one daytime study of an adult that has been carried out. The straightforward nature of wearing the HD-DOT technology was pictured in Figure 7.1.

As should be clear at this point, there are many parallels between the three daytime sessions that were carried out in a sleep-dream laboratory in the 1970s and early 1980s, which lasted from 10–15 minutes to 35–40 minutes, and the home study using the HD-DOT in 14 sessions that each lasted for 12 minutes. Moreover, a new study could go one step further by studying all four of the mental states identified in the second of the three earlier studies. In other words, such a study might make it possible to examine a range of conscious states (see Table 9.4) as well as any brief episodes of dreaming during mind-wandering or daydreaming.

The only new condition that needs to be added to the instructions to participants is that they should keep their eyes closed while in a reclining position throughout the session. Closed eyes and lying in a reclined position

TABLE 9.1 Four kinds of cognition during waking

	Networks	
Alert consciousness	Frontoparietal control network (FPCN) fully active	**waking thought**
Deep concentration	FPCN internal component active	
Mind-wandering	Default network more active than FPCN	
Dreaming(?)	Default network much more active than FPCN	

would be important not only because this condition more closely parallels sleep. There is neuroimaging evidence that the eyes-closed condition changes functional connectivity patterns, especially with regard to the relationships among the primary visual cortex, the salience network, and the default network (Costumero et al., 2020; Ingram et al., 2024).

As a starting point, and in an attempt to create individual baselines, the initial 15–20-minute sessions could begin with uninterrupted HD-DOT mappings of the five association networks. At that point, the HD-DOT records could be examined to determine how many different network configurations can be identified. Once individual baselines were established, participants could be asked in later sessions of perhaps as long as 25–30 minutes what was going through their minds when they were asked to do so. On the basis of their responses, and drawing on the categories in Table 9.4, it might be possible to establish neurocognitive signatures for one or more of the four cognitive states found in the second of the two 1970s studies: full reality contact, deep thought on a particular topic, mind-wandering, and dreaming (Foulkes & Fleisher, 1975).

It might even be possible that glimpses of the sleep-onset process would be captured from time to time with resting-state participants who are on the verge of falling asleep. As noted with some degree of alarm in a re-analysis of several resting-studies using fMRI, one-third of the participants in those studies in one sleep-dreams laboratory unexpectedly showed evidence that at certain points they were in one of the stages of sleep onset (Tagliazucchi & Laufs, 2014). Within the context of the larger purposes of the possible study that is being discussed here, carefully following the sleep-onset process without interruption might provide an excellent incidental opportunity to examine the gradual deactivation of the FPCN and the ascendancy of portions of the default network.

Once the network patterns for each of these mind states were established, the neurocognitive theory of dreaming predicts that during states of alert attention the FPCN, along with the two attention networks, would be relatively activated in relation to the default network and thus would constrain any mind-wandering or daydreaming. When participants reported they were thinking about a topic in a focused way, the theory predicts that the internally oriented subsystem of the FPCN would be ascendant. During mind-wandering or daydreaming, there would be increasing activity in the default network, but other brain areas would remain relatively activated, as shown in a meta-analysis of studies of spontaneous thought, including daydreaming (Fox et al., 2015). As for the brief episodes of dreaming, the neurocognitive theory of dreaming predicts that there would be increased activation of portions of the default network, along with the relative deactivation of the FPCN and the attention networks.

If high-density EEG were to be used instead of the HD-DOT headcap, then the neurocognitive theory of dreaming predicts that each of these four mental states would be accompanied by specific EEG patterns. The two main states of alert attention and concentrated thought would be indicated by varying amounts of gamma (30–100 Hz) waves and beta (13–30 Hz), which are shown in Table 9.5, along with the brain waves that appear during mind-wandering, dreaming, and sleep onset.

TABLE 9.5 The main EEG patterns of waking, dreaming, and the sleep-onset process

Name of pattern	*Frequency*	*Description*	*Illustration*
Gamma	30–100 Hz	Gamma waves are present during intense thinking and concentrating.	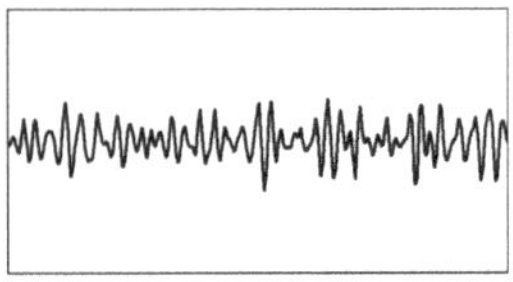
Beta	13–30 Hz	Beta waves are present during directed thinking and attention to external stimuli.	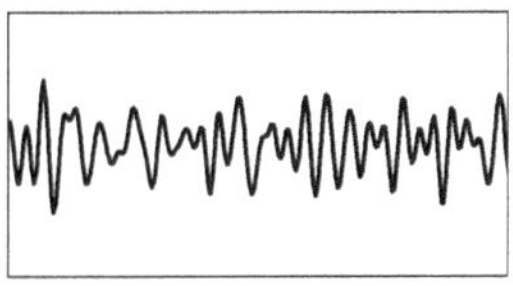
Alpha	8–13 Hz	Alpha waves are often present in drifting waking thought. They are also found in the sleep-onset process and sometimes in REM.	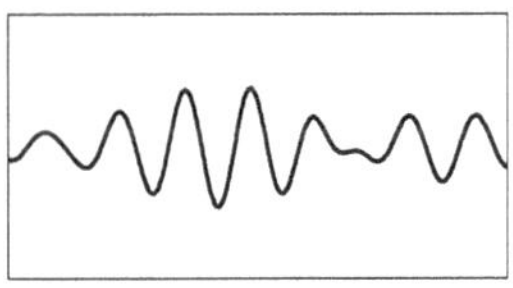
Theta	4–8 Hz	Theta waves are sometimes present in drifting waking thought, are present in the later half of the sleep-onset process, and are prominent in REM sleep.	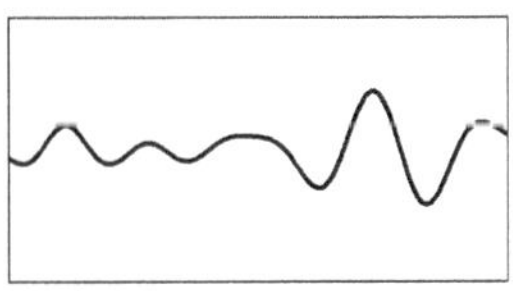
Vertex	n/a	Vertex waves (V waves) are brief, sharp, V-shaped waves that can be detected in some parts of the brain during sleep onset.	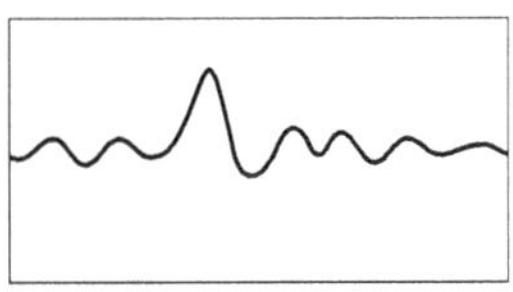
Sleep spindles	12–15 Hz	Sleep spindles (sometimes called Sigma waves) occur in half-second bursts, at sleep onset and in N2, early in the sleep process.	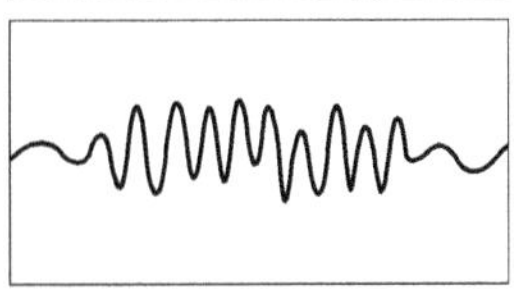

As participants drifted into mind-wandering, there would be an increasing frequency of alpha waves in the lower ranges (8–9 Hz) of the full alpha band (8–13 Hz), and the alpha waves would come to be more concentrated in the frontal regions of the brain. That is, the anterior/posterior (A/P) ratio of alpha would change (e.g., De Gennaro et al., 2001; Hori et al., 1994; Vecchio et al., 2017). During the brief episodes of dreaming, there would be an increase in the appearance of theta.

The possibility that dreaming can occur during waking (albeit when alone and lying down with eyes closed) brings the analysis in this book full circle. Dreaming during waking is plausible within the context of the neurocognitive theory of dreaming whenever the FPCN reduces its control of the default network enough for dreaming to inadvertently occur. According to the neurocognitive theory of dreaming, and the evidence to date, adult-like dreaming thereby may be present in preadolescents, adolescents, and adults at the following times: (1) at varying times during the sleep-onset process; (2) during REM sleep periods throughout the night; (3) in the 1.5–2.5 hours before spontaneous morning awakenings during N2 sleep; and (4) perhaps even during quiet solitary moments during waking. However, more and better evidence would be needed to assert that dreaming occurs during waking.

Conclusion

This chapter most importantly demonstrates that a specific higher-order theory of consciousness, called the multistate hierarchical model of consciousness, can provide a network-based account of autonoetic consciousness that is consistent with many findings on memory, focused thinking, and top-down commands. In addition, the theory's emphasis on the importance of emotions in creating conscious evaluative meaning is supported by the emphasis on emotional reactions in understanding the three main dimensions of meaning—the good-bad dimension, the powerful-powerlessness dimension, and the liveliness-quietness dimension. These three dimensions of evaluative meaning were discovered to be universal by means of several decades of research using the semantic differential in 30 different cultures that speak 21 different languages (Heise, 2010, 2014; Kervyn et al., 2013; Mukherjee & Heise, 2017; Osgood et al., 1959, 1975). The multistate hierarchical model of consciousness, in turn, provides a larger theoretical framework for encompassing the cross-national and cross-cultural findings on the importance of these three dimensions.

The multistate hierarchical model also makes it possible to understand how dreaming relates to consciousness and at the same times explains the cognitive deficiencies that have been found in dreaming and dream content. These cognitive deficiencies explain the rarity of episodic memories in dreaming, for example, as well as the lack of figurative thinking and emotion. The multistate hierarchical framework makes clear that dreaming is a form of fact-knowing (noetic) consciousness and is therefore not a form of self-knowing (autonoetic) consciousness. In doing so, it brings the neurocognitive theory of dreaming within the framework of memory theorist Endel Tulving's seminal theorizing (e.g., Tulving, 2005; Tulving & Thomson, 1973). Moreover, when combined with the multistate hierarchical model of consciousness, and the evidence that supports it, the neurocognitive theory of dreaming can explain and encompass the hybrid sleep state that sometimes includes lucid dreaming.

Then too, the somewhat parallel, and very likely partially overlapping, developmental trajectories of dreaming and consciousness, provide further context and support for the unexpected developmental dimension of dreaming that was discovered in longitudinal and cross-sectional sleep-dream laboratory studies of children and adolescents ages 3–16 (Foulkes, 1982; Foulkes et al., 1990; Strauch, 2005; Strauch & Lederbogen, 1999). In the process, the developmental findings on dreaming may help to encourage greater attention to the processes through which consciousness develops.

Finally, this chapter has provided a possible starting point for studies of dreaming during drifting waking thought. However, these very general suggestions would have to be improved upon and expanded by neurocognitive experts who have carried out somewhat similar waking studies for their own reasons. The types of studies that are suggested here with regard to the possibility of noetic dreaming during waking also might be relevant to studies of autonoetic waking consciousness. But once again it would be necessary for those neuroscientists who are experts on consciousness to find ways to make these possibilities feasible and useful for their own purposes.

10

RETROSPECT AND PROSPECTS

In taking stock of the accomplishments that can be credited to the scientific study of dreams, which began in earnest in 1953, it can be safely concluded that a great deal is now known about dreaming and dream content. There are numerous enduring achievements from the first 40 years of laboratory-oriented dream research. They include the discovery of rapid eye movement (REM) sleep in 1953, the discovery of the complex pan-mammalian non-REM/REM sleep cycle in 1957, the development of detailed and reliable categories for the quantitative study of dream content in the 1960s, and the discovery of the gradual development of dreaming in children in the 1970s. However, the scientific study of dreams was declining by the late 1960s and reached an impasse by the mid-1980s and early 1990s (Foulkes, 1996, for a frank account by a pioneer laboratory dream researcher who began working on dream studies in the late 1950s).

It was at this point that the neuroimaging studies of REM sleep in the mid-1990s provided new vistas for dream researchers (Braun et al., 1997, 1998; Maquet et al., 1996; Nofzinger et al., 1997). Their discoveries were complemented by new findings on the impact of lesions in specific areas of the brain on dreaming, along with a compilation of previous studies, which made it clear that lesion studies were valuable to understanding dreaming (Solms, 1997).

However, new lesion studies were few and far between thereafter, and the REM neuroimaging findings might not have had a useful long-term impact on the psychological study of dreaming if the default network had not been discovered and eventually linked to dreaming (Andrews-Hanna, Reidler, Huang, et al., 2010; Andrews-Hanna, Reidler, Sepulcre, et al., 2010; Buckner, 2012; Buckner et al., 2008; Gusnard et al., 2001; Gusnard & Raichle, 2001;

DOI: 10.4324/9781003732969-10

Raichle et al., 2001; Seeley et al., 2007). Thanks to these network studies, there is good reason to believe that we know where dreaming occurs in the brain, even though detailed neuroimaging studies of the brain regions that are activated and functionally connected during the night are yet to be done. Nevertheless, the neuroimaging studies of REM sleep that were carried out between 1995 and the early 2000s are no small achievement by the neurocognitive researchers who were involved, as were the neuroimaging studies of the sleep-onset process and the first hour of sleep that occurred later.

As detailed in Chapters 2 and 3, much is now known about dream content from childhood to old age (Domhoff, 2022, Chapters 3, 4, and 7; Foulkes, 1982, 1985, 1999; Strauch, 2004, 2005). Adult dream content is more similar than different across nation-states and in the indigenous societies that have been studied (e.g., Domhoff, 1996, Chapter 6; Mazandarani et al., 2013; Pires & Paiva, 2021). At the same time, there are age and gender differences, as also discussed in Chapter 3. In addition, there are very wide individual differences among the people who write down their dreams over years and decades, as discussed in Chapter 4. There is also a strong tendency toward consistency in what people about, as best demonstrated in this book by the findings from the Barb Sanders series presented in Chapter 4. Based on a variety of studies, we also know that dreams contain a large degree of content that is continuous with the dreamer's waking conceptions, personal concerns, and avocational interests (Domhoff, 2022, Chapters 3 and 4). Nevertheless, as shown in both Chapters 3 and 4, a significant minority of dreams appear to be adventure dreams that do not seem to have any clear connections to waking personal concerns.

What We Know about Old Ideas That Should Be Discarded

Research over the past 70+ years also reveals which of the many past ideas about dreams should be abandoned. Put another way, many well-done studies that led to dead ends were nonetheless extremely useful because they helped researchers understand what ideas and methods were worth pursuing and which were not. These studies and the theories they impacted are discussed in the next several subsections.

Freudian Dream Theory: Proven to Be Wrong

The first dream theory of the 20th century, Sigmund Freud's wish fulfillment theory of dreaming, was the first to state that dreams had "psychological meaning" in the full modern sense of the term. However, he saw the psychological meaning in dreams as a form of neurosis (Freud, 1900). Later he stated more directly that "dreams are themselves a neurotic symptom," and therefore dreams are "the best preparation for the study of neurosis"

(Freud, 1916, p. 83). In this regard, the Freudian theory of dreaming provides an ideal example of what medical sociologists mean when they discuss the strong tendency in psychology and sociology to "medicalize" ordinary human cognitive processes and conditions (e.g., Conrad, 2007).

The Freudian theory of dreams was also the first multilevel theory of dreaming in that physiologically based needs were turned into psychological wishes, which in turn were partially satisfied through a cognitively complex set of processes called "the dreamwork" (Freud, 1900; Hall, 1954). The comprehensiveness of Freud's theory, including its attention to the details in the dream reports that his patients provided, inspired numerous later researchers to study dreams, including dream content. Many of them then made systematic methodological and empirical contributions to dream research that were independent of Freudian theory (e.g., Dement & Kleitman, 1957; Hall, 1951, 1956; Hall & Van de Castle, 1966; Solms, 1997).

However, the discovery of REM sleep and the non-REM/REM sleep cycle undercut many of Freud's basic assumptions, and subsequent studies of the content of REM dream reports led to findings that were very different than what the theory expected. As a result, no evidence supports any of the many specific hypotheses offered by Freud or any of the clinical theories that arose from his theory (Domhoff, 2000a, 2003, pp. 136–147; 2018, Chapter 9; 2022, pp. 241–248; Fisher & Greenberg, 1977, 1996; Popp et al., 1992). (For a critique of Jungian dream theory from the perspective of the neurocognitive theory of dreaming and the empirical findings on dream content, see Domhoff (2003, pp. 144–147).)

Despite the many systematic findings that refuted Freudian theory, there was a sustained attempt, beginning in the mid-1990s, to revive it as "neuropsychoanalysis." This effort was notable for ignoring the large literature that did not fit with the theory, including the irrefutable maturational and developmental findings cited in Chapter 2 (see, for example, Solms, 2000, 2004, 2018 for this futile attempt at a restoration project, which sidetracked his own innovative research on the impact of focal brain lesions on dreaming). The revised Freudian theory went beyond Freud's claim that dreams have the same structure as neurotic symptoms. Instead, they are a form of psychosis: "The functional anatomy of dreaming is almost identical to that of schizophrenic psychosis, as revealed by functional-imaging studies" (Solms & Turnbull, 2002, p. 213).

In addition to ignoring the developmental findings on dreaming and claiming dreams are a form of psychosis, the restoration project was scornful, even derisive, in discussing quantitative studies of dream content. In a Hall/Van de Castle analysis of dreams collected from REM awakenings of patients with mild and severe chronic brain syndrome, the researchers found several content differences between the two groups (Kramer et al., 1975). The founder of neuropsychoanalysis concluded that the researchers "arrived at some rather absurd conclusions in this way," which "do not warrant serious scientific consideration" (Solms, 1997, p. 70).

Ironically, the lead author on the article that the founder of neuropsychoanalysis belittled was a psychiatrist who was highly partial to Freudian dream theory. Contrary to being "absurd," this psychiatrist's use of the Hall/Van de Castle coding system in this and several other research projects he was involved in provides further evidence that quantitative content analysis can be put to use by researchers with different theoretical orientations (Domhoff, 2004, for a detailed critique of Solms' claims, including his complete misreading of the history of laboratory dream research and his misunderstanding of the reasons why Freudian theory was generally abandoned by scientifically oriented dream researchers by the early 1970s, at the latest).

The Rise and Fall of a Neurophysiological Theory of Dreaming

The continuing visibility of Freudian dream theory into the 1960s and early 1970s was reflected in the arrival in the late 1970s of a neurophysiological theory—called "activation-synthesis" theory—that was cast as a categorical rejection of Freudian dream theory. It was developed by a psychiatrist who had received some psychoanalytic training, J. Allan Hobson, on the basis of his subsequent co-authored laboratory work on the brainstem basis of REM sleep in cats (e.g., Hobson et al., 1975; McCarley & Hobson, 1975). Extrapolating from this animal work, he and his co-worker concluded that dreaming is simply the forebrain's make-shift reaction to brainstem activation. Dreaming occurs because the forebrain is "making the best of a bad job in producing even partially coherent dream imagery from the relatively noisy signals sent up to it from the brain stem" (Hobson & McCarley, 1977, p. 1347).

According to the three main advocates of this theory after the 1990s, dreaming can be compared to "religious conversion, near-death experience, functional psychosis, delirium, drug-induced conditions, and other altered states of consciousness" (Hobson et al., 2000, p. 802). These claims are completely wrong if the dozens of neuroimaging studies that soon appeared are taken seriously. The activation-synthesis theorists also cited flawed work, beginning in the mid-1990s, that revived the discarded idea that the jerky eye movements that occur in random bursts during REM sleep were attempts to track dream content (Hong et al., 1995, 1997). They did so because this work seemed to vindicate their claim that the random electrical signals originating in the brainstem impact areas in the primary visual cortex and thereby cause the imagery that is the basis for the forebrain's attempt to create dream content that is consistent with the signals it is receiving (Hobson & McCarley, 1977, pp. 1337–1338).

However, this initial 1990s eye-movement study was immediately criticized methodologically as "not ideal for independently characterizing the shorter-lived sleep stages" because "this technique necessitates the integration of data collected over a period of 30 minutes or longer" (Braun et al., 1997, p. 1174). The same team of PET-scan researchers soon thereafter stated that their results relating to activation levels in secondary visual cortices disagree with those provided by the eye-movement theorists. This is because Hong et al.'s (1995) measure "reflects physiological responses over a longer time period," which "may not be comparable" with the time-sensitive measures in a PET-scan study (Braun et al., 1998). In other words, the Hong et al. (1995) study was superseded by a study that was more methodologically sound. This critique was not addressed by the REM eye-movement researchers in any of their later articles.

In addition, the other eye-movement study cited by Hobson et al. (2000) is a pilot study based on several instances of apparent matches in one of the participants (Hong et al., 1997). Nor did the group results with 11 participants reach statistical significance (Domhoff, 2022, pp. 282–285, for a critique of this study, and for the fact that the findings with the group data did not reach statistical significance; Hong et al., 2021, pp. 7, 15). Contrary to these unsupported claims, the detailed studies cited in Chapter 2 fully demonstrate that the random jerky eye movements are not "visually targeted saccades" (pace Hong et al., 2009, p. 7117). More generally, numerous psychophysiological studies in the 1980s and early 1990s showed that "assumptions about how the pons determines the features of dreams are completely without empirical support" (Antrobus, 2000, p. 905; Pivik, 1991, for a summary of this work).

Then, too, neurophysiological researchers who specialize in the study of REM sleep, also using animal models similar to those used by the original activation-synthesis theorists, showed very shortly after the activation-synthesis theory first appeared that every aspect of it was wrong at the brainstem level, due to methodological mistakes in the theorists' work on cats (Jones, 1980; Jones et al., 1977; Sakai et al., 1976; Sastre et al., 1981; Siegel & McGinty, 1977; Siegel et al., 1977). The case against the claims by the activation-synthesis theory at the brainstem level was fully summarized by the mid-1980s (Jones, 1986; Siegel & McGinty, 1986). However, the main author of the theory did not acknowledge these mistakes until more than 20 years later: "The apparent REM discharge selectivity of the large paramedian reticular cells was a function of the head restraint required to allow long-term recording," and "the original attribution of cholinergic neuromodulation to the REM-on cells of the pontine reticular formation was incorrect" (Hobson, 2007, p. 75). Apparently, activation-synthesis theorists seem to think that these basic errors do not matter in terms of the overall thrust of the theory.

This brainstem-reduction theory also led its advocates to a complete rejection of the findings in the longitudinal and cross-sectional studies of children's dreaming, which show that dreaming is a gradual cognitive achievement that is minimally present, if present at all, in preschool children (Foulkes, 1982, 1999; Foulkes et al., 1990). Instead, activation-synthesis theorists claimed that dreaming is already occurring in neonates:

> Similarly, we specifically suggest that the human neonate, spending as it does more than 50 percent of its time in REM sleep, is having indescribable but nevertheless real oneiric experiences.... For us, it is not at all difficult to imagine that an infant might be experiencing hallucinosis, emotions, and fictive kinesthetic sensations during REM sleep.
>
> *(Hobson et al., 2000, p. 803)*

In the face of lab studies revealing the gradual development of dreaming in young children between ages 3 and 9, the activation-synthesis theorists claimed that the children in these studies might be disoriented by the lab setting and therefore forget their dreams, or else they might not feel comfortable reporting their dreams to an alleged stranger (Hobson et al., 2000; Resnick et al., 1994, p. 31). In making these assertions, they ignored the strong evidence that the preschoolers in the longitudinal study were very comfortable in the lab setting and knew the main investigator well, as discussed in Chapter 2 (Foulkes, 1982). Still other inaccurate statements that they made about children's dreams are discussed in detail elsewhere, so there is no need to recount them here (Domhoff, 2018, Chapter 6; 2022, pp. 252–255).

Activation-synthesis theorists also rejected any approach to dreams that "begins with dream content" because the study of dream content is "fraught with conceptual, methodological, and analytic problems..." These problems make it necessary to start with the "details of brain physiology (of REM sleep) in animals" and then make "inferences back up to the psychological level (of dreaming) in humans" (Hobson, 1988, pp. 157–158, with the parenthetical remarks included in the original text that is cited). Despite the many quantitative findings on dream content that had accumulated in the previous 40 years, the primary developer of this theory claimed it is "at least possible that dream content is as much dross as gold, as much cognitive trash as treasure, and as much informational noise as a signal of something" (Hobson, 2002, p. 101).

Hobson and one of his co-workers further asserted that dream content is "generic," so there are not even any gender or individual differences (Hobson & Kahn, 2007). This determination was made on the basis of the inability of "six board-certified psychiatrists (four male and two female), one Ph.D. level clinical psychologist (female), and one Ph.D. level physicist (male)" to correctly sort a set of 50 dream reports from five different individuals (Hobson & Kahn, 2007, p. 851). The results were said to support the conclusion that "chaotic cerebral activation processes" lead to "visuomotor hallucinations, delusional beliefs, thought impairments, emotional storms, and memory defects" that are "so strong that they overwhelm and dilute the individual historical components of dream plot construction" (Hobson & Kahn, 2007, p. 857). In rejecting both developmental studies of dreaming and quantitative studies of dream content, activation-synthesis theorists followed the same pathway as did the founder of neuropsychoanalysis, even while engaging in a running battle with him (Domhoff, 2005, for a discussion of the similarities between the two sets of theorists, as well as their differences).

The new claims about the generic nature of dream content made by Hobson and one of his co-workers in the 2000s were quickly refuted in a study using approximate randomization to analyze thousands of resamples of dream reports of varying sizes. The study showed once again that it takes far more than ten dreams from each of several individuals to detect individual or gender differences (Domhoff & Schneider, 2008a). The study made use of the Hall/Van de Castle codings of the extant 491 female and 500 male dream reports discussed in Chapter 3, along with the 250 coded dream reports from the Barb Sanders series discussed in Chapter 4. It confirmed that it takes 125 dream reports for statistically significant individual and gender differences to appear using a reliable and validated coding system. The attempt to characterize dream content as generic was also refuted anew by the discovery that the character networks in individual dream series are small-world networks (Han, 2014; Han et al., 2015).

More generally, the many failings of this neurophysiological theory, as documented by both sleep researchers and those neurocognitively oriented dream researchers who study dreaming and dream content, have been compiled with increasing detail and updated evidence (Domhoff, 2018, Chapter 6; 2022, pp. 250–261). The discovery of a well-delineated neurocognitive network that has to be mature and intact for dreaming to occur, along with the discovery that the character networks in dreams are small-world networks, provide the final refutations of this reductionistic theory from the pre-neuroimaging era (Han, 2014; Han et al., 2015; Schredl & Schweickert, 2022).

However, the penchant for neurophysiological reductionism that is the main feature of the theory persists in the tendency of several dream researchers to discuss the neural correlates of dreaming instead of thinking in terms of the portions of the default network and secondary visual cortex that are supported by these neural substrates. This tendency persists despite the clear understanding that neurocognitive theories have "three distinct, but fundamentally interrelated, levels of analysis," which consist of the underlying neural substrates, the cognitive processes that the underlying neural substrates support, and the behavioral level (Ochsner & Kosslyn, 2014a, p. 2).

The Daytime Incorporation Theory of Dreaming

The findings in this book also raise serious doubts about claims that waking activities directly shape dreams, an issue that was alluded to in Chapter 4 in the context of the many completely imaginative activities in the dreams about Derek in the Barb Sanders series. According to incorporation theories, the dreamer's activities during the day, such as playing sports or creating music, are the primary basis for dreams (Schredl, 2022; Schredl & Hofmann, 2003). However, an incorporation theory cannot explain dreams such as those that Barb Sanders had about Derek.

Nor can an incorporation theory explain the dreams of individuals who are not involved in aggressive interactions in waking life but nonetheless have frequent dreams of violent and even murderous aggression, as shown in the dream series kept for a three-year period by "Karl." Although the dreamer reports that he had never been involved in aggressive physical interactions in waking life, he readily stated he had great anger and resentment toward his father, mother, and ex-wife and had violent dreams about them. Karl also had sexual intercourse in his dreams with 38 different women that he felt attracted to in waking life, but his sex life consisted of masturbation, which was often accompanied by fantasies about the women to whom he felt attracted (Domhoff, 1996, pp. 178–181).

Similarly, incorporation theories cannot explain continued dreaming about deceased loved ones they miss very much. For example, Merri lost her sister due to a hit-and-run driver three years before she started her dream series. Nonetheless, her deceased sister appeared in 34.4% of her dream reports and is at the center of the character network constructed on the basis of her dream series (Bulkeley, 2009, p. 98; Han et al., 2015). Merri's sister is no longer a part of her waking environment, but she is very much a part of Merri's waking thoughts and dreams.

Nor are events of great concern at the societal level always dreamt about at the time the events first begin to occur. The study of Beverly's delayed inclusion of concerns about covid in her dreams provides an excellent example of this point. This detailed analysis was possible because she kept a brief daytime diary as well as a record of the dreams she recalled. As discussed in Chapter 4, she did not incorporate the pandemic, and then her making of masks for low-income people, into her dreams until several days after she was highly involved in covid-related issues in waking life.

Based on these examples, and many more that could be drawn upon, an incorporation theory cannot explain the full range of events in dreams. A wider theory is therefore needed. As shown throughout this book, the neurocognitive theory of dreaming can explain the full range of events in dreams because it demonstrates that dreams are based on imagination. According to this more comprehensive theory, people most often dream about the issues they think about and worry about during waking, along with the activities that are of personal interest to them.

Thus, a neurocognitive theory rooted in the importance of imagination in human life more parsimoniously and fully explains why people dream about certain activities that they frequently engage in during waking life. The theory is then further supported by the fact that people rarely dream about daily activities that they take part in that are not of personal interest to them—including their jobs in many instances. The theory is also supported by the fact that studies focused on the issue of incorporation, whether inside or outside a laboratory setting, find only low levels of incorporations of stimuli that are administered before bedtime or during REM sleep; similarly, routine aspects of waking life and the minor hassles that are part of many people's daytime hours are less likely to be included (e.g., Arkin & Antrobus, 1991; Domhoff, 2017, pp. 29–33; Foulkes, 1996; Roussy, Brunette, et al., 2000; Roussy et al., 1996; Roussy, Raymond, et al., 2000; van Rijn et al., 2018).

Nor is there evidence of episodic memories in dreams, a topic that also was discussed in Chapter 9, as one part of the evidence of the cognitive deficiencies that are present during dreaming. Here it can be recalled that the researchers who studied 299 spontaneously recalled dreams concluded that there is a "functional dissociation" between dreams and episodic memory (Fosse et al., 2003, p. 1). In the other study discussed in Chapter 9, only one of 186 dreams recalled outside of a laboratory setting by 32 participants included an episodic memory (Malinowski & Horton, 2014, p. 444). Recall, too, that several of the neural substrates that are involved in supporting episodic memory during waking are relatively deactivated during dreaming (Cooper & Simons, 2019; Simons et al., 2022, pp. 174–175; Yoo et al., 2021).

The Many Shortcomings of All Adaptive Theories of Dreaming

All of the several adaptive theories of dreaming, each of which is narrowly focused, are flawed in several ways. Although they all have specific problems, they are also challenged by several general findings, most of which have been mentioned at relevant points in earlier chapters. First, the majority of people recall only 2%–4% of their dreams, which is much lower than would be expected if dream content is in some way important for people to know. Second, it is likely that most of the dreams that are "forgotten" are in fact never encoded in the first place, with the exception of those that are followed by an immediate arousal just as the dream ends. Thus, claims about the usefulness of unrecalled dreams for waking thought no longer seem plausible until adaptation theorists can demonstrate that forgotten dreams are encoded into memory in such a way that they can have an influence on semantic memories and cognitive processes that are important during waking.

Third, the fact that the small amount of dreaming that occurs between ages 3 and 9 lacks complexity and emotions limits any adaptive function for dreaming to the preadolescent, adolescent, and adult years. Fourth, lesion studies of the loss of dreaming are a challenge for most adaptive theories because they show that people can lose dreaming without necessarily losing waking cognitive capacities. Fifth, the consistency of dream content over years and decades, along with the fact that dream content does not change rapidly when it does change, raises very strong doubts about any adaptive theory asserting that dreams deal with new problems or prepare people for future waking situations.

Sixth, and finally, the several cognitive deficiencies that are inherent to dreaming, due to the truncated natured of the neurocognitive network that supports dreaming, make it unlikely that dreaming has adaptive value in relation to waking thought. For example, the relative lack of emotions makes it unlikely that dreaming can generate the affective meaning that is essential to autonoetic consciousness in evaluating the personal meaning of the events that occur during waking.

The Problem-Solving Theory of Dreams

The oldest of the non-clinical adaptive theories, the problem-solving theory, is immediately called into question by the low frequency of dream recall mentioned in the previous paragraph. The fact that 96%–98% of dreams are forgotten, many of which are not even encoded, seems far too large for dreaming to be the result of a series of conserved genetic adaptations that led to a neurocognitive network that produces dreams as an aid in problem-solving (e.g., Barrett, 2007, Chapter 6; D. Barrett, 2017; Cohen, 1979, Chapter 10, for presentations of the theory).

Further doubts about the idea that dreams have a problem-solving function arise from the many studies showing that the relatively few dreams that are recalled do not contain solutions to problems or new creative thoughts. The famous anecdotal examples from the past, which contributed to the development of this theory, turn out to involve any one of several non-dream factors, such as insights during mind-wandering, new thoughts during drowsiness, or taking recreational drugs (Baylor, 2001; Bell, 1992; Rudofsky & Wotiz, 1988; Schneider, 1953; Weisberg, 1986).

Systematic studies in the 1970s and 1980s raised the possibility that dreaming might have a problem-solving function, but they were far from convincing and were never replicated (e.g., Cartwright, 1974, 1977, 1986). As the author of several of these studies later stated, her most important study, which suggested that the dreams of divorced women about their ex-husbands might be helpful, was only "suggestive." This is because "there was only one night of dream collection, and some who did not dream of the spouse that night might well be experiencing a great deal of incorporation on other nights." Moreover, "there was a long gap between that one night of dreaming and the follow-up interview, during which many new reality factors would have intervened" (Cartwright, 1996, p. 185; see Domhoff, 2003, pp. 157–162, for critiques of this and other studies purporting to demonstrate problem-solving during dreaming).

Finally, the problem-solving theory is especially vulnerable to the finding that dream content does not change unless conceptions, personal concerns, and/or avocational interests change. Even then, dream content does not change rapidly, as best seen in this book by the fact that Beverly's growing concern with COVID-19, and then with making masks, did not appear for several days after these new personal concerns were expressed in her waking diary. Dreaming in general is not responsive enough to events in waking life to provide solutions to problems.

The many negative findings from several different kinds of studies strongly suggest that there has been no evolutionary selection for dreaming as a problem-solving aid. Within this context, a more likely and parsimonious explanation—based on reflective thoughts about recalled dreams during waking—has been developed. This alternative explanation suggests that any problem-solving related to dreaming is based on waking reflections about the dream, not on solutions that appear in the dream (Blagrove, 1992, 1996). This alternative explanation fits well with the findings on the gradual return of alertness after waking, and on the large amount of mind-wandering that can occur during this groggy period of sleep inertia. It is also consistent with the findings that incidental cues may bring about dream recall, which in turn can lead to further reflection on the dream during periods of drifting waking thought. It is also consistent with the fact that new post-awakening ideas and insights often occur without any recall of a dream (Wagner et al., 2004).

Dreaming as an Adaptive Form of Rehearsal for Waking Life

Two parallel theories developed by the same research group suggest that dreams provide rehearsals of actions that are useful in waking life and thereby improve reproductive fitness. In the first and most developed of the two theories, dreaming serves a threat-simulation function. This adaptation developed in a dangerous ancestral environment that lasted from about 1.8 million years ago to 11,000 years ago, which included predators, poisonous animals, and aggressive men (Revonsuo, 2000b, p. 892). This evolutionary emphasis leads to the hypothesis that humans may have inherited threat scripts that are triggered by "ecologically valid cues" (Revonsuo, 2000b, p. 878). More recently, these theorists suggest that dreams may have a function in improving social-interaction skills through social simulations (Revonsuo et al., 2015; Tuominen et al., 2019).

The concept of a threat is so wide that it includes virtually every negative event that occurs in dreams, including any worry, mistake, or personal failure. The examples in the coding instructions, developed on the basis of 592 dream reports collected from 52 young adults at the University of Turku, include a girl whose dog is sick, two women who leave their bags on a bus, and a man who can't get into his cabin on a passenger ship (Revonsuo & Valli, 2000, pp. 23–25). As the researchers who developed the theory noted, "our criteria for what should count as a threatening event may have been fairly liberal, which explains why threatening events were found to be so abundant in the dreams" (Revonsuo & Valli, 2000, p. 16).

When it comes to the actual events in dreams that are undoubtedly threatening, a study of 212 recurrent dreams collected for an earlier study did indeed include many threatening events. However, a close examination of the many threats in these dreams determined that 81% of the threats "belonged to the realm of fantasy or fiction" or would be "very unlikely to occur in the subject's waking life." Moreover, only 17% of the recurrent dreams that contained a threat had a positive outcome (Zadra et al., 2006, p. 457). Instead, these dreams ended with the threat being fulfilled (40%) or with the participant waking up (37%). Another 6% of the dreams "changed abruptly in terms of the imminent threat and the outcome was absent or remained vague" (Zadra et al., 2006, p. 457). The researchers concluded that useful rehearsals were rare.

Still another study reported negative results in a comparison of 208 dreams collected from students attending the University of Cape Town, which is located in the most violent and crime-ridden area in South Africa, with 116 dreams collected at the University of Wales in Bangor, a low-crime area in Northern Wales. Although the students at the University of Cape Town reported many more waking-life threatening events within the past four years than did those at the University of Wales at Bangor (49.2% vs. 21.6%), the students in Wales nonetheless had a higher percentage of dream reports with life-threatening events than did those in South Africa (18.6% vs. 8.7%) (Malcolm-Smith et al., 2008, pp. 1285–1286). An earlier study of threat simulation carried out at the University of Cape Town, using a different methodology, also reported results that were inconsistent with the threat simulation theory (Malcolm-Smith & Solms, 2004).

Although the focus of the threat-simulation theory is on the negative events in adult dreams and their potential usefulness in the future, the theory does not address the fact that many of the negative events in dreams concern past events and continuing concerns related to loved ones. For example, the high levels of aggression in the Barb Sanders dream series, which were discussed in Chapter 4, often involve her ongoing annoyances and frustrations concerning her mother, middle daughter, teenage granddaughter, and her ex-husband. It is difficult to conceive of any of these interactions as threat simulations that might be useful in her interactions with any of these individuals in waking life in the future. Similarly, her many positive interactions with her two best friends do not seem to be aimed at improving her social-interaction skills, as would be expected by the same research group's social-simulation theory.

It is also striking that there is little by way of threat simulation or social-interaction simulation in the relatively infrequent and less complex dreams of elementary school children. However, threat-simulation theorists claim that dreaming can mature more rapidly in highly threatening environments, which can lead to threat-simulating dreams (Revonsuo, 2000b, p. 889n5). This claim seems even more unlikely in light of the discovery that the neural substrates that support the default network mature only gradually, as discussed in Chapter 2 (Fair et al., 2008).

On the other hand, and showing that dreams are not necessary to learn to avoid threatening situations, it is notable how quickly children learn about threat avoidance in waking life through one-trial learning, a topic that has been well understood for over 80 years (e.g., Postman, 1963, for the history). There is also evidence that toddlers and preschool children also learn to avoid specific dangerous situations almost as soon as they are encountered in waking life (Burris et al., 2020; LoBue et al., 2014; LoBue & Rakison, 2013).

At the same time, children are learning social skills during waking by playing with other children from an early age in all cultures. By way of contrast, the dreams of young children include very few social interactions or threatening situations until preadolescence and early adolescence, so it seems extremely unlikely that their dreams provide any occasions to rehearse behaviors that might prove useful in waking life.

The threat-simulation and social-simulation theories are also called into doubt because they rest on two untested assumptions related to learning during sleep, which have never been empirically supported. Specifically, the two theories assume there can be "implicit" learning during sleep—that is, learning without any intention or directed attention. As two of the theorists involved in the development of both theories acknowledge, implicit learning that affects waking performance is a difficult assumption to test (Revonsuo, 2000a, pp. 890, 1081; Valli & Revonsuo, 2009, p. 33). Second, the theorists assume that this new implicit learning can be "transferred" to waking-life situations, a process that is called the "transfer of learning," or the "transfer of training," by researchers who study waking memory. The transfer of learning seems especially unlikely in light of a neuroimaging study showing that the transfer of training during waking requires the activation of the dorsolateral prefrontal cortex, which is an essential basis for the frontoparietal control network (FPCN) (Verghese et al., 2016).

Moreover, the transfer of learning during waking has proven to be very narrow in its scope (Gobet & Sala, 2023; Sala & Gobet, 2017). In this regard, it is especially noteworthy that there is no transfer of training from highly visual, fast-action video games—which may be vaguely comparable to dreams—to other cognitive tasks. "Importantly, we found no evidence of a causal relationship between playing video games and enhanced cognitive ability. Video game training thus represents no exception to the general difficulty of obtaining far transfer" (Sala et al., 2018, p. 111).

In the end, most aspects of this theory appear to be untestable because of the conditions that rehearsal theorists set for what is a relevant study. Even though the theorists' coding categories for threat simulation and social simulation were developed on the basis of everyday dream reports, they reject the many contradictory findings reported in studies of dream content by other researchers. They do so because they claim the dreams were not collected in ecologically valid contexts. As for the low levels of dreaming in elementary school children and the anodyne nature of their content, which do not fit with either version of the rehearsal theory, they are waved aside with the unproven assertion that children in highly threatening environments might dream more frequently. The fact that there is no evidence for any type of learning during sleep is admitted to be a difficult issue for the theory, but no attempts have been made by its proponents to show that any form of learning can occur during sleep.

Finally, the threat-simulation and social-simulation theories face a new problem because of their assumption that dreams do not have to be recalled to carry out their putative rehearsal functions. The advocates of these theories now have to bring forth evidence and arguments showing that most dreams have been encoded into memory, which seems to be a necessary condition for them to have any influence on waking cognition. Or else they need to show that dreams have their impacts while they are occurring, which seems unlikely based on the fact that the FPCN and the two attention networks are relatively deactivated throughout sleep.

Is There Memory Consolidation during REM Sleep? Is It the Basis for Dreaming?

The idea that memory consolidation may occur during REM sleep was first proposed in the late 1960s as part of a study of 18 REM-deprived human participants. It led to mixed results in a serial learning task (Feldman & Dement, 1968; Fowler et al., 1973, for a follow-up study that found no evidence for memory consolidation in humans in REM sleep). Studies in the late 1970s and 1980s of both humans and animals also led to mixed results. In the case of the REM deprivation studies using animal models, they were strongly criticized because of the likely confounds that are introduced by the stress produced by the sleep-deprivation methodologies that were used and were eventually abandoned (e.g., Born & Gais, 2000; Horne & McGrath, 1984; Vertes, 1995). More wide-ranging critiques, which also included studies of the fact that anti-depressant medications can eliminate REM sleep in humans for months and years without any apparent effect on memory, soon followed (Siegel, 2001; Vertes & Eastman, 2000).

The possibility of memory consolidation as an important function of REM sleep was re-introduced by activation-synthesis theorists in the late 1990s (Stickgold, 1998; Stickgold et al., 1999, 2000). Leaving behind the REM-deprivation methodologies, they revived the theory in part on the basis of a new line of studies based on animal models. These studies traced the persistence of very specific waking brain-wave patterns in rodents, which occurred as a result of a spatial learning task, into the sleep period (Wilson & McNaughton, 1994).

These and related studies soon led to the further hypothesis that dreaming is based on memory consolidation (e.g., Stickgold, 2005; Stickgold & Wamsley, 2017; Wamsley & Stickgold, 2011). More exactly, dreaming is "*simply* the conscious perception of the stream of images, thoughts, and feelings evoked in the brain by one or more of the many forms of off-line learning and memory processing that occur during sleep" (Stickgold & Wamsley, 2017, p. 514, italics added). This conclusion provides the basis for a functional theory that encompasses dreaming: "the function of dreaming may be *reducible* to a question of the function of the sleep-dependent memory processes that result in the conscious experience of dreaming" (Stickgold & Wamsley, 2017, p. 513, italics added). Put another way, dreaming is a "by-product of mechanisms that evolved to facilitate sleep-dependent memory consolidation and integration" (Stickgold & Wamsley, 2017, p. 513).

This reductive memory consolidation theory of dreaming is first of all refuted by the complete lack of evidence for memory consolidation during REM sleep in the rodent-based studies that began in 1994, as well as the earlier studies of humans going back to the late 1960s (e.g., Feldman & Dement, 1968; Fowler et al., 1973). Instead, the sharp-wave ripples in the hippocampal region, which are the brain waves used to indicate memory consolidation, do not show a "firing-rate correlation" that is related to memory consolidation during REM sleep (Chen & Wilson, 2017, p. 3). On the other hand, these sharp-wave ripples are frequent and related to new daytime learning in slow-wave sleep and quiet wakefulness (Chen & Wilson, 2017, p. 3).

A similar lack of support for the claim of memory consolidation during REM sleep is also reported in a large-scale study of human participants. It concluded that "Contrary to our expectation, REM sleep deprivation did not affect encoding in general.... Altogether, these findings indicate an importance of Non-REM rather than REM sleep for the encoding of information..."

(Kaida et al., 2015, p. 72). These conclusions are similar to those in other studies by the same core research group (Born & Wilhelm, 2012; Rasch & Born, 2015; Rasch et al., 2009). These results thereby disagree with earlier studies, some of which were carried out by the same researchers who came to new conclusions based on new studies.

Similarly, a well-controlled study that used anti-depressant medications to reduce REM sleep by as much as 39% found "no association of REM sleep diminution with decreases in memory performance or cognitive flexibility," which supports the earlier clinical findings on the lack of any negative effects from the loss of REM sleep on memory (Göder et al., 2011, p. 544). The theory of memory consolidation during REM sleep was directly challenged by the same sleep researchers who had written critiques of the earlier studies of memory consolidation during REM sleep (Vertes & Siegel, 2005).

The conclusion that memory consolidation does not occur during REM sleep in humans is supported by two independent meta-analyses. Both reported evidence for memory consolidation in non-REM sleep, but no evidence for memory consolidation in REM sleep (Hu et al., 2020; Hudachek & Wamsley, 2023). The second of the two meta-analyses is especially interesting for how it handles the fact that it found no evidence that recently acquired learning is solidified during REM sleep. The co-authors of the second meta-analysis first of all note that they had found a "strong and statistically significant association between task-related dreaming and memory performance" in "sixteen studies qualified for inclusion" (Hudachek & Wamsley, 2023, p. 1).

However, as they then note, "Among studies *using polysomnography*, this relationship was statistically significant for dreams collected from non-rapid eye movement (Non-REM) sleep (n = 10) but not for dreams collected from rapid eye movement (REM) sleep (n = 12)" (Hudachek & Wamsley, 2023, p. 1, italics added). Moreover, the "moderating effect of sleep stage did not reach statistical significance in a model that combined both REM and Non-REM reports" (Hudachek & Wamsley, 2023, p. 7). And yet they conclude:

> Integrating *all* available studies, this meta-analysis suggests that dreaming of newly learned information is indeed *robustly associated* with improved information following sleep. This is consistent with the hypothesis that dream content *reflects* the reactivation and consolidation of newly formed memory traces, a process *well-established* to occur during sleep and result in improved memory retention.
>
> *(Hudachek & Wamsley, 2023, pp. 9–10, italics added)*

What is striking about this conclusion is that dreaming occurs most frequently during REM sleep, but the meta-analytic findings only provide evidence for memory consolidation during non-REM sleep. The evidence therefore does not support the memory consolidation theory of dreaming (e.g., Stickgold, 2005; Stickgold & Wamsley, 2017).

Meanwhile, the weak and contradictory nature of the findings on memory consolidation during sleep in general has not gone unnoticed by sleep researchers (Cordi & Rasch, 2021a). In recognition of these difficulties, 19 sleep researchers concerned with the topic of memory consolidation during sleep joined together to address the fact that "the role of sleep in human memory consolidation is still under considerable debate, and numerous contradictory and non-replicable findings have been reported" (Németh et al., 2024, p. 123). They suggest several ways to address various methodological issues "related to experimental designs, task characteristics and measurements, and data-analysis...." Then they suggest "constructive solutions" to address the various problems this research field faces. They state their belief that "implementing these solutions in future sleep and memory research will substantially advance the field and improve understanding of the specific role of sleep in memory consolidation" (Németh et al., 2024, p. 123).

This is a striking degree of uncertainty for a research literature that has been a work in progress since 1968. Whether any agreed-upon procedures and rules of evidence can be established in this contentious field of research remains to be seen.

More generally, the idea that dreaming is reducible to the functions of sleep-dependent memory processes is not credible. It does not fit with the lack of evidence in animal models or humans that there is memory consolidation during REM sleep, nor with the minimal amounts of declarative memory consolidation that is found during non-REM sleep in recent studies using better controls (Cordi & Rasch, 2021b). Nor does it fit with the fact that dreaming occurs during the sleep-onset process, REM sleep, and in N2 sleep in the 1.5–2.5 hours before the morning awakening. Dreaming occurs for too long at too many different times for it to be plausible that memory consolidation is the basis for dreaming. Moreover, as Chapter 2 shows, there is compelling evidence that the neurocognitive network that supports dreaming has been identified by a combination of replicated neuroimaging, lesion, and developmental studies. This network cannot be realistically based in the process of memory consolidation.

Two Emotion-Related Adaptive Theories of Dream Function

Finally, there are two slightly differing theories suggesting that dreaming has an important adaptive function in relation to emotions. First, one of the activation-synthesis theorists who re-introduced the idea of memory consolidation during REM sleep soon thereafter added emotion regulation as an important function of dreaming during REM sleep (Stickgold, 2005). The second of the two emotion-related theories, the emotion-assimilation theory, which appeared ten years after the emotion-regulation theory, differs in that it does not prioritize REM sleep dreaming and instead places its emphasis on the assimilation and integration of thoughts into the memory system during dreaming. In this theory, "emotions act as a marker for information to be selectively processed during sleep, including consolidation into long term memory structures and integration into pre-existing memory networks" (Malinowski & Horton, 2015, p. 3).

Both theories face four insurmountable obstacles based on evidence presented at various points in this book. First, as shown in detail in the previous subsection, there is no evidence that any form of memory consolidation occurs during REM sleep, the sleep stage that accounts for the lion's share of dreaming. Thus, both theories are limited to N2 dreaming. Second, the finding that dreams are not likely to be encoded into memory if they are not immediately recalled means that a majority of dreams do not become part of the memory system for most people. Unencoded dreams therefore cannot contribute to regulation or assimilation because they have no cognitive remnants that can be drawn upon.

Third, there are very few emotions in the less frequent and less complex dreams of children and young adolescents aged from 3 to 11–12. This means that most emotional regulation that takes place during these years has to be carried out by waking processes, which is a major research topic in developmental psychology and educational psychology. Thus, both sets of theorists who claim that dreaming has adaptive functions with regard to emotions would have to explain why this putative adaptive function is important enough to be selected for as part of the evolutionary process but does not become operative until preadolescence. Since humans are notable for their extended periods of infancy, childhood, and adolescence, why is there so little dreaming until ages 9–11, and why do those few and simple dreams contain very few emotions? Neither set of theorists has chosen to address this longstanding omission in their respective theories.

Fourth, and finally, these theories need to explain why the regulation or assimilation of emotions is a function of dreaming even though 50%–75% of *recalled* adult dreams do not contain an emotion in the ten large samples that were discussed in Chapter 9. This relatively small amount of emotions in recalled dreams, when placed within the context of the small percentage of adult dreams that are encoded, makes the claims by both of these theories all the more unlikely.

The minimal amount of emotional regulation that might occur in adult dreams is further revealed by a study showing that the alleged amount of emotion regulation during REM sleep occurs just as frequently during slow-wave non-REM sleep during naps: "Although prior evidence has connected negative emotional memory formation to REM sleep *physiology*, we found that Non-REM delta activity and the amount of slow wave sleep in the nap were robustly related to the selective consolidation of negative information" (Payne et al., 2015, p. 176, italics added in order to document the emphasis on REM sleep in the emotion-regulation theory). The researchers added that the "magnitude of the emotional memory benefit" conferred by REM sleep "can be economically achieved by taking a nap" (Payne et al., 2015, p. 176). This conclusion might seem devastating to a theory that emphasizes the importance of REM sleep in the regulation of emotions, but it has had no apparent impact on the theory.

The Continuing Interest in Dreaming and Dream Content

Although there is no evidence that supports any past theory related to dreaming, a conclusion that includes all of the adaptive theories of dreaming, dreaming will nonetheless continue to be fascinating and useful to people in general and to cognitive neuroscientists in particular. As noted in Chapter 1, and in the conclusion to Chapter 3, dreams have had important uses in many indigenous societies and throughout the history of Western civilization, including in their contributions to religious experiences. It therefore seems unlikely that their usefulness would be diminished if they do not have an evolutionary adaptive value.

As recent decades have shown, dreams will continue to serve as a starting point for people to talk about their personal conceptions and concerns in counseling, clinical, and group discussion sessions, as noted in the conclusion to Chapter 3 (Hill et al., 1997; Hill & Spangler, 2007). There is also evidence that new insights can arise for people when they share their dreams in a dream group (e.g., Blagrove et al., 2019; Edwards et al., 2013). And of course, dreams will continue to be a source of new ideas and imagery for writers, painters, and musicians, as they have throughout history.

Moreover, the findings on individual dream series presented in Chapter 4 suggest that some individuals will continue to find insights about themselves as well as enjoyment in keeping a dream series (Bulkeley, 2023, pp. 5–7, for one personal example). In the process, they may continue to contribute to dream research in new and unexpected ways. Further, dreaming has to be understood more fully in order to provide another vantage point for finding new ways to help people who suffer from nightmares.

Finally, cognitive neuroscientists need to study dreaming and dream content for important theoretical reasons. Dreaming is a pervasive cognitive process that must be examined in order to fully understand the range of human cognition. No general theory of mind can be complete if it cannot explain why we dream, as well as the nature of dream content. The final section of this chapter therefore suggests an empirically based research agenda, which might make it possible to determine how dreams fit into the general picture of human perception and cognition developed by cognitive neuroscientists. In the process of carrying out this agenda, the virtues and shortcomings of the neurocognitive theory of dreaming should become apparent.

Plausible Ways Forward

Several new technologies and systematic empirical findings developed in recent decades provide overlapping opportunities to revolutionize the empirical study of dream recall, dreaming, and dream content. Such a large enterprise could involve the separate areas of expertise brought to the table by a wide range of researchers. However, these comments are made with the full realization that scientists prefer to develop their own agendas, although they sometimes come up with their new ideas and projects by building off of commentaries by others about future possibilities.

This hypothetical general agenda begins with cell phones and voice-to-text technologies, which were mentioned in Chapter 8. A study of everyday recall that relied on these technologies, and recruited paid volunteers to report their dreams on a 24/7 basis for a period of one or two weeks, could provide ecologically valid data on the contexts in which dream recall occurs. In addition to providing new information on morning recall and the relative importance of various retrieval cues, it might reveal how frequently people awaken during the night after a period of dreaming. In the process, one-week or two-week studies of this kind might provide large samples of dream reports for automated coding, as well as pools of participants known to be frequent or infrequent recallers.

As a next step, still other researchers might be interested in interviewing the participants at length about their history of remembering and discussing dreams, which might provide information about their earliest memories of dream recall, the origin of any interest they may have in their dreams, their history of nightmares, their history of lucid dreaming, and many other questions. It also might be useful to administer a battery of cognitive, visual imagery, and personality tests, which would be chosen by the investigators on the basis of the specific issues they wanted to address.

The interviews and tests, in turn, might provide pools of participants for laboratory-oriented dream researchers. For example, samples of frequent and infrequent dream recallers could be studied in either comfortable apartment-based laboratory settings or their own home settings, using instruments that detect REM sleep and perhaps N2 sleep. The use of such instrumentation would allow researchers to contact the participants at their homes and collect detailed voice-to-text dream reports. With the reports from awakenings in hand, the researchers could compare the content of freely recalled dreams and those collected via awakenings.

At that point, waking neuroimaging researchers might be interested in running trials to see if wearable high-density diffuse optical tomography (HD-DOT) headcaps make it possible to distinguish focused thought, mind-wandering, and brief episodes of dreaming while participants are reclining alone for 20–30 minutes in a dimly lighted room with their eyes closed. This approach may be feasible because wearable headcaps have been shown to be comfortable during waking use, and both the FPCN and the default network were detected in the study of one person (Uchitel et al., 2022; Vidal-Rosas et al., 2023). Such trials might be especially revealing if they included individuals from the pool of participants who are frequent dream recallers or who score high on openness to new experiences or fantasy proneness.

Then, too, daytime studies using an HD-DOT headcap may provide the opportunity to study the sleep-onset process in more detail with greater ecological validity if some of the participants unexpectedly drifted off to sleep. These opportunistic sleep-onset findings might be especially useful in tracing the relative deactivation of the FPCN and the two attention networks, along with the ascendancy of the neurocognitive network that produces dreaming.

It also could be that at this point sleep-dream laboratory researchers might become interested in testing the feasibility of using HD-DOT to study brain activation levels during sleep. In initial trials, it might be useful to begin by attaching the headcap during a brief period of spontaneous arousal in the 2–3 hours before morning, or after an early-morning trip to the bathroom. The first studies of sleep with this new technology therefore could focus on intriguing empirical questions about the frequency and nature of dreaming and dream content in the 1.5–2.5 hours before the spontaneous morning awakening.

If the headcap proved to be comfortable enough to allow normal sleep in the early-morning hours, neuroimaging researchers might be more inclined to carry out all-night studies of frequent dream recallers. Indeed, nothing is needed more than sustained neuroimaging studies of full nights of sleep in order to firmly establish what neural substrates are and are not functionally connected during periods of adequate activation during sleep. Then, too, neuroimaging studies that continue throughout several nights of sleep might make it possible to determine the degree to which frequent dream recallers experience the post-dream arousals that may lead to the encoding of dreams into memory.

For researchers without access to HD-DOT technology or a sleep laboratory, there are many other avenues for new research. For example, Artificial Intelligence (AI)-based solutions like the DreamCoder could be employed to carry out coding of dream samples that have not been studied before (Bongalon, 2025). Such studies could draw on the samples collected by means of cell phone reports to voice-to-text recorders. However, researchers would not have to rely exclusively on newly acquired samples, because there are thousands of dream reports available on the DreamBank that have not yet been studied in any detail.

For example, a pair of dream series were kept independently in the early 1960s by a wife ("Melora," $n = 211$) and husband ("Melvin," $n = 128$), which was also the year in which their first child was born. "Sally" is a forester in a very extensive wooded area in the Western United States, whose 249 dreams often involve her intense concern with preventing and fighting forest fires. There are also 593 dreams from a Vietnam veteran—a medic who was involved in the intense daily fighting in the Cambodian highlands in 1969–1970. He suffers from a very serious case of PTSD, which has often required hospitalization. However, he was able to write down his nightmares for several years after he left the Army. Later, he wrote down every dream he remembered over the space of 12 months in 2016–2017, when he was 67 years old. He also provided a large amount of information about his life over the course of many years (Levy, 2016, 2018).

Then, too, the availability of automated coding tools, along with the search programs and statistical routines that are part of the DreamBank and DreamSAT, may energize present and future dream researchers to gather bigger and better collections of dream reports using the Most Recent Dream methodology. (As shown in Chapter 3, this method leads to findings that are very similar to the Hall/Van de Castle normative findings with dream reports containing 50 or more words. It therefore can be used to compare dreams from different societies and from subgroups that may have different avocational interests or sexual preferences.) Researchers may also be motivated to keep their own dream journals for automated coding.

In addition, these technological advances might spur dream researchers to carry out their own versions of one or more of the aforementioned studies. Such new research would make it possible to re-examine all past findings on dream content, and to determine if there have been any historical changes in what people dream about.

Due to this abundance of new possibilities, the scientific study of dreaming could prosper if scientific studies continue to be valued and supported by the institutions within large-scale and prosperous societies. However, even if science continues to be valued and supported, scientific studies of dreaming could fall by the wayside once again, if scientifically oriented individuals continue to focus most of their attention on other topics. It is therefore impossible to predict the future of scientific dream research.

APPENDIX

Methodological Issues in Assessing the Frequency of Emotions in Dream Reports

This appendix provides a methodological critique of two studies carried out under the auspices of the Central Institute of Mental Health in Mannheim, which conclude that emotions are frequent in dream reports (Röver & Schredl, 2017; Schredl & Doll, 1998). They do so on the basis of self-ratings by the participants of their own dream reports, as well as ratings by one independent rater in each of the two studies. Some of the methodological criticisms that follow hold for rating scales relating to emotions in general (Domhoff, 2022, pp. 221–224, for a comparison of rating scales and coding categories for emotions). However, most of the critiques in this appendix specifically concern these two emotion-focused studies.

The participants in these two studies were instructed to include "implicit" emotions and "moods" in making their self-ratings, which exacerbates several of the general problems with rating scales when they are applied to dreams. In particular, the instructions to use implicit emotions and moods reinforce the problem that participants and researchers alike tend to have a "wake-state bias" in rating dream reports.

The concept of a wake-state bias is premised upon the observation that people generally tend to assume that dreaming and waking thought are based on similar cognitive processes. They therefore further assume that dreams can be understood by comparing them with waking thought. More specifically, the wake-state bias has been defined as "The practice of projecting beliefs about waking experience onto dreaming without critical reflection or solid empirical evidence" (Windt, 2015, p. 200).

This bias is understandable due to the seeming parallels between dreaming and waking, such as "seeing" in both instances, even though in fact visual imagery is not the same as visual perception. Then, too, the experience of dreaming sometimes feels very "real" after waking, and the contents of the dreams that people recall often include familiar people and familiar settings. More generally, dreams create a "subjective impression of verisimilitude" (Windt, 2015, pp. 309–310).

This emphasis on the wake-state bias seems even more relevant in considering the issue of emotions in dreams: self-raters very likely assume there must have been emotions in their dream because emotions almost certainly would have been experienced in similar situations in waking life. Contrary to this general assumption, one sleep-dream laboratory study of emotions found that emotions that would have been present in similar situations in waking life were absent in 17.4% of the laboratory dreams they collected (Foulkes et al., 1988, pp. 34–35).

Moreover, it is one thing to recall a dream during the morning awakening, which is based on the memory of a recent experience. On the other hand, judgments about memories are based on "metamemory." Metamemory arises from a more complex neurocognitive network than recall does, and it includes several of the most recently evolved prefrontal and parietal areas, including the lateral frontal pole (Mansouri et al., 2017; Saccenti et al., 2024; Wirebring et al., 2018). Most importantly for the purposes of this appendix, waking studies of people's judgments about their memories also show that these judgments are often incorrect (Gaynor & Chua, 2018).

The weaknesses of self-ratings are first of all revealed in the degree of difference in the self-ratings and the ratings by the independent raters. In the first of the two studies by the researchers affiliated with the Central Institute of Mental Health in Mannheim, the 964 self-ratings by the 263 participants (190 women and 73 men) led to the finding that only 7.3% of the dream reports lacked an emotion. Ratings by the independent rater, based on one dream report from each of 180 participants, led to the conclusion that 14.4% of the dream reports contained no emotions, a gap of 7.1 percentage points (Schredl & Doll, 1998, p. 640, Table 1).

Here readers may recall from Chapter 9 that the two researchers who conducted the 1998 research study discussed in the previous paragraph also carried out Hall/Van de Castle codings of the same subset of 180 dream reports that was used by the independent rater. This analysis led to the conclusion that 60.6% of these dream reports lacked an emotion, a difference of 46.2 percentage points from the independent rater. In addition, their conclusion that 60.6% of the dream reports had no emotions is very similar to the Hall/Van de Castle combined norms for non-lab dream reports, 58.3%, a difference of only 2.3 percentage points (Schredl & Doll, 1998, p. 640, Table 1). Moreover, as also noted in Chapter 9, very similar results were obtained by two other researchers using their own nominal categories for coding emotions (McCarley & Hoffman, 1981; Snyder, 1970).

This similarity between findings in both Germany and the United States using the Hall/Van de Castle coding system is very strong evidence that its coding categories can be reliably used. Thus, it can be inferred that the rating studies greatly underrate the percentage of dream reports that did not contain any emotion; otherwise, the studies using the Hall/Van de Castle coding system, including the one by the researchers at the Central Institute of Mental Health, are wrong.

The second Central Institute of Mental Health study, which was carried out by the lead researcher and a different co-worker, found even larger differences between the participants' self-ratings of their own dreams and the ratings by the independent rater, who made independent ratings of the same 1207 diary dreams rated by the participants. According to the 413 participants (350 women and 63 men), only 4.7% of their own dream reports did not include an emotion. However, the independent rater reported a No-Emotions Percent of 17.5%, a difference of 12.8 percentage points (Röver & Schredl, 2017, Table 3, for the no-emotions findings).

The large differences between the self-ratings by participants and those by the independent rater raise questions about both the reliability and the validity of this rating system. They also raise the possibility that any one or more of several factors are biasing the self-ratings by participants. In addition to the wake-state bias discussed above, the self-ratings may be influenced by the inadvertent "demand characteristics" created by the researchers by asking self-raters to include "implicit emotions" and "moods." More generally, at least some of the participants may be among the subset of participants in psychological studies who have a general desire to provide ratings and replies that they think will please the experimenters, which is known as "social-desirability bias" ("Social-desirability bias," 2025).

Further evidence related to these large differences between self-ratings and the codings by researchers is provided by two of three studies of emotions that were carried out at the University of Turku, which were overviewed in Chapter 9 with a focus on the codings by the two independent coders. Here it is relevant to add that these two studies also included self-ratings using the same 10 categories for positive emotions and the same 10 categories for negative emotions—20 emotion categories in all—that were used by the independent coders. (The third of the three studies discussed in Chapter 9 did not use self-ratings, so it is not relevant here; Sikka et al., 2018).

The participants examined the dream reports for the presence or absence of any of the 20 emotions on a scale that included five categories. These five categories ranged from (0) "I did not experience any of these feelings at all," to "I experienced these feelings" (1) a little bit; (2) moderately; (3) quite a bit; (4) extremely. The participants were asked to rate the dream they just had experienced, not the dream report itself, an instruction that has parallels with the instructions in the Mannheim studies to consider implicit emotions and moods in making their ratings.

The University of Turku researchers therefore stress that participants may be drawing upon both their memory of the experience, including mood states, as well as the report they provided to the researchers. In the case of the independent coders, on the other hand, they were relying exclusively on the transcriptions of the spoken dream reports. Further, the independent coders made note of each of the emotions they coded in each dream. They also met to resolve differences when they had finished with their independent codings. It is therefore possible to make direct comparisons of self-ratings with a coding system *other than the Hall/Van de Castle coding system*. The fact that the independent coders are using a different coding system provides an ideal comparison for determining whether or not the self-raters and the independent raters still differ. Generally speaking, there are very large differences between the results derived from the participants' self-ratings and the codings by independent researchers.

The first study was based on 115 lab dream reports from 17 participants, 10 women and 7 men (Sikka et al., 2014, pp. 54–55). The participants judged that none of their dream reports lacked an emotion, so the No-Emotions Percent was 0%, as compared to 71.3% according to the coders. This is an extremely large difference (Sikka et al., 2014, pp. 56–57). The second study used 552 non-lab dream reports provided by 44 participants, 28 women and 16 men. The participants self-rated that only 2.5% of their dream reports did not include an emotion. The two coders, on the other hand, concluded that 52.2% of the dream reports did not contain any of the 20 emotions, a difference of 49.7 percentage points.

These results demonstrate once again that independent coders differ greatly from the self-ratings provided by participants. In effect, these results thereby provide a conceptual replication of the several different coding studies that were overviewed in Chapter 9. It is therefore highly unlikely, contrary to the Central Institute of Mental Health researchers, that self-ratings of dream reports are accurate.

Within the context of the overall findings from the several studies discussed in this appendix, a further point can be added. Self-ratings that find emotions in 92.7%–100% of dream reports—i.e., No-Emotion Percents that ranged from 7.3% to 0%—seem even more unlikely and implausible if the neuroimaging findings on the five association networks that support emotions during waking are taken into account (L. F. Barrett, 2017; Polner-Clark et al., 2016; Raz et al., 2016; Touroutoglou et al., 2015). This is because all of these association networks, with the partial exception of portions of the default network, are relatively deactivated throughout the sleep period, as discussed in several earlier chapters, including Chapter 9.

Conclusion

For several reasons, then, self-ratings by participants cannot provide useful information on emotions in dream reports. The evidence suggests that participants provide very large over-estimations of the frequency of emotions in dream reports, not underestimations. Self-raters are very likely subject to several of the factors that can lead to inaccurate judgments. They include a wake-state bias, inadvertent demand characteristics created by the researchers (e.g., in this case asking self-raters to include "implicit emotions" and "moods"), and social-desirability bias.

Moreover, the large percentage of dreams that lack emotions in the ten studies overviewed in Chapter 9, including the Hall/Van de Castle coding study by Schredl and Doll (1998), is entirely consistent with what would be expected by the neurocognitive theory of dreaming. This is because the theory emphasizes the cognitive deficiencies during dreaming, which are due to the relative deactivation of four of the five association networks, as well as the relative deactivation of portions of the default network.

REFERENCES

Abdallah, C., Averill, C., Ramage, A., Averill, L., Young-McCaughan, S., Fox, P., & Peterson, A. (2019). Salience network disruption in U.S. army soldiers with posttraumatic stress disorder. *Chronic Stress*, *3*, 1–10. https://doi.org/10.1177/2470547019850467

Abraham, A. (2013). The world according to me: Personal relevance and the medial prefrontal cortex. *Frontiers in Human Neuroscience*, *7*, 341–344.

Abraham, A. (2016). The imaginative mind. *Human Brain Mapping*, *37*, 4197–4211.

Aguerre, N. V., Gómez-Ariza, C. J., Ibáñez-Molina, A. J., & Bajo, M. T. (2023). Electrophysiological correlates of dispositional mindfulness: A quantitative and complexity EEG study *British Journal of Psychology*, *114*, 566–579. https://doi.org/10.1111/bjop.12636

Allen, E., Laroi, F., McGuire, P., & Aleman, A. (2008). The hallucinating brain: A review of structural and functional neuroimaging studies of hallucinations. *Neuroscience & Biobehavioral Reviews*, *32*, 175–191. https://doi.org/10.1016/j.neubiorev.2007.07.012

Allison, T., & Van Twyver, H. (1970a). The evolution of sleep. *Natural History*, *79*, 56–65.

Allison, T., & Van Twyver, H. (1970b). Sleep in the opossum Didelphis marsupialis. *Electroencephalography and Clinical Neurophysiology*, *29*(2), 181–189. https://doi.org/10.1016/0013-4694(70)90121-5

Allport, G. (1942). *The use of personal documents in psychological science*. Social Science Research Council.

Al-Shama, R., Uleman, J., Mariana Pereira, M., Jurgen A.H.R. Claassen, J., & Dresler, M. (2024). Cerebral blood flow in sleep: A systematic review and meta-analysis. Sleep Medicine Reviews, 77, 1–13.

Amft, M., Bzdok, D., Laird, A., Fox, P., & Schilbach, L. (2015). Definition and characterization of an extended social-affective default network. *Brain Structure & Function*, *220*, 1031–1049.

Andrews-Hanna, J. (2012). The brain's default network and its adaptive role in internal mentation. *The Neuroscientist*, *18*, 251–270.

Andrews-Hanna, J., Reidler, J., Huang, C., & Buckner, R. (2010). Evidence for the default network's role in spontaneous cognition. *Journal of Neurophysiology*, *104*, 322–335.

Andrews-Hanna, J., Reidler, J., Sepulcre, J., Poulin, R., & Buckner, R. (2010). Functional-anatomic fractionation of the brain's default network *Neuron*, *65*, 550–562.

Andrews-Hanna, J., Smallwood, J., & Spreng, R. N. (2014). The default network and self-generated thought: Component processes, dynamic control, and clinical relevance. *Annals of the New York Academy of Science*, *1316*, 29–52.

Antrobus, J. (1983). REM and NREM sleep reports: Comparisons of word frequencies by cognitive classes. *Psychophysiology*, *20*, 562–568.

Antrobus, J. (1993). Dreaming: Could we do without it? In A. Moffitt, M. Kramer, & R. Hoffmann (Eds.), *The functions of dreaming* (pp. 549–558). State University of New York Press.

Antrobus, J. (2000). How does the dreaming brain explain the dreaming mind? *Behavioral and Brain Sciences*, *23*(6), 904–907.

Antrobus, J., Kondo, T., & Reinsel, R. (1995). Dreaming in the late morning: Summation of REM and diurnal cortical activation. *Consciousness & Cognition*, *4*, 275–299.

APA. (2023). Natural Experiment. *APA Dictionary of Psychology*, March 14, 2023, https://dictionary.apa.org/natural-experiment.

APA. (2024). Affective Meaning. *APA Dictionary of Psychology*. https://dictionary.apa.org/affective-meaning

Aquino, G., Benz, F., Dressle, R. J., Gemignani, A., Alfì, G., Palagini, L., & Feige, B. (2024). Towards the neurobiology of insomnia: A systematic review of neuroimaging studies. *Sleep Medicine Reviews*, *73*. https://doi.org/10.1016/j.smrv.2023.101878

Arkin, A., & Antrobus, J. (1991). The effects of external stimuli applied prior to and during sleep on sleep experience. In S. J. Ellman & J. S. Antrobus (Eds.), *The mind in sleep: Psychology and psychophysiology* (2nd ed., pp. 265–307). Wiley.

Armitage, R. (1995). The distribution of EEG frequencies in REM and NREM sleep stages in healthy young adults. *Sleep*, *18*, 334–341 https://doi.org/10.1093/sleep/18.5.334

Aserinsky, E. (1996). Memories of famous neuropsychologists: The discovery of REM sleep. *Journal of the History of the Neurosciences*, *5*(3), 213–227.

Aserinsky, E., & Kleitman, N. (1953). Regularly occurring periods of eye motility, and concomitant phenomena, during sleep. *Science*, *118*, 273–274.

Aserinsky, E., Lynch, J., Mack, M., Tzankoff, S., & Hurn, E. (1985). Comparison of eye motion in wakefulness and REM sleep. *Psychophysiology*, *22*(1), 1–10. https://doi.org/10.1111/j.1469-8986.1985.tb01551.x

Avidan, A. (2017). Non-rapid eye movement parasomnias: Clinical spectrum, diagnostic features, and management. In M. Kryger, T. Roth, & W. Dement (Eds.), *Principles and practices of sleep medicine* (6th ed., pp. 981–1001). Elsevier.

Avila-White, D., Schneider, A., & Domhoff, G. W. (1999). The most recent dreams of 12–13 year-old boys and girls: A methodological contribution to the study of dream content in teenagers. *Dreaming*, *9*, 163–171.

Avram, M., Fortea, L., Wollner, L., Coenen, R., Korda, A., & al., e. (2024). Large-scale brain connectivity changes following the administration of lysergic acid diethylamide, d-amphetamine, and 3,4-methylenedioxyamphetamine. *Molecular Psychiatry*, *30*, 1297–1307. https://doi.org/10.1038/s41380-024-02734-y

Badia, P., Wright, K., & Wauquier, A. (1994). Fluctations in single-hertz EEG activity during the transition to sleep. In R. Ogilvie & J. Harsh (Eds.), *Sleep onset: Normal and abnormal processes* (pp. 201–218). American Psychological Association.

Baird, B., Castelnovo, A., Gosseries, O., & Tononi, G. (2018). Frequent lucid dreaming associated with increased functional connectivity between frontopolar cortex and temporoparietal association areas. *Science Reports*, *8*(17798). https://doi.org/10.1038/s41598-018-36190-w

Baird, B., Tononi, G., & LaBerge, S. (2022). Lucid dreaming occurs in activated rapid eye movement sleep, not a mixture of sleep and wakefulness. *Sleep*, *45*(4), 1–15. https://doi.org/10.1093/sleep/zsab294

Baker, E., Young, M. P., Gauld, D. M., & Fleming, J. F. (1970). A new look at bimedial prefrontal leukotomy. *Canadian Medical Association Journal*, *102*, 37–41.

Balkin, T., Braun, A., Wesensten, N., Jeffries, K., & Varga, M. (2002). The process of awakening: A PET study of regional brain activity patterns mediating the re-establishment of alertness and consciousness. *Brain*, *125*, 2308–2319.

Bar, M. (2011). The proactive brain. In M. Bar (Ed.), *Predictions in the brain: Using our past to generate a future* (pp. 13–26). Oxford University Press.

Barrett, D. (2001). *The committee of sleep: How artists, scientists, and athletes use dreams for creative problem-solving—and how you can too.* Crown/Random House.

Barrett, D. (2007). An evolutionary theory of problem-solving. In D. Barrett & P. McNamara (Eds.), *The new science of dreaming: Cultural and theoretical perspectives* (Vol. 3, pp. 133–153). Praeger.

Barrett, D. (2017). Dreams and creative problem-solving. *Annals of the New York Academy of Sciences*. *1406*(1), 60–67.

Barrett, D., Juarez, E., Ruby, C., & Grayson, M. (2024). Dreams of three 20th century novelists: Comparisons to normative dreams, to each other, and to their fiction. *Psychology of Consciousness*, *11*(1), 111–121. https://doi.org/10.1037/cns0000390

Barrett, L. F. (2017). The theory of constructed emotion: An active inference account of interoception and categorization. *Social Cognitive and Affective Neuroscience*, *12*, 1–23.

Barrett, L. F., Atzil, S., Bliss-Moreau, E., Chanes, L., Gendron, M., Hoemann, K., & Westlin, C. (2025). The theory of constructed emotion: More than a feeling. *Perspectives on Psychological Science*, *20* (3), 392–420. https://doi.org/10.1177/17456916251319045

Bassett, D. S., & Bullmore, E. T. (2017). Small-world brain networks revisited. *The Neuroscientist*, *5*, 499–516. https://doi.org/10.1177/1073858416667720

Bauer, P., Burch, M., Scholin, S., & Güler, E. (2007). Using cue words to investigate the distribution of autobiographical memories in childhood. *Psychological Science*, *18*, 910–916.

Baylor, G. (2001). What do we really know about Mendeleev's dream of the periodic table? A note on dreams of scientific problem solving. *Dreaming*, *11*, 89–92.

Beaty, R., & Silvia, P. J. (2013). Metaphorically speaking: Cognitive abilities and the production of figurative language. *Memory & Cognition*, *41*, 255–267.

Beaty, R., Silvia, P. J., & Benedek, M. (2017). Brain networks underlying novel metaphor production. *Brain and Cognition, 111,* 163–170.

Beaulieu-Prévost, D., & Zadra, A. (2005a). Dream recall frequency and attitude towards dreams: A reinterpretation of the relation. *Personality and Individual Differences, 38,* 919–927.

Beaulieu-Prévost, D., & Zadra, A. (2005b). How dream recall frequency shapes people's beliefs about the content of their dreams. *North American Journal of Psychology, 7,* 253–264.

Beaulieu-Prévost, D., & Zadra, A. (2007). Absorption, psychological boundaries, and attitude towards dreams as correlates of dream recall: Two decades of research seen through a meta-analysis. *Journal of Sleep Research, 16,* 51–59.

Beaulieu-Prévost, D., & Zadra, A. (2015). When people remember dreams they never experienced: A study of the malleability of dream recall over time. *Dreaming, 25,* 18–31.

Bell, I. 1992. *Robert Louis Stevenson: Dreams of exile.* Edinburg: Mainstream Publishing.

Bell, A., & Hall, C. (1971). *The personality of a child molester: An analysis of dreams.* Aldine.

Benedek, M., Beaty, R., Jauk, E., Koschutnig, K., Fink, A., Silvia, P. J., & Neubauer, A. (2014). Creating metaphors: The neural basis of figurative language production. *Neuroimage, 90,* 99–106.

Benington, J. H. (2004). Homeostatic and circadian influences. In C. A. Kushida (Ed.), *Sleep deprivation: Basic science, physiology, & behavior.* Dekker.

Benjamin, G. (2014). *Temiar religion, 1964–2012: Enchantment, disenchantment, and re-enchantment in Malaysia's uplands.* NUS Press.

Berger, R., & Phillips, N. (1995). Energy conservation and sleep. *Behavioural Brain Research, 69,* 65–73.

Berkovitch, L., Fauvel, B., Preller, K. H., & Gaillard, R. (2025). Neurocognitive effects of psilocybin: A systematic and comprehensive review of neuroimaging studies in humans. *Neuroscience and Biobehavioral Reviews,* 175. https://doi.org/10.1016/j.neubiorev.2025.106239

Bernstein, D. M., & Belicki, K. (1995-1996). On the psychometric properties of retrospective dream content questionnaires. *Imagination, Cognition and Personality, 15,* 351–364.

Bertolero, M., Yeo, B., Bassett, D. S., & D'Esposito, M. (2018). A mechanistic model of connector hubs, modularity and cognition. *Nature of Human Behavior, 10,* 765–777. https://doi.org/10.1038/s41562-018-0420-6

Bertolini, L., Elce, V., Michalak, A., Bernardi, G., & Weeds, J. (2024). Automatic scoring of dream reports' emotional content with large language models. In *Proceedings of the 9th Workshop on Computational Linguistics and Clinical Psychology (CLPsych 2024)* (pp. 92–107). https://aclanthology.org/2024.clpsych-1.7/

Binder, J. R., & Desai, R. H. (2011). The neurobiology of semantic memory. *Trends in Cognitive Sciences, 15*(11), 527–536. https://doi.org/10.1016/j.tics.2011.10.001

Bischof, M., & Basset, C. (2004). Total dream loss: A distinct neuropsychological dysfunction after bilateral PCA stroke. *Annals of Neurology, 56,* 583–586.

Blagrove, M. (1992). Dreams as a reflection of our waking concerns and abilities: A critique of the problem-solving paradigm in dream research. *Dreaming,* 2, 205–220.

Blagrove, M. (1996). Problems with the cognitive psychological modeling of dreaming. *Journal of Mind and Behavior*, *17*, 99–134.

Blagrove, M. (2007). Dreaming and personality. In D. Barrett & P. McNamara (Eds.), *The new science of dreaming: Content, recall, and personality correlates* (Vol. 2, pp. 115–158). Preager.

Blagrove, M., & Akehurst, L. (2000). Personality and dream recall frequency: Further negative findings. *Dreaming*, *10*, 139–148.

Blagrove, M., Edwards, C., van Rijn, E., Reid, A., & Malinowski, J. (2019). Insight from the consideration of REM dreams, non-REM dreams, and daydreams. *Psychology of Consciousness: Theory, Research, and Practice*, *6*, 138–162. https://doi.org/10.1037/cns0000167

Blake, Y., Terburg, D., Balchin, R., van Honk, J., & Solms, M. (2019). The role of the basolateral amygdala in dreaming. *Cortex*, *113*, 169–183. https://doi.org/10.1016/j.cortex.2018.12.016

Bogdan, P. C. (2025). One decade into the replication crisis, how have psychological results changed? *Advances in Methods and Practices in Psychological Science*, *8*(2). https://doi.org/10.1177/25152459251323480

Boly, M., Massimini, M., Tsuchiya, N., Postle, B. R., Koch, C., & Tononi, G. (2017). Are the neural correlates of consciousness in the front or in the back of the cerebral cortex? Clinical and neuroimaging evidence. *Journal of Neuroscience*, *37*, 9603–9613.

Bongalon, B. (2025). *Leveraging large language models for automated HVdC dream content coding* [Conference presentation]. International Association for the Study of Dreams. https://TheDreamCoder.com/downloads/IASD2025.pdf

Born, J., & Gais, S. (2000). REM sleep deprivation: The wrong paradigm leading to wrong conclusions. *Behavioral and Brain Sciences*, *23*(6), 912.

Born, J., & Wilhelm, I. (2012). System consolidation of memory during sleep. *Psychological Research*, *76*, 192–203.

Branstetter, B. K., Finneran, J. J., Fletcher, E. A., Weisman, B. C., & Ridgway, S. H. (2012). Dolphins can maintain vigilant behavior through echolocation for 15 days without interruption or cognitive impairment. *PLoS One*, 1–10. https://doi.org/10.1371/journal.pone.0047478

Braun, A., Balkin, T., Wesensten, N., Carson, R., Varga, M., Baldwin, P., & Herscovitch, P. (1997). Regional cerebral blood flow throughout the sleep-wake cycle: An $H_2{}^{15}O$ PET study. *Brain*, *120*, 1173–1197.

Braun, A., Balkin, T., Wesensten, N., Gwadry, F., Carson, R., Varga, M., & Herscovitch, P. (1998). Dissociated pattern of activity in visual cortices and their projections during human rapid eye movement sleep. *Science*, *279*, 91–95.

Bresser, T., Blanken, T. F., de Lange, S. C., Leerssen, J., Foster-Dingley, J. C., Lakbila-Kamal, O., ..., & Van Someren, E. J. W. (2025). Insomnia subtypes have differentiating deviations in brain structural connectivity. *Biological Psychiatry*, *97*(3), 302–312.

Broughton, R. (1968). Sleep disorders: Disorders of arousal? *Science*, *159*, 1070–1078.

Broughton, R. (2015). Psi and biology: An evolutionary perspective. In E. Cardeña, J. Palmer, & D. Marcusson-Clavertz (Eds.), *Parapsychology: A handbook for the 21st century* (pp. 139–148). MacFarland.

Brown, R., Lau, H., & LeDoux, J. (2019). Understanding the higher-order approach to consciousness. *Trends in Cognitive Sciences*, *23*, 754–768. https://doi.org/10.1016/j.tics.2019.06.009

Brydges, C. R., Fox, A., Reid, C. L., & Anderson, M. (2014). The differentiation of executive functions in middle and late childhood: A longitudinal latent-variable analysis. *Intelligence*, *47*, 34–43.

Buckner, R. (2012). The serendipitous discovery of the brain's default network. *Neuroimage*, *62*, 1137–1145.

Buckner, R., Andrews-Hanna, J., & Schacter, D. (2008). The brain's default network: Anatomy, function, and relevance to disease. *Annals of the New York Academy of Sciences*, *1124*, 1–38. https://doi.org/10.1196/annals.1440.011

Buckner, R., Roffman, J. L., & Smoller, J. W. (2014). Brain Genomics Superstructure Project (GSP) Dataverse, version 10.5. *Harvard Dataverse*. https://dataverse.harvard.edu/dataset.xhtml?persistentId=doi:10.7910/DVN/25833

Bulgarelli, C., Klerk, C. C. J. M., Richards, J., Southgate, V., Hamilton, A., & al, e. (2020). The developmental trajectory of fronto-temporoparietal connectivity as a proxy of the default mode network: A longitudinal fNIRS investigation. *Human Brain Mapping*, *41*, 2717–2740. https://doi.org/10.1002/hbm.24974

Bulkeley, K. (2008). *Dreaming in the world's religions: A comparative history*. New York University Press.

Bulkeley, K. (2009). The religious content of dreams: A new scientific foundation. *Pastoral Psychology*, *58*, 93–106.

Bulkeley, K. (2018). The meaningful continuities between dreaming and waking: Results of a blind analysis of a woman's 30-year dream journal. *Dreaming*, *28*, 337–350. https://doi.org/10.1037/drm0000083

Bulkeley, K. (2023). *The scribes of sleep: Insights from the most important dream journals in history*. Oxford University Press.

Bullmore, E., & Sporns, O. (2009). Complex brain networks: Graph theoretical analysis of structural and functional systems. *Nature Reviews Neuroscience*, *10*, 186–198.

Bunce, L., & Boerger, E. A. (2022). Openness to experience mediates the relation between fantasy proneness and creative thinking. *Imagination, Cognition and Personality*, *42*(2), 192–214. https://doi.org/10.1177/02762366221120214

Burger, A., Fennessy, J., Fennessy, S., & Dierkes, P. (2020). Nightly selection of resting sites and group behavior reveal antipredator strategies in giraffe. *Ecology*, *10*(6), 2917–2927. https://doi.org/10.1002/ece3.6106

Burgess, P. W., Dumontheil, I., & Gilbert, S. J. (2007). The gateway hypothesis of rostral prefrontal cortex (area 10) function. *Trends in Cognitive Sciences*, *11*. https://doi.org/10.1016/j.tics.2007.05.004

Burris, J. L., Oleas, D., Reider, L., Buss, K. A., Pérez-Edgar, K., & LoBue, V. (2020). Biased attention to threat: Answering old questions with young infants. *Current Directions in Psychological Science*, *28*(6), 534–539. https://doi.org/10.1177/0963721419861415

Bussey, K. (2013). Gender development. In M. Ryan & N. Branscombe (Eds.), *Sage handbook of gender and psychology* (pp. 81–99). Sage.

Campbell, I., Grimm, K., de Bie, E., & Feinberg, I. (2012). Sex, puberty, and the timing of sleep EEG measured adolescent brain maturation. *Proceedings of the*

National Academy of Sciences of the United States of America, 109, 5740–5743. https://doi.org/10.1073/pnas.1120860109

Carbonell, F., Bellec, P., & Shmuel, A. (2014). Quantification of the impact of a confounding variable on functional connectivity confirms anti-correlated networks in the resting-state. *Neuroimage, 86*, 343–353.

Carr, M. (2025, January). Engineering our dreams. *Scientific American*, 46–51.

Carr, M., Haar, A., Amores, J., Lopes, P., Bernal, G., Vega, T., Maes, P. (2020). Dream engineering: Simulating worlds through sensory stimulation. *Consciousness and Cognition, 82*, 1–19. https://doi.org/10.1016/j.concog.2020.102955

Cartwright, R. (1974). Problem solving: Waking and dreaming. *Journal of Abnormal Psychology, 83*, 451–455.

Cartwright, R. (1977). *Night life: Explorations in dreaming*. Prentice-Hall.

Cartwright, R. (1986). Affect and dream work from an information processing point of view. *Journal of Mind & Behavior, 7*, 411–427.

Cartwright, R. (1996). Dreams and adaptation to divorce. In D. Barrett (Ed.), *Trauma and dreams* (pp. 179–185). Harvard University Press.

Cartwright, R., & Ratzel, R. (1968). NonREM dreaming and auditory thresholds. *Psychophysiology, 5*, 231.

Cavallero, C., Cicogna, P., Natale, V., & Occhionero, M. (1992). Slow wave sleep dreaming. *Sleep, 15*, 562–566.

Cerri, M., & Amici, R. (2021). Thermoregulation and sleep: Functional interaction and central nervous control. *Comprehensive Physiology, 11*(2), 1591–1604. https://doi.org/10.1002/cphy.c140012

Chang, C., Liu, Z., Chen, M., Liu, X., & Duyn, J. (2013). EEG correlates of time-varying BOLD functional connectivity. *Neuroimage, 72*, 227–236.

Chavez, R. S., Guthrie, T. D., & Kapustka, J. M. (2025). Person knowledge is independently encoded by allocentric and egocentric reference frames within separate brain systems. *Psychological Science, 36*(4), 265–277. https://doi.org/10.1177/09567976251328430

Chen, A., Oathes, D., Chang, C., Bradley, T., & Zhou, Z.-W. (2013). Causal interactions between fronto-parietal central executive and default-mode networks in humans. *Proceedings of the National Academy of Sciences, 110*, 19944–19949.

Chen, Z., & Wilson, M. (2017). Deciphering neural codes of memory during sleep. *Trends in Neuroscience, 40*, 260–275. https://doi.org/10.1016/j.tins.2017.03.005

Cheyne, J. A., & Pennycook, G. (2013). Sleep paralysis post-episode distress: Modeling potential effects of episode characteristics, general psychological distress, beliefs, and cognitive style. *Clinical Psychological Science, 1*, 135–148.

Childs, M. K., & Polich, J. M. (1979). Developmental differences in mental rotation. *Journal of Experimental Child Psychology, 27*, 339–351.

Chow, H., Horovitz, S., Picchioni, D., Balkin, T., & Braun, A. (2013). Rhythmic alternating patterns of brain activity distinguish rapid eye movement sleep from other states of consciousness. *Proceedings of the National Academy of Sciences, 110*, 10300–10305.

Christensen, J., Aubin, S., Nielsen, T., Ptito, M., Kupers, R., & Jennum, P. (2019). Rapid eye movements are reduced in blind individuals. *Journal of Sleep Research, 28*, Article e12866. https://doi.org/10.1111/jsr.12866

Christoff, K. (2014). Thinking. In K. Ochsner & S. Kosslyn (Eds.), *The Oxford handbook of cognitive neuroscience* (pp. 318–333). Oxford University Press.

Christoff, K., & Gabrieli, J. D. (2000). The frontopolar cortex and human cognition: Evidence for a rostrocaudal hierarchical organization within the human prefrontal cortex. *Psychobiology*, *28*, 168–186.

Christoff, K., Irving, Z., Fox, K., Spreng, R. N., & Andrews-Hanna, J. (2016). Mind-wandering as spontaneous thought: A dynamic framework. *Nature Reviews Neuroscience*, *17*, 718–731.

Christoff, K., Prabhakaran, V., Dorfman, J., Zhao, Z., Kroger, J. K., Holyoak, K., & Gabrieli, J. D. (2001). Rostrolateral prefrontal cortex involvement in relational integration during reasoning. *Neuroimage*, *14*, 1136–1149. https://doi.org/10.1006/nimg.2001.0922

Christoff, K., Ream, J. M., Geddes, L. P., & Gabrieli, J. D. (2003). Evaluating self-generated information: anterior prefrontal contributions to human cognition. *Behavioral Neuroscience*, *117*, 1161–1168. https://doi.org/10.1037/0735-7044.117.6.1161

Cicogna, P., Natale, V., Occhionero, M., & Bosinelli, M. (1998). A comparison of mental activity during sleep onset and morning awakening. *Sleep*, *21*(5), 462–470.

Cipolli, C., Calasso, E., Maccolini, S., Pani, R., & Salzarulo, P. (1984). Memory processes in morning recall after multiple night awakenings. *Perceptual and Motor Skills*, *59*, 435–446.

Cipolli, C., Salazarulo, P., & Calabrese, A. (1981). Memory processes involved in morning recall of mental REM-sleep experience: A psycholinguistic study. *Perceptual and Motor Skills*, *52*(2), 391–406. https://doi.org/10.2466/pms.1981.52.2.391

Clancy, S. (2005). *Abducted: How people come to believe they were kidnapped by aliens*. Harvard University Press.

Cohen, D. (1974). Toward a theory of dream recall. *Psychological Bulletin*, *38*, 122–138.

Cohen, D. (1979). *Sleep and dreaming: Origins, nature, and function*. Pergamon Press.

Cohen, D., & Wolfe, G. (1973). Dream recall and repression: Evidence for an alternative hypothesis. *Journal of Consulting and Clinical Psychology*, *41*(3), 349–355. https://doi.org/10.1037/h0035333

Cohen, J. (1962). The statistical power of abnormal-social psychological research: A review *Journal of Abnormal and Social Psychology*, *65*(3), 145–153

Cohen, J. (1977). *Statistical power analysis for the behavioral sciences*. Academic Press.

Colombo, M. A., Comanducci, A., Casarotto, S., Derch, C.-C., Annen, J., Viganò, A., & Rosanova, M. (2023). Beyond alpha power: EEG spatial and spectral gradients robustly stratify disorders of consciousness. *Cerebral Cortex*, *33*(11), 7193–7210. https://doi.org/10.1093/cercor/bhad031

Conrad, P. (2007). *The medicalization of society: On the transformation of human conditions into treatable disorders*. John Hopkins University Press

Conway, M. A., Justice, L. V., & D'Argembeau, A. (2019). The self-memory system revisited. In J. Mace (Ed.), *The organization and structure of autobiographical memory* (pp. 28–51). Oxford University Press. https://doi.org/10.1093/oso/9780198784845.001.0001

Cooper, R., & Simons, J. S. (2019). Exploring the neurocognitive basis of episodic recollection in autism. *Psychonomic Bulletin & Review*, *26*, 163–181. https://doi.org/10.3758/s13423-018-1504-z

Cordi, M., & Rasch, B. (2021a). How robust are sleep-mediated memory benefits? *Current Opinion in Neurobiology*, *67*, 1–7. https://doi.org/10.1016/j.conb.2020.06.002

Cordi, M., & Rasch, B. (2021b). No evidence for intra-individual correlations between sleep mediated declarative memory consolidation and slow wave sleep. *Sleep*, *44*(8), 1–10. https://doi.org/10.1093/sleep/zsab034

Corneille, O., & Lush, P. (2023). Sixty years after Orne's American psychologist article: A conceptual framework for subjective experiences elicited by demand characteristics. *Personality and Social Psychology Review*, *27*(1), 83–101. https://doi.org/10.1177/10888683221104368

Cortal, G. (2024). Sequence-to-sequence language models for character and emotion detection in dream narratives. *Proceedings of the 2024 Joint International Conference on Computational Linguistics, Language Resources and Evaluation (Torino, Italy)*. https://aclanthology.org/2024.lrec-main.1282/

Costumero, V., Bueichekú, E., Adrián-Ventura, J., & Avila, C. (2020). Opening or closing eyes at rest modulates the functional connectivity of V1 with default and salience networks. *Science Reports*, *10*. https://doi.org/10.1038/s41598-020-66100-y

Coughlin, C., Robins, R. W., & Ghetti, S. (2019). Development of episodic prospection: Factors underlying improvements in middle and late childhood. *Child Development*, *90*(4), 1109–1122. https://doi.org/10.1111/cdev.13001

Craig, A. R., & Fisher, W. W. (2019). Randomization tests as alternative analysis methods for behavior-analytic data. *Journal of the Experimental Analysis of Behavior*, *11*(2), 309–328. https://doi.org/10.1002/jeab.500

Crawford, L. (2022). The salience network. *Omniscient Neurotechnology Blog*. www.o8t.com/blog/salience-network

Cronbach, L., & Meehl, P. (1955). Construct validity in psychological tests. *Psychological Bulletin*, *52*(4), 281–302. https://doi.org/10.1037/h0040957

Crugnola, C., Maggiolini, A., Caprin, C., Martini, C., & Giudici, F. (2008). Dream content of 10- to 11-year-old preadolescent boys and girls. *Dreaming*, *18*, 201–218.

Csernai, M., Borbély, S., Kocsis, K., Burka, D., Fekete, Z., Balogh, V., & Barthó, P. (2019). Dynamics of sleep oscillations is coupled to brain temperature on multiple scales. *Journal of Physiology*, *597*(15), 4069–4086. https://doi.org/10.1113/JP277664

Curot, J., Valton, L., Denuelle, M., Vignal, J.-P., Maillard, L., Pariente, J., Trébuchon, A., Bartolomei, F., & Barbeau, E. J. (2018). Déjà-rêvé: Prior dreams induced by direct electrical brain stimulation. *Brain Stimulation*, *11*, 875–885. https://doi.org/10.1016/j.brs.2018.02.016

D'Andrade, R. (1961). Anthropological studies in dreams. In F. Hsu (Ed.), *Psychological anthropology* (pp. 296–332). Dorsey Press.

Dale, A., Lortie-Lussier, M., Wong, C., & De Koninck, J. (2016). Dreams of Canadian students: Norms, gender differences, and comparison with American norms. *Journal of Cross Cultural Psychology*, *47*(7), 941–955. https://doi.org/10.1177/0022022116655788

Darwin, C. (1872/1998). *The expression of the emotions in man and animals* (3rd ed.). Harper Collins.

Davimes, J. G., Alagaili, A. N., Bhagwandin, A., Bertelsen, M. F., Mohammed, O. B., Bennett, N. C., & Gravett, N. (2018). Seasonal variations in sleep of free-ranging

Arabian oryx (Oryx leucoryx) under natural hyperarid conditions. *Sleep*, *41*(5), 1–16. https://doi.org/10.1093/sleep/zsy038

de Chazal, P., Mazzotti, D. R., & Cistulli, P. A. (2022). Automated sleep staging algorithms: Have we reached the performance limit due to manual scoring? *Sleep*, *45*(9), zsac159. https://doi.org/10.1093/sleep/zsac159

De Gennaro, L., Ferrara, M., Curcio, G., & Cristiani, R. (2001). Antero-posterior EEG changes during the wakefulness-sleep transition. *Clinical Neurophysiology*, *112*, 1901–1911.

De Gennaro, L., Vecchio, F., Ferrara, M., Curcio, G., Rossini, P., & Babiloni, C. (2004). Changes in fronto-posterior functional coupling at sleep onset in humans. *Journal of Sleep Research*, *13*, 209–217.

Dean, A. L., & Harvey, W. O. (1979). An information-processing analysis of a Piagetian imagery task. *Developmental Psychology*, *15*, 474–475.

Dean, A. L., Duhe, D. A., & Green, D. A. (1983). The development of children's mental tracking strategies on a rotation task. *Journal of Experimental Child Psychology*, *36*, 226–240.

Dement, W. (1965). An essay on dreams: The role of physiology in understanding their nature. In F. Barron, W. Dement, J. Olds, & M. Olds (Eds.), *New directions in psychology II* (pp. 135–257). Holt, Rinehart, and Winston.

Dement, W. (1968). The biological role of REM sleep. In A. Kales (Ed.), *Sleep: physiology and pathology*. Lippincott.

Dement, W. (1973). Commentary on "The biological role of REM sleep". In W. B. Webb (Ed.), *Sleep: An active process* (pp. 48–58). Scott, Foresman and Company.

Dement, W., & Kleitman, N. (1957). Cyclic variations in EEG during sleep and their relation to eye movements, body motility, and dreaming. *Electroencephalography and Clinical Neurophysiology*, *9*, 673–690.

Dement, W., Kahn, E., & Roffwarg, H. (1965). The influence of the laboratory situation on the dreams of the experimental subject. *Journal of Nervous & Mental Disease*, *140*(2), 119–131.

Di, X., & Biswal, B. B. (2015). Dynamic brain functional connectivity modulated by resting-state networks. *Brain Structure & Function*, *220*, 37–46.

Diamond, E. (1962). *The Science of Dreams*. Doubleday.

Ditta, A., & Storm, B. C. (2018). A consideration of the seven sins of memory in the context of creative cognition. *Creativity Research Journal*, *30*, 402–417.

Dixon, M. L., Andrews-Hanna, J., Spreng, R. N., Christoff, K., & Irving, Z. (2017). Interactions between the default network and dorsal attention network vary across default subsystems, time, and cognitive states. *Neuroimage*, *147*, 632–649.

Dixon, M. L., Fox, K., & Christoff, K. (2014a). Evidence for rostro-caudal functional organization in multiple brain areas related to goal-directed behavior. *Brain Research*, *1572*, 26–39. https://doi.org/10.1016/j.brainres.2014.05.012

Dixon, M. L., Fox, K., & Christoff, K. (2014b). A framework for understanding the relationship between externally and internally directed cognition. *Neuropsychologia*, *62*, 321–330.

Dixon, M. L., Moodie, C. A., Goldin, P. R., Farb, N., Heimberg, R. G., Zhang, J., & Gross, J. J. (2022). Frontoparietal and default mode network contributions to self-referential processing in social anxiety disorder. *Cognitive, Affective, & Behavioral Neuroscience*, *22*, 187–198.

Dixon, M. L., Vega, A., Andrews-Hanna, J., Mills, C., Spreng, R. N., Cole, M. W., & Christoff, K. (2018). Heterogeneity within the frontoparietal control network and its relationship to the default and dorsal attention networks. *Proceedings of the National Academy of Sciences of the United States of America*, *115*(7), E1598–E1607. https://doi.org/10.1073/pnas.1715766115

Domhoff, G. W. (1969). Home dreams and laboratory dreams: Home dreams are better. In M. Kramer (Ed.), *Dream psychology and the new biology of dreaming* (pp. 119–217). C. C. Thomas.

Domhoff, G. W. (1996). *Finding meaning in dreams: A quantitative approach*. Plenum. http://dreamresearch.net/FMID/

Domhoff, G. W. (2000a). The misinterpretation of dreams. *American Scientist*, *88*, 175–178.

Domhoff, G. W. (2000b). A new neurocognitive theory of dreams [Conference presentation]. *Annual Meeting of the Association for Psychological Science*, Miami Beach, Florida.

Domhoff, G. W. (2003). *The scientific study of dreams: Neural networks, cognitive development, and content analysis*. American Psychological Association. http://dreamresearch.net/TSSOD/

Domhoff, G. W. (2004). Why did empirical dream researchers reject Freud? A critique of historical claims by Mark Solms. *Dreaming*, *14*, 3–17.

Domhoff, G. W. (2005). Refocusing the neurocognitive approach to dreams: A critique of the Hobson vs. Solms debate. *Dreaming*, *15*, 3–20.

Domhoff, G. W. (2011). The neural substrate for dreaming: Is it a subsystem of the default network? *Consciousness and Cognition*, *20*, 1163–1174.

Domhoff, G. W. (2015). Dreaming as embodied simulation: A widower dreams of his deceased wife. *Dreaming*, *25*, 232–256.

Domhoff, G. W. (2016). *We need bigger and better samples of dream reports: Most recent dream reports and dream journals are the answers* [Conference presentation]. International Association for the Study of Dreams. http://dreamresearch.net/Library/domhoff_2016.html

Domhoff, G. W. (2017). The invasion of the concept snatchers: The origins, distortions, and future of the continuity hypothesis. *Dreaming*, *27*, 14–39.

Domhoff, G. W. (2018). *The emergence of dreaming: Mind-Wandering, embodied simulation, and the default network*. Oxford University Press. http://dreamresearch.net/TEOD/

Domhoff, G. W. (2022). *The neurocognitive theory of dreaming: The where, how, when, what, and why of dreams*. MIT Press. http://dreamresearch.net/NCTD/

Domhoff, G. W. (2023). The relationship between dreaming and autonoetic consciousness: The neurocognitive theory of dreaming gains in explanatory power by drawing upon the multistate hierarchical model of consciousness. *Dreaming*, *33*(1), 1–18. https://doi.org/10.1037/drm0000233

Domhoff, G. W., & Fox, K. (2015). Dreaming and the default network: A review, synthesis, and counterintuitive research proposal. *Consciousness and Cognition*, *33*, 342–353.

Domhoff, G. W., & Kamiya, J. (1964). Problems in dream content study with objective indicators: II. The influence of the laboratory setting. *Archives of General Psychiatry*, *11*, 525–528.

Domhoff, G. W., & Schneider, A. (1999). Much ado about very little: The small effect sizes when home and laboratory collected dreams are compared. *Dreaming*, *9*, 139–151.

Domhoff, G. W., & Schneider, A. (2008a). Similarities and differences in dream content at the cross-cultural, gender, and individual levels. *Consciousness and Cognition*, *17*, 1257–1265.

Domhoff, G. W., & Schneider, A. (2008b). Studying dream content using the archive and search engine on DreamBank.net. *Consciousness and Cognition*, *17*, 1238–1247.

Domhoff, G. W., & Schneider, A. (2015). Assessing autocorrelation in studies using the Hall and Van de Castle coding system to study individual dream series. *Dreaming*, *25*, 70–79.

Domhoff, G. W., & Schneider, A. (2018). Are dreams social simulations? Or are they enactments of conceptions and personal concerns? An empirical and theoretical comparison of two dream theories. *Dreaming*, *28*, 1–23.

Domhoff, G. W., & Schneider, A. (2020). From adolescence to young adulthood in two dream series: The consistency and continuity of characters and major personal interests. *Dreaming*, *30*, 140–161. https://doi.org/10.1037/drm0000133

Domhoff, G. W., Meyer-Gomes, K., & Schredl, M. (2005-2006). Dreams as the expression of conceptions and concerns: A comparison of German and American college students. *Imagination, Cognition & Personality*, *25*, 269–282.

dos Santos, R., Osório, F., Crippa, J., & Hallak, J. (2016). Classical Hallucinogens and neuroimaging: A systematic review of human studies: Hallucinogens and neuroimaging. *Neuroscience and Biobehavioral Reviews*, *71*, 715–728.

Dresler, M., Wehrle, R., Spoormaker, V., Koch, S., Holsboer, F., Steiger, A., & Czisch, M. (2012). Neural correlates of dream lucidity obtained from contrasting lucid versus non-lucid REM sleep: A combined EEG/fMRI case study. *Sleep*, *35*, 1017–1020.

Duff, M. C., Covington, N. V., Hilverman, C., & Cohen, N. J. (2020). Semantic memory and the hippocampus: Revisiting, reaffirming, and extending the reach of their critical relationship. *Frontiers in Human Neuroscience*, *13*. https://doi.org/10.3389/fnhum.2019.00471

Ebdlahad, S., Nofzinger, E., James, J. A., Buysse, D., Price, J., C., & Germain, A. (2013). Comparing neural correlates of REM sleep in posttraumatic stress disorder and depression: A neuroimaging study. *Psychiatry Research*, *214*, 422–428.

Edlow, B., Olchanyi, M., Folkerth, R., Fischl, B., & Kinney, H. (2024). Multimodal MRI reveals brainstem connections that sustain wakefulness in human consciousness. *Science Translational Medicine*, *16*(745). https://doi.org/10.1126/scitranslmed.adj4303

Edwards, C., Ruby, P., Malinowski, J., Bennett, P., & Blagrove, M. (2013). Dreaming and insight. *Frontiers in Psychology*, *4*. https://doi.org/10.3389/fpsyg.2013.00979

Eichenlaub, J.-B., Bertrand, O., Morlet, D., & Ruby, P. (2014). Brain reactivity differentiates subjects with high and low dream recall frequencies during both sleep and wakefulness. *Cerebral Cortex*, *24*, 1206–1215. https://doi.org/10.1093/cercor/bhs388

Eisbach, A. O. (2013). *"Catching" a wandering mind: Developmental changes in the reporting of off-task thoughts* [Conference presentation]. Biennial Meeting of the Society for Research on Child Development, Seattle, Washington.

Elce, V., Bergamo, D., Bontempi, G., Pedreschi, B., Bellesi, M., Handjaras, G., & Bernardi, G. (2025). The individual determinants of morning dream recall. *Communications Psychology*, *3*(25), 1–12. https://doi.org/10.1038/s44271-025-00191-z

Epel, N., & Nichols, J. T. (1993). *Writers dreaming*. Carol Southern Books.

Estes, D. (1998). Young children's awareness of their mental acitvity: The case of mental rotation. *Child Development*, *69*, 1345–1360.

Fair, D., Cohen, A. L., Dosenbach, N., Church, J. A., Miezin, F. M., Barch, D. M., & Schlaggar, B. L. (2008). The maturing architecture of the brain's default network. *Proceedings of the National Academy of Sciences*, *105*, 4028–4032.

Fair, D., Cohen, A. L., Power, J. D., Dosenbach, N., Church, J. A., Miezin, F. M., & Peterson, S. (2009). Functional brain networks develop from a "local to distributed" organization. *PLoS Biology*, *5*, 1–14. https://doi.org/10.1371/journal.pcbi.1000381

Fair, D., Dosenbach, N., Church, J. A., Cohen, A. L., Brahmbhatt, S., Miezin, F. M., & Schlaggar, B. L. (2007). Development of distinct control networks through segregation and integration. *Proceedings of the National Academy of Sciences*, *104*, 13507–13512.

Falk, C. F., Huang, A., & Ilagan, M. J. (2025). Unsupervised randomly responding survey bot detection: In search of high classification accuracy. *Psychological Methods*. https://doi.org/10.1037/met0000746

Fan, F., Liao, X., Lei, T., Tao, S., & He, Y. (2021). Development of the default-mode network during childhood and adolescence: A longitudinal resting-state fMRI study. *Neuroimage*, *226*, Article 117581. https://doi.org/10.1016/j.neuroimage.2020.117581

Fan, L., Zhong, Q., Qin, J., Li, N., Su, J., Zeng, L. L., Shen, H. (2021). Brain parcellation driven by dynamic functional connectivity better capture intrinsic network dynamics. *Human Brain Mapping*, *42*, 1416–1433. https://doi.org/10.1002/hbm.25303

Feldman, R., & Dement, W. (1968). Possible relationships between REM sleep and memory consolidation. *Psychophysiology*, *5*, 243.

Fernández-Espejo, D., A., S., Cruse, D., Palacios, E., Junque, C., Vanhaudenhuyse, A., & Owen, A. (2012). A role for the default mode network in the bases of disorders of consciousness. *Annals of Neurology*, *72*, 335–343.

Fisher, C., Kahn, E., Edwards, A., & Davis, D. (1973). A psychophysiological study of nightmares and night terrors: Physiological aspects of the Stage 4 night terror. *Journal of Nervous and Mental Disease*, *157*, 75–98.

Fisher, S., & Greenberg, R. (1977). *The scientific credibility of freud's theories and therapy*. Basic Books.

Fisher, S., & Greenberg, R. (1996). *Freud scientifically appraised*. John Wiley.

Fisher-Hicks, S., Lovett, V., Wood, R. L., & Blagrove, M. (2025). The association of brain injury severity with dream cessation and nightmares. *Neuropsychologia*, Article 109209. https://doi.org/10.1016/j.neuropsychologia.2025.109209

Fivush, R. (2020). The emergence of autobiographical consciousness and the construction of an autobiographical self. In S. Gülgöz & B. Sahin-Acar (Eds.), *Autobiographical memory development: Theoretical and methodological approaches* (pp. 6–21). Routledge. https://doi.org/10.4324/9780429022791-2

Flannery, T. F., Rich, T. H., Vickers-Rich, P., Ziegler, T., Veatch, E. G., & Helgen, K. M. (2022). A review of monotreme (Monotremata) evolution. *Alcheringa: An Australasian Journal of Palaeontology*, *46*(1), 3–20. https://doi.org/10.1080/03115518.2022.2025900

Ford, J., Roach, B., Jorgensen, K., Turner, J., & al, e. (2009). Tuning in to the voices: A multisite fMRI study of auditory hallucinations. *Schizophrenia Bulletin*, *35*, 58–66. https://doi.org/10.1093/schbul/sbn140

Fosse, M. J., Fosse, R., Hobson, J. A., & Stickgold, R. (2003). Dreaming and episodic memory: A functional dissociation? *Journal of Cognitive Neuroscience*, *15*, 1–9.

Fosse, R., Stickgold, R., & Hobson, J. A. (2004). Thinking and hallucinating: Reciprocal changes in sleep. *Psychophysiology*, *41*, 298–305.

Foulkes, D. (1962). Dream reports from different states of sleep. *Journal of Abnormal and Social Psychology*, *65*, 14–25.

Foulkes, D. (1982). *Children's dreams: Longitudinal studies*. Wiley.

Foulkes, D. (1985). *Dreaming: A cognitive-psychological analysis*. Erlbaum.

Foulkes, D. (1993). Data constraints on theorizing about dream function. In A. Moffitt, M. Kramer, & R. Hoffmann (Eds.), *The functions of dreaming* (pp. 11–20). State University of New York Press.

Foulkes, D. (1996). Dream research: 1953–1993. *Sleep*, *19*, 609–624.

Foulkes, D. (1999). *Children's dreaming and the development of consciousness*. Harvard University Press.

Foulkes, D. (2017). Dreaming, reflective consciousness, and feelings in the preschool child. *Dreaming*, *27*, 1–13.

Foulkes, D., & Fleisher, S. (1975). Mental activity in relaxed wakefulness. *Journal of Abnormal Psychology*, *84*, 66–75. https://doi.org/10.1037/h0076164

Foulkes, D., & Rechtschaffen, A. (1964). Presleep determinants of dream content: Effects of two films. *Perceptual and Motor Skills*, *19*, 983–1005.

Foulkes, D., & Schmidt, M. (1983). Temporal sequence and unit comparison composition in dream reports from different stages of sleep. *Sleep*, *6*, 265–280.

Foulkes, D., & Scott, E. (1973). An above-zero baseline for the incidence of momentarily hallucinatory mentation. *Sleep Research*, *2*, 108.

Foulkes, D., & Vogel, G. (1965). Mental activity at sleep onset. *Journal of Abnormal Psychology*, *70*, 231–243.

Foulkes, D., Hollifield, M., Sullivan, B., Bradley, L., & Terry, R. (1990). REM dreaming and cognitive skills at ages 5–8: A cross-sectional study. *International Journal of Behavioral Development*, *13*, 447–465.

Foulkes, D., Spear, P., & Symonds, J. (1966). Individual differences in mental activity at sleep onset. *Journal of Abnormal and Social Psychology*, *71*, 280–286.

Foulkes, D., Sullivan, B., Hollifield, M., & Bradley, L. (1989). Mental rotation, age, and conservation. *Journal of Genetic Psychology*, *150*, 449–451.

Foulkes, D., Sullivan, B., Kerr, N., & Brown, L. (1988). Appropriateness of dream feelings to dreamed situations. *Cognition and Emotion*, *2*, 29–39.

Fowler, M. J., Sullivan, M. J., & Ekstrand, B. R. (1973). Sleep and memory. *Science*, *179*, 302–304.

Fox, K. (2018). Neural origins of self-generated thought: Insights from intracranial electrical stimulations and recordings in humans. In K. Fox & K. Christoff (Eds.), *The Oxford handbook of spontaneous thought: Mind-wandering, creativity, and dreaming* (pp. 165–179). Oxford University Press.

Fox, K., Dixon, M. L., Nijeboer, S., Girn, M., Floman, J., Lifshitz, M., & Christoff, K. (2016). Functional neuroanatomy of meditation: A review and meta-analysis of 78 functional neuroimaging investigations. *Neuroscience Behavioral Review*, *65*, 208–228.

Fox, K., Girn, M., Parro, C. C., & Christoff, K. (2018). Functional neuroimaging of psychedelic experience: An overview of psychological and neural effects and their relevance to research on creativity, daydreaming, and dreaming. In R. E. Jung & O. Vartanian (Eds.), *The Cambridge handbook of the neuroscience of creativity* (pp. 92–113). Cambridge University Press.

Fox, K., Nijeboer, S., Solomonova, E., Domhoff, G. W., & Christoff, K. (2013). Dreaming as mind wandering: Evidence from functional neuroimaging and first-person content reports *Frontiers in Human Neuroscience*, *7*, Article 412.

Fox, K., Spreng, R. N., Ellamil, M., Andrews-Hanna, J., & Christoff, K. (2015). The wandering brain: Meta-analysis of functional neuroimaging studies of mind-wandering and related spontaneous thought processes. *Neuroimage*, *111*, 611–621.

Frank, M. (2012). Erasing synapses in sleep: is it time to be SHY? *Neural Plasticity*, *2012*, Article 264378. https://doi.org/10.1155/2012/264378

Frank, M. (2020). The ontogenesis of mammalian sleep: Form and function. *Current Sleep Medicine Reports*, *6*(4), 267–279. https://doi.org/10.1007/s40675-020-00190-y

Frank, M. (2021). Renormalizing synapses in sleep: The clock is ticking. *Biochemical Pharmacology*, *191*. https://doi.org/10.1016/j.bcp.2021.114533

Franklin, R., Allison, D., & Gorman, B. (1997). *Design and analysis of single-case research*. Erlbaum.

Freud, S. (1900). *The interpretation of dreams*. Oxford University Press.

Freud, S. (1916). *Introductory lectures on psychoanalysis* (Vol. 15). Hogarth Press.

Frick, A., Hansen, M., & Newcombe, N. (2013). Development of mental rotation in 3- to 5-year-old children. *Cognitive Development*, *28*, 386–399.

Frick, A., Möhring, W., & Newcombe, N. S. (2014). Development of mental transformation abilities. *Trends in Cognitive Sciences*, *18*, 536–542.

Gao, W., Zhu, H., Giovanello, K., Smith, J. K., Shen, D., Gilmore, J., & Lin, W. (2009). Evidence on the emergence of the brain's default network from 2-week-old to 2-year-old healthy pediatric subjects. *Proceedings of the National Academy of Sciences*, *106*, 6790–6795.

Garin, C., Hori, Y., Everling, S., Whitlow, C., Calabro, F., Luna, B., & Constantinidis, C. (2022). An evolutionary gap in primate default mode network organization. *Cell Press*, *39*, Article 110669. https://doi.org/10.1016/j.celrep.2022.110669

Garrison, K. A., Zeffiro, T. A., Scheinost, D., Constable, R. T., & Brewer, J. A. (2015). Meditation leads to reduced default mode network activity beyond an active task. *Cognitive, Affective & Behavioral Neuroscience*, *15*, 712–720.

Gavrilov, V. M., Golubeva, T. B., & Bushuev, A. V. (2023). Metabolic rate, sleep duration, and body temperature in evolution of mammals and birds: The influence of geological time of principal groups divergence. *ZooKeys*, *1148*, 1–27. https://doi.org/10.3897/zookeys.1148.93458

Gaynor, A., & Chua, E. (2018). Transcranial direct current stimulation over the prefrontal cortex alters encoding and judgments of learning based on fluency.

Journal of Cognitive Neuroscience, *31*, 1710–1725. https://doi.org/10.1162/jocn_a_01449

Gelman, S. (2013). Concepts in development. In P. Zelazo (Ed.), *The Oxford handbook of developmental psychology (Vol 1): Body and mind* (pp. 542–563). Oxford University Press.

Germain, A. (2013). Sleep disturbances as the hallmark of PTSD: Where are we now?. *American Journal of Psychiatry*, *170*, 372–382.

Germain, A., James, J., Salvatore, I., Herringa, R. J., Mammen, O., Price, J., & Nofzinger, E. (2013). A window into the invisible wound of war: Functional neuroimaging of REM sleep in returning combat veterans with PTSD. *Psychiatry Research: Neuroimaging*, *211*, 176–179.

Gibbs, R. (1994). *The poetics of mind: Figurative thought, language, and understanding*. Cambridge University Press.

Gibbs, R. (2014). Conceptual metaphor in thought and social action. In M. Landau, M. Robinson, & B. Meier (Eds.), *The power of metaphor: Examining its influence on social life* (pp. 17–40). American Psychological Association.

Gifuni, A., Kendal, A., & Jollant, F. (2017). Neural mapping of guilt: a quantitative meta-analysis of functional imaging studies. *Brain Imaging and Behavior*, *11*, 1164–1178.

Girn, M., Setton, R., Turnerd, G., & Spreng, R. (2024). The "limbic network", comprising orbitofrontal and anterior temporal cortex, is part of an extended default network: Evidence from multi-echo fMRI *Network Neuroscience*. https://doi.org/10.1162/netn_a_00385

Gobet, F., & Sala, G. (2023). Cognitive training: A field in search of a phenomenon. *Perspectives on Psychological Science*, *18*, 125–141. https://doi.org/10.1177/17456916221091830

Göder, R., Seeck-Hirschner, M., Stingele, K., Huchzermeier, C., Kropp, C., Palaschewski, M., & Koch, J. (2011). Sleep and cognition at baseline and the effects of REM sleep diminution after 1 week of antidepressive treatment in patients with depression. *Journal of Sleep Research*, *20*, 544–551. https://doi.org/10.1111/j.1365-2869.2011.00914.x

Gold, S., & Henderson, B. B. (1990). Daydreaming and curiosity: Stability and change in gifted children and adolescents. *Adolescence*, *25*, 701–708.

Gold, S., & Reilly, J. (1985/1986). Daydreaming, current concerns, and personality. *Imagination, Cognition and Personality*, *5*, 117–125.

Goodenough, D. (1991). Dream recall: History and current status of the field. In S. Ellman & J. Antrobus (Eds.), *The mind in sleep: Psychology and psychophysiology* (2nd ed., pp. 143–171). Wiley & Sons.

Goodenough, D., Shapiro, A., Holden, M., & Steinschriber, L. (1959). A comparison of "dreamers" and "nondreamers": Eye movements, electroencephalograms, and the recall of dreams. *Journal of Abnormal and Social Psychology*, *59*, 295–302.

Gopnik, A. (2009). *The philosophical baby: What children's minds tell us about truth, love, and the meaning of life*. Picador.

Gordon, E. M., Laumann, E., Adeyemo, B., Huckins, J. F., Kelley, W. M., & Petersen, S. E. (2016). Generation and evaluation of a cortical area parcellation from resting-state correlations. *Cerebral Cortex*, *26*(1), 288–303. https://doi.org/10.1093/cercor/bhu239

Gordon, E. M., Lee, P. S., Maisog, J. M., Foss-Feig, J., Billington, M. E., Van-Meter, J., & Vaidya, C. J. (2011). Strength of default mode resting-state connectivity relates to white matter integrity in children. *Developmental Science*, *14*, 738–751.

Gorgoni, M., D'Atri, A., Scarpelli, S., Ferrara, M., & De Gennaro, L. (2019). Timing and topography of sleep onset: Asynchronies and regional changes of brain activity. In H. C. Dringenberg (Ed.), *Handbook of sleep research* (pp. 19–31). Elsevier Academic Press. https://doi.org/10.1016/B978-0-12-813743-7.00002-5

Gravett, N., Bhagwandin, A., Sutcliffe, R., Landen, K., Chase, M. J., Lyamin, O. I., & Manger, P. (2017). Inactivity/sleep in two wild free-roaming African elephant matriarchs – Does large body size make elephants the shortest mammalian sleepers? *PLoS One*, *12* (3). https://doi.org/10.1371/journal.pone.0171903

Green, C. (1968). *Lucid dreaming*. Institute of Psychophysical Research.

Greenblatt, M., & Solomon, H. C. (1952). Survey of nine years of lobotomy investigations. *American Journal of Psychiatry*, *109*(4), 262–265.

Gregor, T. (1981a). A content analysis of Mehinaku dreams. *Ethos*, *9*, 353–390.

Gregor, T. (1981b). "Far, far away my shadow wandered…": The dream symbolism and dream theories of the Mehinaku Indians of Brazil. *American Ethnologist*, *8*, 709–720.

Guldenmund, P., Demertzi, A., Boveroux, P., Boly, M., Vanhaudenhuyse, A., Bruno, M., Gosseries, O., Noirhomme, Q., Brichant, J., Bonhomme, V., Laureys, S., & Soddu, A. (2013). Thalamus, brainstem and salience network connectivity changes during propofol-induced sedation and unconsciousness. *Brain Connectivity*, *3*, 273–285. https://doi.org/10.1089/brain.2012.0117

Gusnard, D. A., & Raichle, M. E. (2001). Searching for a baseline: Functional imaging and the resting human brain. *Nature Reviews Neuroscience*, *2*, 685–694.

Gusnard, D. A., Akbudak, E., Shulman, G. L., & Raichle, M. E. (2001). Medial prefrontal cortex and self-referential mental activity: Relation to a default mode of brain function. *Proceedings of the National Academy of Sciences*, *98*, 4259–4264.

Hall, C. (1951). What people dream about. *Scientific American*, *184*(5), 60–63.

Hall, C. (1953). A cognitive theory of dream symbols. *Journal of General Psychology*, *48*, 169–186.

Hall, C. (1954). *A primer of Freudian psychology*. World Publishing.

Hall, C. (1956). Current trends in research on dreams. In D. Brower & L. Abt (Eds.), *Progress in clinical psychology* (pp. 239–257). Grune and Stratton.

Hall, C. (1966a). A comparison of the dreams of four groups of hospitalized mental patients with each other and with a normal population. *Journal of Nervous and Mental Diseases*, *143*, 135–139.

Hall, C. (1966b). *Studies of dreams collected in the laboratory and at home*. Institute of Dream Research. http://dreamresearch.net/Library/hall_1966.pdf

Hall, C. (1967). Representation of the laboratory setting in dreams. *Journal of Nervous and Mental Disease*, *144*, 198–206.

Hall, C. (1980). Pegasus: An elemental man. *DreamBank*. https://dreambank.net/search.html

Hall, C. (1984). A ubiquitous sex difference in dreams, revisited. *Journal of Personality and Social Psychology*, *46*, 1109–1117.

Hall, C., & Domhoff, G. W. (1963). Aggression in dreams. *International Journal of Social Psychiatry*, *9*, 259–267.

Hall, C., & Domhoff, G. W. (1964). Friendliness in dreams. *Journal of Social Psychology*, *62*, 309–314.
Hall, C., & Lind, R. (1970). *Dreams, life and literature: A study of Franz Kafka*. University of North Carolina Press.
Hall, C., & Van de Castle, R. (1966). *The content analysis of dreams*. Appleton-Century-Crofts.
Hall, C., Domhoff, G. W., Blick, K., & Weesner, K. (1982). The dreams of college men and women in 1950 and 1980: A comparison of dream contents and sex differences. *Sleep*, *5*, 188–194.
Hallett, E. Y., Leonardi, M., Cerasoni, J. N., Will, M., Beyer, R., Krapp, M., Kandel, A. W., Manica, A., & Scerri, E. M. L. (2025). Major expansion in the human niche preceded out of Africa dispersal. *Nature*. https://doi.org/10.1038/s41586-025-09154-0
Han, H. J. (2014). *Structural and longitudinal analysis of cognitive social networks in dreams* [Ph.D. Dissertation]. Purdue University.
Han, H. J., & Schweickert, R. (2016). Continuity: Knowing each other, emotional closeness, and appearing together in dreams *Dreaming*, *26*, 299–307. https://doi.org/10.1037/drm0000038
Han, H. J., Schweickert, R., Xi, Z., & Viau-Quesnela, C. (2015). The cognitive social network in dreams: Transitivity, assortativity, and giant component proportion are monotonic. *Cognitive Science*, *40*, 671–696.
Harari, G., Lane, N., Wang, R., Crosier, B., Campbell, A., & al, e. (2016). Using smartphones to collect behavioral data in psychological science: Opportunities, practical considerations, and challenges. *Perspectives on Psychological Science*, *11*, 838–854. https://doi.org/10.1177/1745691616650285
Hare, B. (2017). Survival of the friendliest: Homo sapiens evolved via selection for prosociality. *Annual Review of Psychology*, *68*, 155–186. https://doi.org/10.1146/annurev-psych-010416-044201
Hare, B., & Woods, V. (2020). *Survival of the friendliest*. Random House.
Hartmann, E. (2011). *The nature and functions of dreaming*. Oxford University Press.
Hartmann, E., Elkin, R., & Garg, M. (1991). Personality and dreaming: The dreams of people with very thick or very thin boundaries. *Dreaming*, *1*, 311–324.
Hartogsveld, B., Bramson, B., Vijayakumara, S., Dilenevan, A., Campena, J. P., Marques, K., & Marsab, R. B. (2018). Lateral frontal pole and relational processing: Activation patterns and connectivity profile. *Behavioural and Brain Research*, *355*, 2–11. https://doi.org/10.1016/j.bbr.2017.08.003
Hayashi, M., Katoh, K., & Hori, T. (1999). Hypnagogic imagery and EEG activity. *Perceptual and Motor Skills*, *88*, 676–678.
He, W., Sowman, P., Brock, J., Etchell, A., Stam, C., & al., e. (2019). Increased segregation of functional networks in developing brains. *Neuroimage*, *200*, 607–620. https://doi.org/10.1016/j.neuroimage.2019.06.055
Heise, D. (2010). *Surveying cultures: Discovering shared conceptions and sentiments*. Wiley.
Heise, D. (2014). Cultural variations in sentiments. *SpringerPlus*, *3*, 1–11. www.springerplus.com/content/3/1/170
Henn, B., Gignoux, C. R., & Jobin, M. (2011). Hunter-gatherer genomic diversity suggests a southern African origin for modern humans. *PNAS: Proceedings of the*

National Academy of Sciences of the United States of America, *108*(13), 5154–5162. https://doi.org/10.1073/pnas.1017511108

Henseler, I., Krüger, S., Dechent, P., & Gruber, O. (2011). A gateway system in rostral PFC? Evidence from biasing attention to perceptual information and internal representations. *Neuroimage*, *56*, 1666–1676. https://doi.org/10.1016/j.neuroimage.2011.02.056

Hill, C. E., & Spangler, P. (2007). Dreams and psychotherapy. In D. Barrett & P. McNamara (Eds.), *The new science of dreaming: Volume 2. Content, recall, and personality correlates* (pp. 159–186). Praeger /Greenwood Publishing Group.

Hill, C. E., Diemer, R. A., & Heaton, K. J. (1997). Dream interpretation sessions: Who volunteers, who benefits, and what volunteer clients view as most and least helpful. *Journal of Counseling Psychology*, *44*(1), 53–62.

Hobson, J. A. (1988). *The dreaming brain*. Basic Books.

Hobson, J. A. (2002). *Dreaming: An introduction to the science of sleep*. Oxford University Press.

Hobson, J. A. (2007). Current understanding of cellular models of REM expression. In D. Barrett & P. McNamara (Eds.), *The new science of dreaming: Biological aspects* (Vol. 1, pp. 71–84). Praeger/Greenwood.

Hobson, J. A., & Kahn, D. (2007). Dream content: Individual and generic aspects. *Consciousness and Cognition*, *16*, 850–858.

Hobson, J. A., & McCarley, R. (1977). The brain as a dream state generator: An activation-synthesis hypothesis of the dream process. *American Journal of Psychiatry*, *134*, 1335–1348.

Hobson, J. A., McCarley, R., & Wyzinski, P. (1975). Sleep cycle oscillation: Reciprocal discharge by two brainstem neuronal groups. *Science*, *189*, 55–58.

Hobson, J. A., Pace-Schott, E., & Stickgold, R. (2000). Dreaming and the brain: Toward a cognitive neuroscience of conscious states. *Behavioral and Brain Sciences*, *23*(6), 793–842.

Hoffman, R., & Hampson, M. (2012). Functional connectivity studies of patients with auditory verbal hallucinations. *Frontiers in Human Neuroscience*. https://doi.org/10.3389/fnhum.2012.00006

Holyoak, K., & Stamenkovic, D. (2018). Metaphor comprehension: A critical review of theories and evidence. *Psychological Bulletin*, *144*, 641–671. https://doi.org/10.1037/bul0000145

Hong, C. C., Fallon, J., & Friston, K. (2021). fMRI evidence for default mode network deactivation associated with rapid eye movements in sleep. *Brain Sciences*, *11*(1528), 1–21. https://doi.org/10.3390/brainsci11111528

Hong, C. C., Gillin, J. C., Dow, B. M., Wu, & Buchsbaum, M. S. (1995). Localized and lateralized cerebral glucose metabolism associated with eye movements during REM sleep and wakefulness: A positron emission tomography (PET) study. *Sleep*, *18*(7), 570–580. https://doi.org/10.1093/sleep/18.7.570

Hong, C. C., Harris, J. C., Pearlson, G. D., Kim, J.-S., Calhoun, V. D., Fallon, J. H., van Zijl, P. (2009). fMRI evidence for multisensory recruitment associated with rapid eye movements during sleep. *Human Brain Mapping*, *30*(5), 1705–1722. https://doi.org/10.1002/hbm.20635

Hong, C. C., Potkin, S., Antrobus, J., Dow, B., Callaghan, G., & Gillin, J. (1997). REM sleep eye movement counts correlate with visual imagery in dreaming: A pilot study. *Psychophysiology*, *34*, 377–381.

Hori, T., Hayashi, M., & Morikawa, T. (1994). Topographic EEG changes and the hypnagogic experience. In R. Ogilvie & J. Harsh (Eds.), *Sleep onset: Normal and abnormal processes* (pp. 237–253). American Psychological Association.

Horne, J., & McGrath, M. (1984). The consolidation hypothesis for REM sleep function: Stress and other confounding factors: A review. *Biological Psychology*, *18*, 165–184. https://doi.org/10.1016/0301-0511(84)90001-2

Horovitz, S., Braun, A., Carr, W., Picchioni, D., Balkin, T., Fukunaga, M., & Duyn, J. (2009). Decoupling of the brain's default mode network during deep sleep. *Proceedings of the National Academy of Sciences of the United States*, *106*, 11376–11381.

Horton, C. (2009). Applying memory theory to dream recall: Are dreams and waking memories the same? In M. Kelley (Ed.), *Applied memory* (pp. 275–303). Nova Science Publishers.

Horton, C. (2015). Correlates of dream recall: Implications for confabulation *Imagination, Cognition and Personality*, *34*(2), 163–177. https://doi.org/10.2190/IC.34.2.e

Hu, X., Cheng, L., Chiu, M., & Paller, K. (2020). Promoting memory consolidation during sleep: A meta-analysis of targeted memory reactivation. *Psychological Bulletin*, *148*(3), 218–244. https://doi.org/10.1037/bul0000223

Hudachek, L., & Wamsley, E. J. (2023). A meta-analysis of the relation between dream content and memory consolidation. *Sleep*, *46*(12), 1–13. https://doi.org/10.1093/sleep/zsad111

Hurovitz, C., Dunn, S., Domhoff, G. W., & Fiss, H. (1999). The dreams of blind men and women: A replication and extension of previous findings. *Dreaming*, *9*, 183–193.

Hyde, J. S. (2014). Gender similarities and differences. *Annual Review of Psychology*, *65*, 373–398.

Hyman, I., & Loftus, E. (2002). False childhood memories and eyewitness memory errors. In M. L. Eisen, J. A. Quas, & G. S. Goodman (Eds.), *Memory and suggestibility in the forensic interview* (pp. 63–84). Erlbaum.

Incelli, N. A., & Gallagher, S. P. (2022). Pandemic dreams are susceptible to priming and unrelated to COVID-19 exposure. *Journal of Evidence-Based Psychotherapies*, *21*(2), 191–208. https://doi.org/10.24193/jebp.2021.2.18

Ingram, B. T., Mayhew, S. D., & Bagshaw, A. P. (2024). Brain state dynamics differ between eyes open and eyes closed rest. *Human Brain Mapping*, *45*(10). https://doi.org/10.1002/hbm.26746

Iranzo, A. (2022). Other parasomnias. In M. Kryger, B. J. Roth, C. Goldstein, & W. Dement (Eds.), *Principles and practices of sleep medicine* (7th ed., pp. 1110–1118). Elsevier.

Jackson, J. J., Connolly, J. J., Garrison, S. M., Leveille, M. M., & Connolly, S. L. (2015). Your friends know how long you will live: A 75-year study of peer-rated personality traits. *Psychological Science*, *26*(3), 335–340. https://doi.org/10.1177/0956797614561800

Jacobs, L., Feldman, M., & Bender, M. (1970). The pattern of human eye movements during sleep. *Transactions of the American Neurological Association*, *95*, 114–119.

Jacobs, L., Feldman, M., & Bender, M. (1972). Are the eye movements of dreaming sleep related to the visual images of dreams? *Psychophysiology*, *9*, 393–401.

Johnston, C. D., & Madson, G. J. (2022). Negativity bias, personality and political ideology. *Nature Human Behaviour*, *6*(5), 666–676. https://doi.org/10.1038/s41562-022-01327-5

Jones, B. E. (1980). Projections from the pontine gigantocellur tegmental field in the rat. *Neuroscience Abstracts*, *6*, 59.

Jones, B. E. (1986). The need for a new model of sleep cycle generation. *Behavioral and Brain Sciences*, *9*, 409–411.

Jones, B. E. (2018). The mysteries of sleep and waking unveiled by Michel Jouvet. *sleep Medicine*, *44*, 14–19.

Jones, B. E. (2020). Arousal and sleep circuits. *Neuropsychopharmacology*, *45*, 14–19. https://doi.org/10.1038/s41386-019-0444-2

Jones, B. E., Harper, S., & Halaris, A. (1977). Effects of locus coeruleus lesions upon cerebral monamine content, sleep-wakefulness states and the response to amphetamine in the cat. *Brain Research*, *124*, 473–496.

Jouvet, M., Buda, C., & Sastre, J. (1990). Progressive hypothermia is accompanied by an almost permanent paradoxical sleep in pontine cats. *Sleep Research*, *19*, 38.

Jung, C. M., Melanson, E. L., Frydendall, E. J., Perreault, L., Eckel, K., & Wright, K. P. (2011). Energy expenditure during sleep, sleep deprivation and sleep following sleep deprivation in adult humans. *Journal of Physiology*, *589*, 235–244.

Jus, A., Jus, K., Gautier, J., Villeneuve, A., Pires, P., Lachance, R., & Villeneuve, R. (1973). Dream reports after reserpine in chronic lobotomized schizophrenic patients. *Vie Medicale au Canada Français*, 2, 843–848.

Jus, A., Jus, K., Villeneuve, A., Pires, A., Lachance, R., Fortier, J., & Villeneuve, R. (1973). Studies of dream recall in chronic schizophrenic patients after prefrontal lobotomy. *Biological Psychiatry*, *6*, 275–293.

Kaida, K., Niki, K., & Born, J. (2015). Role of sleep for encoding of emotional memory. *Neurobiology of Learning and Memory*, *121*, 72–79.

Kail, R., Pelligrino, J., & Carter, P. (1980). Developmental changes in mental rotation *Journal of Experimental Child Psychology*, *29*, 102–116.

Kamberov, Y. G., Guhan, S. M., DeMarchis, A., Jiang, J., Wright, S. S., Morgan, B. A., & Lieberman, D. E. (2018). Comparative evidence for the independent evolution of hair and sweat gland traits in primates. *Journal of Human Evolution*, *125*, 99–105. https://doi.org/10.1016/j.jhevol.2018.10.008

Kamiya, J. (1961). Behavioral, subjective, and physiological aspects of drowsiness and sleep. In D. W. Fiske & S. R. Maddi (Eds.), *Functions of varied experience* (pp. 145–174). Dorsey.

Karagianni, M., Papadopoulou, A., Kallini, A., Dadatsi, A., & Abatzoglou, G. (2013). Dream content of Greek children and adolescents. *Dreaming*, *23*, 91–96.

Kass, W., Preiser, G., & Jenkins, A. (1970). Inter-relationship of hallucinations and dreams in spontaneously hallucinating patients. *Psychiatric Quarterly*, *44*(3), 488–499.

Kaufmann, C., Wehrle, R., Wetter, T. C., Holsboer, F., Auer, D., Pollmacher, T., & Czisch, M. (2006). Brain activation and hypothalamic functional connectivity during human non-rapid eye movement sleep: An EEG/fMRI study. *Brain*, *129*, 655–667.

Kay, D. B., Karim, H. T., Soehner, A. M., Hasler, B. P., Kupfer, D. J., Germain, A., & Buysse, D. (2016). Sleep-wake differences in relative regional cerebral metabolic rate for glucose among patients with insomnia compared with good sleepers. *Sleep*, *39*(1779). https://doi.org/10.5665/sleep.6154.

Kendall-Bar, J. M., Vyssotski, A. L., Mukhametov, L. M., Siegel, J. M., & Lyamin, O. I. (2019). Eye state asymmetry during aquatic unihemispheric slow wave sleep in northern fur seals (Callorhinus ursinus). *PLoS One*, *14*(5), 1–13. https://doi.org/10.1371/journal.pone.0217025

Kendall-Bar, J. M., Williams, T. M., Mukherji, R., Lozano, D. A., Pitman, J. K., Holser, R. R., Costa, D. P. (2023). Brain activity of diving seals reveals short sleep cycles at depth. *Science*, *380*, 260–265.

Kerr, N. (1993). Mental imagery, dreams, and perception. In D. Foulkes & C. Cavallero (Eds.), *Dreaming as cognition* (pp. 18–37). Harvester Wheatsheaf.

Kerr, N., & Domhoff, G. W. (2004). Do the blind literally "see" in their dreams? A critique of a recent claim that they do. *Dreaming*, *14*, 230–233.

Kerr, N., & Foulkes, D. (1981). Right hemispheric mediation of dream visualization: A case study. *Cortex*, *17*, 603–610.

Kerr, N., Foulkes, D., & Jurkovic, G. (1978). Reported absence of visual dream imagery in a normally sighted subject with Turner's syndrome. *Journal of Mental Imagery*, *2*, 247–264.

Kerr, N., Foulkes, D., & Schmidt, M. (1982). The structure of laboratory dream reports in blind and sighted subjects. *Journal of Nervous and Mental Disease*, *170*, 286–294.

Kervyn, N., Fiske, S. T., & Yzerbyt, V. Y. (2013). Integrating the stereotype content model (warmth and competence) and the Osgood semantic differential (evaluation, potency, and activity) . *European Journal of Social Psychology*, *43*, 673–681.

Kihlstrom, J. (2002). Demand characteristics in the laboratory and the clinic: Conversations and collaborations with subjects and patients. *Prevention & Treatment*, *5*, Article 36. https://doi.org/10.1037/1522-3736.5.1.536c

Kirtley, D. (1975). *The psychology of blindness*. Nelson-Hall.

Kiyatkin, E. A. (2019). Brain temperature and its role in physiology and pathophysiology: Lessons from 20 years of thermorecording. *Temperature*, *6*(4), 271–333. https://doi.org/10.1080/23328940.2019.1691896

Klinger, E. (1971). *Structure and functions of fantasy*. Wiley-Interscience.

Klinger, E. (2009). Daydreaming and fantasizing: Thought flow and motivation. In K. Markman, W. Klein, & J. Suhr (Eds.), *Handbook of imagination and mental simulation* (pp. 225–239). Psychology Press.

Körner, R., & Schütz, A. (2023). Friends know us even when they are different from us: Accuracy and bias in self–other perceptions of the Big Five. *Journal of Individual Differences*, *44*(3), 181–189 https://doi.org/10.1027/1614-0001/a000391

Kosslyn, S., Margolis, J., Barrett, A., Goldknopfan, E., & Daly, P. (1990). Age differences in imagery abilities. *Child Development*, *61*, 995–1010. https://doi.org/10.1111/j.1467-8624.1990.tb02837.x

Kosslyn, S., Thompson, W. L., & Alpert, N. (1997). Neural systems shared by visual imagery and perception: A positron emission tomography study. *Neuroimage*, *6*, 320–334.

Kramer, M., Roth, T., & Trinder, J. (1975). Dreams and dementia: A laboratory exploration of dream recall and dream content in chronic brain syndrome patients. *International Journal of Aging and Human Development*, 6, 169–178. https://doi.org/10.2190/X9A5-12D7-MV2A-TQ7E

Krippner, S. (2011). The parapsychological odyssey of Stanley Krippner: An interview with Rosemary Pilkington. *NeuroQuantology*, *9*(2), 322–332.
Krueger, J., Frank, M., Wisor, J., & Roy, S. (2016). Sleep function: Toward elucidating an enigma. *Sleep Medicine Reviews*, *28*, 46–54.
LaBarre, W. (1972). *The ghost dance: Origins of religion*. Dell Publishing.
LaBerge, S. (1980). *Lucid dreaming: An exploratory study of consciousness during sleep* [Ph.D.]. Stanford University.
LaBerge, S., Nagel, L., Dement, W., & Zarcone, V. (1981). Lucid dreaming verified by volitional communication during REM sleep. *Perceptual and Motor Skills*, *52*, 727–732.
Lacaux, C., Strauss, M., Bekinschtein, T. A., & Oudiette, D. (2024). Embracing sleep-onset complexity. *Trends in Neurosciences*, *47*(4), 273–288. https://doi.org/10.1016/j.tins.2024.02.002
Lakoff, G. (1987). *Women, fire, and dangerous things*. University of Chicago Press.
Lakoff, G. (1997). How unconscious metaphorical thought shapes dreams. In D. Stein (Ed.), *Cognitive science and the unconscious* (pp. 89–120). American Psychiatric Press.
Lakoff, G., & Johnson, M. (1999). *Philosophy in the flesh*. Basic Books.
Lau, H., & Rosenthal, D. (2011). Empirical support for higher-order theories of conscious awareness. *Trends in Cognitive Sciences*, *365–373*, 365–373.
Laureys, S., Pellas, F., Van Eeckhout, P., Ghorbel, S., Schnakers, C., Perrin, F., Berré, J., Faymonville, M., Pantke, K., Damas, F., Lamy, M., Moonen, G., & Goldman, S. (2005). The locked-in syndrome: What is it like to be conscious but paralyzed and voiceless? *Progress in Brain Research*, *150*, 495–511. https://doi.org/10.1016/S0079-6123(05)50034-7
Leaper, C., & Farkas, T. (2015). The socialization of gender during childhood and adolescence (2nd, Trans.). In J. Grusec & P. Hastings (Eds.), *Handbook of socialization: Theory and research* (pp. 541–565). Guilford Press.
LeDoux, J. (2015). *Anxious*. Viking.
LeDoux, J. (2019). *The deep history of ourselves: The four-billion year story of how we got conscious brains*. Viking.
LeDoux, J. (2020a). How does the non-conscious become conscious? *Current Biology*, *30*, R1–R4. https://doi.org/10.1016/j.cub.2020.01.033
LeDoux, J. (2020b). Thoughtful feelings. *Current Biology*, *30*(11), R619–R623. https://doi.org/10.1016/j.cub.2020.04.012
LeDoux, J. (2021a). As soon as there was life, there was danger: The deep history of survival behaviours and the shallower history of consciousness. *Philosophical Transactions of the Royal Society B: Biological Sciences*, *377*, Article 20210292. https://doi.org/10.1098/rstb.2021.0292
LeDoux, J. (2021b). What emotions might be like in other animals. *Current Biology*, *31*, R824–R829. https://doi.org/10.1016/j.cub.2021.05.005
LeDoux, J., & Brown, R. (2017). A higher-order theory of emotional consciousness. *Proceeding of the National Academy of Sciences Biological Sciences*, *114*, E2016–E2025. https://doi.org/10.1073/pnas.1619316114
LeDoux, J., & Lau, H. (2020). Seeing consciousness through the lens of memory. *Current Biology*, *30*, R1018–R1022. https://doi.org/10.1016/j.cub.2020.08.008
LeDoux, J., Michel, M., & Lau, H. (2020). A little history goes a long way toward understanding why we study consciousness the way we do today. *Proceedings*

of the National Academy of Sciences, *117*, 6976–6984. https://doi.org/10.1073/pnas.1921623117

Lee, M., Hacker, C., Snyder, A., Corbetta, M., Zhang, D., & Leuthardt, E. (2012). Clustering of resting state networks. *PLoS One*, *7*, Article e40370. https://doi.org/10.1371/journal.pone.0040370

Lesku, J. A., & Schmidt, M. H. (2022). Energetic costs and benefits of sleep. *Current Biology*, *32*, R656–R661. https://doi.org/10.1016/j.cub.2022.04.004

Levin, R., Fireman, G., & Rackley, C. (2003). Personality and dream recall frequency: Still further negative findings. *Dreaming*, *13*, 155–162.

Levorsen, M., Aoki, R., Sedikides, C., & Izuma, K. (2025). Decomposing cognitive processes in the mPFC during self-thinking. *Journal of Neuroscience*, *45*, Article e2378242025. https://doi.org/10.1523/jneurosci.2378-24.2025

Levy, M. (2016). *Vietnam, dreams*. Winter Street Press.

Levy, M. (2018). *Other dreams*. Telegraphos Press.

Levy, R. (2024). The prefrontal cortex: From monkey to man. *Brain*, *147*(3), 794–815.

Lewis, J. (2008). Dream Reports of Animal Rights Activists. *Dreaming*, *18*, 181–200. https://doi.org/doi:10.1037/a0013393

Li, J., Curley, W., Guerin, B., Dougherty, D., Dalca, A., Fischl, B., & Edlow, B. (2021). Mapping the subcortical connectivity of the human default mode network. *Neuroimage*, *245*, Article 118758. https://doi.org/10.1016/j.neuroimage.2021.118758

Li, M., Dahmani, L., Wang, D., Ren, J., Stocklein, S., Lin, Y., & Liu, H. (2021). Co-activation patterns across multiple tasks reveal robust anti-correlated functional networks. *Neuroimage*, *227*, 1–13. https://doi.org/10.1016/j.neuroimage.2020.117680

Libman, J. (1988, November 15). Dr. Dreams: Stanford scientist Stephen LaBerge is sleeping on the idea that dreams are a tool for bettering our lives. *Los Angeles Times*. www.latimes.com/archives/la-xpm-1988-11-15-vw-221-story.html

Lieberman, M. D. (2013). *Social: Why our brains are wired to connect*. Broadway Books.

Lindquist, K., Satpute, A., Wager, T., Weber, J., & Barrett, L. F. (2016). The brain basis of positive and negative affect: Evidence from a meta-analysis of the human neuroimaging literature. *Cerebral Cortex*, *26*, 1910–1922. https://doi.org/10.1093/cercor/bhv001

Lindquist, K., Wager, T., Kober, H., Bliss-Moreau, E., & Barrett, L. F. (2012). The brain basis of emotion: A meta-analytic review. *Behavioral and Brain Sciences*, *35*, 121–143.

Lipnicki, D. M. (2025). "Observer dreams: Criteria and frequency." *Journal of Sleep Research*. Advance online publication. https://doi.org/10.1111/jsr.70201

Lipnicki, D. M., Valentí, M., Valeriano-Lorenzo, E., Vella, A. S., Zea-Sevilla, M., Ricciardi, M., Frades, B., Martinez, M., Wagner, S., Sachdev, P. S., del Ser, T., & Sanchez-Juan, P. (2025). *Poor dream recall associates with Alzheimer's disease biomarkers and dementia risk* [Conference presentation]. Alzheimer's Association International Conference, Toronto, Canada.

Lipnicki, D. M., Vella, A. S., Costa, E., Ritchie, K., Rolandi, E., Kim, K. W., & Sachdev, P. S. (2025). *Associations between disturbing dreams and incident dementia and Alzheimer's disease across diverse international cohort studies: a*

COSMIC collaboration study [Conference presentation]. Alzheimer's Association International Conference, Toronto, Canada.
LoBue, V., & Rakison, D. (2013). What we fear most: A developmental advantage for threat-relevant stimuli. *Developmental Review*, *33*, 285–303. https://doi.org/10.1016/j.dr.2013.07.005
LoBue, V., Matthews, K., Harvey, T., & Thrasher, C. (2014). Pick on someone your own size: The detection of threatening facial expressions posed by both child and adult models. *Journal of Experimental Child Psychology*, *118*, 134–142. https://doi.org/10.1016/j.jecp.2013.07.016
Lortie-Lussier, M., Cote, L., & Vachon, J. (2000). The consistency and continuity hypotheses revisited through the dreams of women at two periods of their lives. *Dreaming*, *10*, 67–76.
Lucidity Newsletter. (1986). A panel discussion of lucid dreaming. *Lucidity Newsletter*, 74–95.
Lyamin, O. I., & Siegel, J. M. (2019). Sleep in aquatic mammals. *Handbook of Behaviorial Neuroscience*, *30*, 375–393. https://doi.org/10.1016/b978-0-12-813743-7.00025-6
Lyamin, O. I., Kosenko, P., Korneva, S., Vyssotski, A., Mukhametov, L., & Siegel, J. M. (2018). Fur seals suppress REM sleep for very long periods without subsequent rebound. *Current Biology*, *28*, 2000–2005.
Lyamin, O. I., Manger, P. R., Ridgway, S. H., Mukhametov, L. M., & Siegel, J. M. (2008). Cetacean sleep: An unusual form of mammalian sleep. *Neuroscience & Biobehavioral Reviews*, *32*, 1451–1484.
Lyamin, O., Borshchenko, V., & Siegel, J. M. (2024). A 108-h total sleep deprivation did not impair fur seal performance in delayed matching to sample task. *Journal of Comparative Physiology and Biology*, *194*(3), 315–333. https://doi.org/10.1007/s00360-023-01511-7
Lyamin, O., Siegel, J. M., Nazarenko, E., & Rozhnov, V. (2022). Sleep in the lesser mouse-deer (Tragulus kanchil). *Sleep*, *45*(7), 1–14. https://doi.org/10.1093/sleep/zsab199
Maccoby, E. (1998). *The two sexes: Growing up apart, coming together*. Harvard University Press.
MacDonald, S., & Culham, J. (2015). Do human brain areas involved in visuomotor actions show a preference for real tools over visually similar non-tools? *Neuropsychologia*, *77*, 35–41.
MacLean, H. N. (1993). *Once upon a time: A true story of memory, murder and the law*. Harper Collins.
Madsen, P. L., Holm, S., Vorstrup, S., Friberg, L., Lassen, N. A., & Wildschidtz, G. (1991). Human regional cerebral blood flow during rapid-eye-movement sleep. *Journal of Cerebral Blood Flow Metabolism*, *11*, 502–507.
Madsen, P. L., Schmidt, F., Holm, S., Vorstrup, S., Lassen, N. A., & Wildschidtz, G. (1991). Cerebral oxygen metabolism and cerebral blood flow in man during light sleep (stage 2). *Brain Research*, *557*(Brain Research), 217–220.
Malcolm-Smith, S., & Solms, M. (2004). Incidence of threat in dreams: A response to Revonsuo's threat simulation theory. *Dreaming*, *14*, 220–229.
Malcolm-Smith, S., Solms, M., Turnbull, O., & Tredoux, C. (2008). Threat in dreams: An adaptation? *Consciouness and Cognition*, *17*, 1281–1291.

Malinowski, J., & Horton, C. (2014). Memory sources of dreams: The incorporation of autobiographical rather than episodic experiences. *Journal of Sleep Research*, *23*, 441–447. https://doi.org/10.1111/jsr.12134

Malinowski, J., & Horton, C. (2015). Metaphor and hyperassociativity: The imagination mechanisms behind emotion assimilation in sleep and dreaming. *Frontiers in Psychology*, *6*, Article 1132. https://doi.org/10.3389/fpsyg.2015.01132

Mallett, R., Konkoly, K. R., Nielsen, T., Carr, M., & Paller, K. A. (2024). New strategies for the cognitive science of dreaming. *Trends in Cognitive Sciences*. https://doi.org/10.1016/j.tics.2024.10.004

Mandler, J. (2004). *The foundations of mind: Origins of conceptual thought*. Oxford University Press.

Mandler, J. (2008). On the birth and growth of concepts. *Philosophical Psychology*, *21*, 207–230.

Mandler, J. (2012). On the spatial foundations of the conceptual system and its enrichment. *Cognitive Science*, *36*, 421–451.

Mansouri, F., Koechlin, E., Rosa, M., & Buckley, M. (2017). Managing competing goals — A key role for the frontopolar cortex. *Nature Reviews Neuroscience*, *18*, 645–657.

Maquet, P. (2000). Functional neuroimaging of normal human sleep by positron emission tomography. *Journal of Sleep Research*, *9*, 207–231.

Maquet, P., Peters, J., Aerts, J., Delfiore, G., Dequerldre, C., Luxen, A., & Franck, G. (1996). Functional neuroanatomy of human rapid-eye-movement sleep and dreaming. *Nature*, *383*, 163–166.

Maquet, P., Ruby, P., Maudoux, A., Albouy, G., Sterpenich, V., Dang-Vu, T., Laureys, S. (2005). Human cognition during REM sleep and the activity profile within frontal and parietal cortices: A reappraisal of functional neuroimaging data. *Progress in Brain Research*, *150*, 219–227.

Markert, B., & Schredl, M. (2024). Music in the "Barb Sanders" dream series. *Dreaming*, *34*(2), 186–194. https://doi.org/10.1037/drm0000263

Markert, B., & Schredl, M. (2025). Dreaming about pain: Dreams series of a chronic pain patient. *Dreaming*, *35*. https://doi.org/doi:10.1037/drm0000313

Marmor, G. S. (1975). Development of kinetic images: When does the child first represent movement in mental images? *Cognitive Psychology*, *7*, 548–559.

Martina, L. S. (2014). Didelphis marsupialis, southern opossum. *Animal Diversity Web*. https://animaldiversity.org/accounts/Didelphis_marsupialis/

Marzano, C., Ferrara, M., Mauro, F., Moroni, F., Gorgoni, M., Tempesta, D., & De Gennaro, L. (2011). Recalling and forgetting dreams: theta and alpha oscillations during sleep predict subsequent dream recall. *Journal of Neuroscience*, *31*, 6647–6683.

Mazandarani, A. A., Aguilar-Vafaie, M. E., & Domhoff, G. W. (2013). Content analysis of Iranian college students' dreams: Comparison with American data. *Dreaming*, *23*, 163–174.

McCaig, R. G., Dixon, M. L., Keramatian, K., Liua, I., & Christoff, K. (2011). Improved modulation of rostrolateral prefrontal cortex using real-time fMRI training and meta-cognitive awareness. *Neuroimage*, *55*, 1298–1305.

McCarley, R., & Hobson, J. A. (1975). Discharge patterns of cat pontine brain stem neurons during desynchronized sleep. *Journal of Neurophysiology*, *38*, 751–766.

McCarley, R., & Hoffman, E. (1981). REM sleep dreams and the activation-synthesis hypothesis. *American Journal of Psychiatry*, *138*, 904–912.

McGinty, D., & Szymusiak, R. (2022). Neural control of sleep in mammals. In M. Kryger, T. Roth, C. Goldstein, & W. Dement (Eds.), *Principles and practices of sleep medicine* (7th ed., pp. 54–67). Elsevier.

McNally, R. J., & Clancy, S. (2005). Sleep paralysis, sexual abuse, and space alien abduction. *Transcultural Psychiatry*, *42*(1), 113–122. https://doi.org/10.1177/1363461505050715

McNamara, P., McLaren, D., & Durso, K. (2007). Representation of the self in REM and NREM dreams. *Dreaming*, *17*, 113–126.

McNamara, P., McLaren, D., Smith, D., Brown, A., & Stickgold, R. (2005). A 'Jekyll and Hyde' within: Aggressive versus friendly interactions in REM and NREM dreams. *Psychological Science*, *16*, 130–136.

Meaidi, A., Jennum, P., Ptito, M., & Kupers, R. (2014). The sensory construction of dreams and nightmare frequency in congenitally blind and late blind individuals. *Sleep Medicine*, *15*(5), 586–595. https://doi.org/10.1016/j.sleep.2013.12.008

Mehl, M. R., Eid, M., Wrzus, C., Harari, G. M., & Ebner-Priemer, U. W. (2024). *Mobile sensing in psychology: Methods and applications*. Guilford Press.

Meier, C., Ruef, H., Ziegler, A., & Hall, C. (1968). Forgetting of dreams in the laboratory. *Perceptual and Motor Skills*, *26*, 551–557.

Menon, V. (2023). 20 years of the default mode network: A review and synthesis. *Neuron*, *111*(16), 2469–2487. https://doi.org/10.1016/j.neuron.2023.04.023

Menon, V., & Uddin, L. (2010). Saliency, switching, attention and control: A network model of insula function. *Brain Structure & Function*, *214*, 655–667.

Meyer, M. L., & Lieberman, M. D. (2018). Why people are always thinking about themselves: Medial prefrontal cortex activity during rest primes self-referential processing. *Journal of Cognitive Neuroscience*, *30*, 714–721. https://doi.org/10.1162/jocn_a_01232

Meyer, S., & Shore, C. (2001). Children's understanding of dreams as mental states. *Dreaming*, *11*, 179–194.

Miyamoto, K., Rushworth, M., & Shea, N. (2023). Imagining the future self through thought experiments *Trends in Cognitive Sciences*, *27*(5), 446–455. https://doi.org/10.1016/j.tics.2023.01.005

Moehlman, T., Chang, C., Duyn, J., & Picchioni, D. (2018). All-night functional magnetic resonance imaging sleep studies. *Journal of Neuroscience Methods*, *316*, 83–98. https://doi.org/10.1016/j.jneumeth.2018.09.019

Möhring, W., & Frick, A. (2013). Touching up mental rotation: Effects of manual experience on 6-month-old infants' mental object rotation. *Child Development*, *8*, 1554–1565.

Montangero, J., & Cavallero, C. (2015). What renders dreams more or less narrative? A microstructural study of REM and Stage 2 dreams reported upon morning awakening. *International Journal of Dream Research*, *8*(2), 105–119.

Montangero, J., Ivanyi, C., & de Saint-Hilaire, Z. (2003). Completeness and accuracy of morning reports after a recall cue: Comparison of dream and film reports. *Consciousness & Cognition*, *12*, 49–62.

Moraczewski, D., Nketia, J., & Redcay, E. (2020). Cortical temporal hierarchy is immature in middle childhood. *Neuroimage*, *216*, 116616. https://doi.org/10.1016/j.neuroimage.2020.116616

Moskowitz, E., & Berger, R. J. (1969). Rapid eye movements and dream imagery: Are they related? *Nature*, *224*, 613–614.

Moulton, S. T., & Kosslyn, S. (2011). Imagining predictions: Mental imagery as mental emulation. In M. Bar (Ed.), *Predictions in the brain: Using our past to generate a future* (pp. 95–106). Oxford University Press.

Mukherjee, S., & Heise, D. R. (2017). Affective meanings of 1,469 Bengali concepts. *Behavior Research Methods*, *49*(1), 184–197. https://doi.org/10.3758/s13428-016-0704-6

Mysliwiec, V., O'Reilly, B., Polchinski, J., Kwon, H., Germain, A., & Roth, B. J. (2014). Trauma associated sleep disorder: A proposed parasomnia encompassing disruptive nocturnal behaviors, nightmares, and REM without atonia in trauma survivors. *Journal of Clinical Sleep Medicine*, *10*, 1143–1148.

Nelson, K. (2005). Emerging levels of consciousness in early human development. In H. S. Terrace & J. Metcalfe (Eds.), *The missing link in cognition: Origins of self-reflective consciousness* (pp. 116–141). Oxford University Press.

Nelson, K. (2007). *Young minds in social worlds: Experience, meaning, and memory.* Harvard University Press.

Nelson, K. (2011). "Concept" is a useful concept in developmental research. *Journal of Theoretical and Philosophical Psychology*, *31*, 96–101.

Nelson, K. (2014). Sociocultural theories of memory development. In P. Bauer & R. Fivush (Eds.), *The Wiley handbook on the development of children's memory* (Vol. I, pp. 87–108). Wiley-Blackwell.

Nelson, K., & Fivush, R. (2020). The development of autobiographical memory, autobiographical narratives, and autobiographical consciousness *Psychological Reports*, *123*, 71–96. https://doi.org/10.1177/0033294119852574

Németh, D., Gerbier, E., Born, J., Rickard, T., Diekelmann, S., Fogel, S., Genzel, L., Prehn-Kristensen, A., Payne, J., Dresler, M., Simor, P., Mazza, S., Hoedlmoser, K., Ruby, P., Spencer, R. M. C., Albouy, G., Vékony, T., Schabus, M., & Janacsek, K. (2024). Optimizing the methodology of human sleep and memory research. *Nature Reviews Psychology*, *3*(2), 123–137. https://doi.org/10.1038/s44159-023-00262-0

Nielsen, T. (2000). A review of mentation in REM and NREM sleep: "Covert" REM sleep as a possible reconciliation of two opposing models. *Behavioral and Brain Sciences*, *23*, 851–866. https://doi.org/10.1017/S0140525X0000399X

Nielsen, T. (2004). Chronobiological features of dream production. *Sleep Medicine Reviews*, *8*(5), 403–424. https://doi.org/10.1016/j.smrv.2004.06.005

Nofzinger, E., Mintun, M., Wiseman, M., Kupfer, D., & Moore, R. (1997). Forebrain activation in REM sleep: An FDG PET study. *Brain Research*, *770*, 192–201.

Noreen, E. (1989). *Computer intensive methods for testing hypotheses: An introduction.* Wiley.

Norris, C. J. (2021). The negativity bias, revisited: Evidence from neuroscience measures and an individual differences approach. *Social Neuroscience*, *16*, 68–82. https://doi.org/10.1080/17470919.2019.1696225

Norris, D. (2017). Short-Term memory and long-term memory are still different. *Psychological Bulletin*, *143*(9), 992–1009. https://doi.org/10.1037/bul0000108

Nunn, C. L., & Samson, D. R. (2018). Sleep in a comparative context: Investigating how human sleep differs from sleep in other primates. *American Journal of Biological Anthropology*, *166*, 601–612.

O'Nell, C., & O'Nell, N. (1977). A cross-cultural comparison of aggression in dreams: Zapotecs and Americans. *International Journal of Social Psychiatry*, *125*, 35–41.

Oberst, U., Charles, C., & Chamarro, A. (2005). Influence of gender and age in aggressive dream content in Spanish children and adolescents. *Dreaming*, *15*, 170–177.

Ochsner, K., & Kosslyn, S. (2014a). Cognitive neuroscience: Where are we now? In K. Ochsner & S. Kosslyn (Eds.), *The Oxford handbook of cognitive neuroscience* (Vol. 2, pp. 1–7). Oxford University Press. https://doi.org/10.1093/oxfordhb/9780199988709.013.0001

Ochsner, K., & Kosslyn, S. (2014b). Cognitive neuroscience: Where are we going? In K. Ochsner & S. Kosslyn (Eds.), *The Oxford handbook of cognitive neuroscience* (Vol. 2, pp. 476–483). Oxford University Press. https://doi.org/10.1093/oxfordhb/9780199988709.013.0030

Odegaard, B. (2019). *Convincing evidence for a role of prefrontal cortex in consciousness* [Conference presentation]. Northern California Consciousness Conference, Davis, CA.

Odegaard, B., Knight, R. T., & Lau, H. (2017). Should a few null findings falsify prefrontal theories of conscious perception? *Journal of Neuroscience*, *37*, 9593–9602.

Ogilvie, R. (2001). The process of falling asleep. *Sleep Medicine Reviews*, *5*, 247–270.

Ogilvie, R., Hunt, H., Tyson, P., Lucescu, M., & Jeakins, D. (1982). Lucid dreaming and alpha activity: A preliminary report. *Perceptual & Motor Skills*, *55*, 795–808.

Open Science Collaboration. (2015). Estimating the reproducibility of psychological science. *Science*, *349*, Article aac4716. https://doi.org/10.1126/science.aac4716

Oreskes, N. (2019). *Why trust science?* Princeton University Press.

Orne, M. (1962). On the social psychology of the psychological experiment: With particular reference to demand characteristics and their implications. *American Psychologist*, *17*, 776–783.

Osgood, C. (1971). Commentary on "the semantic differential and mediation theory". *Linguistics*, *9*(66), 88–96. https://doi.org/10.1515/ling.1971.9.66.88

Osgood, C., May, W., & Miron, M. (1975). *Cross-cultural universals of affective meaning*. University of Illinois Press.

Osgood, C., Suci, G., & Tannenbaum, P. (1959). *The measurement of meaning*. University of Illinois Press.

Pace-Schott, E. (2007). The frontal lobes and dreaming. In D. Barrett & P. McNamara (Eds.), *The new science of dreaming: Biological aspects* (Vol. 1, pp. 115–154). Praeger/Greewood.

Pacheco, D., & Peters, B. (2024). Somniphobia: Understanding the fear of sleep. In *Mental health and sleep*. www.sleepfoundation.org/mental-health/somniphobia. National Sleep Foundation. Washington, DC. https://www.thensf.org/

Pagel, J. F., Blagrove, M., Levin, R., States, B., Stickgold, R., & White, S. (2001). Definitions of dream: A paradigm for comparing field descriptive specific studies of dream. *Dreaming*, *11*(4), 195–202.

Paquola, C., Garber, M., Frässle, S., Royer, J., Zhou, Y., Tavakol, S., & Bernhardt, B. C. (2025). The architecture of the human default mode network explored through cytoarchitecture, wiring and signal flow. *Nature Neuroscience*, *28*, 654–664.

Parmeggiani, P. L. (1977). Interaction between sleep and thermoregulation. *Waking & Sleeping*, *1*(2), 123–132.

Parmeggiani, P. L. (2011). *Systemic homeostasis and poikilostasis in sleep: Is REM sleep a physiological paradox?* Imperial College Press.

Paul, N., Fitzgerald, E., & Greenblatt, M. (1956). Bimedial lobotomy: five-year evaluation. *Journal of Nervous and Mental Disease*, *124*(1), 49–52. https://doi.org/10.1097/00005053-195607000-00007

Paulson, D., & Krippner, S. (2010). *Haunted by combat: Understanding PTSD in war veterans*. Rowman & Littlefield.

Payne, J., Kensinger, E., Wamsley, E., Spreng, R. N., & Alger, S. (2015). Napping and the selective consolidation of negative aspects of scenes. *Emotion*, *15*, 176–186.

Perogamvros, L., Baird, B., Seibold, M., Riedner, B., Boly, M., & Tononi, G. (2017). The phenomenal contents and neural correlates of spontaneous thoughts across wakefulness, NREM sleep, and REM sleep. *Journal of Cognitive Neuroscience*, *29*, 1766–1777.

Picchioni, D., Fukunaga, M., Carr, W., Braun, A., Balkin, T., Duyn, J., & Horovitz, S. (2008). fMRI differences between early and late stage-1 sleep. *Neuroscience Newsletter*, *441*, 81–85.

Picchioni, D., Pixa, M., Fukunaga, M., Carr, W., Horovitz, S., Braun, A., & Duyn, J. (2014). Decreased connectivity between the thalamus and the neocortex during human nonrapid eye movement sleep *Sleep*, *37*(2), 387–397.

Pires, J. R., & Paiva, T. (2021). Dream recall frequency and dream content in women. *International Journal of Dream Research*, *14*(2), 266–271.

Pivik, R. T. (1991). Tonic states and phasic events in relation to sleep mentation. In S. Ellman & J. Antrobus. (Eds.), *The mind in sleep: Psychology and psychophysiology* (2nd ed., pp. 214–247). Wiley.

Pivik, R. T., & Foulkes, D. (1968). NREM mentation: Relation to personality, orientation time, and time of night. *Journal of Consulting and Clinical Psychology*, *32*(2), 144–151.

Polner-Clark, E., Wager, T., Satpute, A., & Barrett, L. F. (2016). Neural fingerprinting: Meta-Analysis, variation, and the search for brain-based essences in the science of emotions. In L. F. Barrett, M. Lewis, & J. Haviland-Jones (Eds.), *Handbook of Emotions* (4th ed., pp. 146–165). Guilford Press.

Popp, C., Lubarsky, L., & Crits, C. (1992). The parallel of the CCRT from therapy narratives with the CCRT from dreams. In L. Lubarsky & C. Crits (Eds.), *Understanding transference* (pp. 158–172). Basic Books.

Poppen, J. L. (1948). Technic of prefrontal lobotomy. *Journal of Neurosurgery*, *5*(6), 514–520. https://doi.org/10.3171/jns.1948.5.6.0514

Postman, L. (1963). One-trial learning. In C. Cofer & B. Musgrave (Eds.), *Verbal behavior and learning: Problems and processes* (pp. 295–335). McGraw-Hill. https://doi.org/10.1037/11178-008

Power, J. D., Cohen, A., Nelson, S., & Petersen, S. (2011). Functional organization of the human brain. *Neuron*, *72*, 665–678.

Poza, J., & Marti-Masso, J. (2006). Total dream loss secondary to left temporo-occipital brain injury. *Neurologia*, *21*, 152–154.

Quinn, P. C., & Liben, L. S. (2014). A sex difference in mental rotation in infants: Convergent evidence. *Infancy*, *19*, 103–116.

Raichle, M. E., MacLeod, A. M., Snyder, A. Z., Powers, W. J., Gusnard, D. A., & Shulman, G. L. (2001). A default mode of brain function. *Proceedings of the National Academy of Sciences*, *98*, 676–682.

Rakison, D., & Lawson, C. (2013). Categorization. In P. Zelazo (Ed.), *The Oxford handbook of developmental psychology (Vol 1): Body and mind* (pp. 591–627). Oxford University Press.

Rapp, A., Mutschler, D., & Erb, M. (2012). Where in the brain is nonliteral language? A coordinate-based meta-analysis of functional magnetic resonance imaging studies. *Neuroimage*, *63*, 600–610.

Rasch, B., & Born, J. (2015). In search of a role of REM sleep in memory formation. *Neurobiology of Learning and Memory*, *122*, 1–3.

Rasch, B., Pommer, J., Diekelmann, S., & Born, J. (2009). Pharmacological REM sleep suppression paradoxically improves rather than impairs skill memory. *Natural Neuroscience*, *12*, 396–397.

Raz, G., Touroutoglou, A., Atzil, S., & Barrett, L. F. (2016). Functional connectivity dynamics during film viewing reveal common networks for different emotional experiences. *Cognitive, Affective & Behavioral Neuroscience*, *16*, 709–723. https://doi.org/10.3758/s13415-016-0425-4

Read, D. W., Manrique, H. M., & Walker, M. J. (2022). On the working memory of humans and great apes: Strikingly similar or remarkably different? *Neuroscience Biobehavioral Review*, *134*. https://doi.org/10.1016/j.neubiorev.2021.12.019

Rechtschaffen, A., & Foulkes, D. (1965). Effect of visual stimuli on dream content. *Perceptual and Motor Skills*, *20*, 1149–1160.

Rechtschaffen, A., & Kales, A. (1968). *A manual of standardized terminology, techniques, and scoring system for sleep stages of human subjects*. Pubic Health Service.

Rechtschaffen, A., Cornwell, P., Zimmerman, W. B., & Bassan, M. (1965). *Brain Temperature Variations with Paradoxical Sleep: Implications for Relationships among EEG, Cerebral Metabolism, Sleep And Consciousness* [Conference presentation]. Lyon Symposium on Sleep and Consciousness, Lyon, France. http://dreamresearch.net/Library/rechtschaffen_1965.pdf

Rechtschaffen, A., Hauri, P., & Zeitlin, M. (1966). Auditory awakening thresholds in REM and NREM sleep stages *Perceptual and Motor Skills*, *22*, 927–942.

Rechtschaffen, A., Verdone, P., & Wheaton, J. (1963). Reports of mental activity during sleep. *Canadian Psychiatric Association Journal*, *8*, 409–414.

Reese, E. (2013). Culture, narrative, and imagination. In M. Taylor (Ed.), *The Oxford handbook of the development of imagination* (pp. 196–211). Oxford University Press.

Reinsel, R., Antrobus, J., & Wollman, M. (1985). The phasic-tonic difference and the time-of-night effect. *Sleep Research*, *14*, 115.

Replication crisis (2025, May 30). In *Wikipedia*. https://en.wikipedia.org/w/?title=Replication_crisis&oldid=1293129732

Resnick, J., Stickgold, R., Rittenhouse, C., & Hobson, J. A. (1994). Self-representation and bizarreness in children's dream reports collected in the home setting. *Consciousness and Cognition*, *3*, 30–45.

Revonsuo, A. (2000a). Did ancestral humans dream for their lives? *Behavioral & Brain Sciences*, *23*, 1063–1082.

Revonsuo, A. (2000b). The reinterpretation of dreams: An evolutionary hypothesis of the function of dreaming. *Behavioral and Brain Sciences*, *23*(6), 877–901.

Revonsuo, A., & Valli, K. (2000). Dreaming and consciousness: Testing the threat simulation theory of the function of dreaming. *Psyche*, *6*, 1–31.

Revonsuo, A., Tuominen, J., & Valli, K. (2015). The avatars in the machine: Dreaming as a simulation of social reality. In T. Metzinger & J. Windt (Eds.), *Open MIND: 32(T)* (pp. 1–28). MIND Group. https://doi.org/10.15502/9783958570375

Reznick, J. S., & Bauer, P. J. (2008). Constructing a mind, one image schema at a time. *Journal of Cognition and Development*, *9*, 253–255.

Robinson, M. F. (1954). *Psychosurgery and the self.* Grune & Stratton.

Roehrs, T. A., & Roth, T. (2015). Sleep disturbance in substance use disorders. *Psychiatric Clinical Journal of North America*, *38*(4), 793–803.https://doi.org/10.1016/j.psc.2015.07.008

Rogoff, B. (1993). Apprenticeship in Thinking: Cognitive Development in Social Context Oxford University Press.

Rogoff, B., Sellers, M. J., Pirrotta, S., Fox, N., & White, S. H. (1975). Age of assignment of roles and responsibilities to children. *Human Development*, *18*, 353–369.

Rolls, E., Deco, G., Huang, C., & Feng, J. (2024). The connectivity of the human frontal pole cortex, and a theory of its involvement in exploit versus explore. *Cerebral Cortex*, *34*(1), 1–19. https://doi.org/10.1093/cercor/bhad416

Rolston, D. (2013, November 21). The dream catcher: Why does the researcher who pioneered the study of lucid dreaming face a future in academic exile? In *Matter.* https://medium.com/matter-archive/the-dream-catcher-c85e3bb29693

Roseman, M. (1991). Healing sounds from the Malaysian rainforest: Temiar music and medicine. University of California Press.

Rosenthal, R., & Ambady, N. (1995). Experimenter effects. In A. Manstead & M. Hewstone (Eds.), *Encyclopedia of social psychology* (pp. 230–235). Blackwell.

Rosenthal, R., & Rosnow, R. L. (2009). *Artifacts in behavioral research.* Oxford University Press.

Rosnow, R. L., & Rosenthal, R. (1997). *People studying people: Artifacts and ethics in behavioral research.* W.H. Freeman.

Ross, J., Hutchison, J., & Cunningham, S. J. (2024). The self-memory system: Exploring developmental links between self and memory across early to late childhood. *Child Development*, *96*, 234–250. https://doi.org/10.1111/cdev.14163

Roussy, F., Brunette, M., Mercier, P., Gonthier, I., Grenier, J., Sirois-Berliss, M., De Koninck, J. (2000). Daily events and dream content: Unsuccessful matching attempts. *Dreaming*, *10*, 77–83.

Roussy, F., Camirand, C., Foulkes, D., De Koninck, J., Loftis, M., & Kerr, N. (1996). Does early-night REM dream content reliably reflect presleep state of mind? *Dreaming*, *6*, 121–130.

Roussy, F., Raymond, I., & De Koninck, J. (2000). Affect in REM dreams: Exploration of a time-of-night effect. *Sleep*, *23*, A174–A175.

Röver, S. A., & Schredl, M. (2017). Measuring emotions in dreams: Effects of dream length and personality. *International Journal of Dream Research*, *10*, 65–68.

Ruby, P., Eskinazi, M., Bouet, R., Rheims, S., & Peter-Derex, L. (2021). Dynamics of hippocampus and orbitofrontal cortex activity during arousing reactions from sleep: An intracranial electroencephalographic study. *Human Brain Mapping*, *42*(16), 5188–5203.

Rudofsky, S., & Wotiz, J. (1988). Psychologists and the dream accounts of August Kekulé. *Journal of Human Behavior & Learning*, *5*, 1–11.

Ryan, M., Whisson, D., Holland, G., & Arnould, J. (2013). Activity patterns of free-ranging koalas (Phascolarctos cinereus) revealed by accelerometry. *PLoS One*, *8*(11). https://doi.org/10.1371/journal.pone.0080366

Saccenti, D., Moro, A., Sassaroli, S., Malgaroli, A., Ferro, M., & Lamanna, J. (2024). Neural correlates of metacognition: Disentangling the brain circuits underlying prospective and retrospective second-order judgments through noninvasive brain stimulation. *journal of Neuroscience Research*, *102*(4), 1–18. https://doi.org/10.1002/jnr.25330

Sakai, K., Petitjean, F., & Jouvet, M. (1976). Effects of ponto-mesencephalic lesions and electrical stimulation upon PGO waves and EMPs in unanesthetized cats. *Electroencephalography and Clinical Neurophysiology*, *41*, 49–63.

Sala, G., & Gobet, F. (2017). Does far transfer exist? Negative evidence from chess, music, and working memory training. *Current Directions in Psychological Science*, *26*, 515–520.

Sala, G., Tatlidil, K. S., & Gobet, F. (2018). Video game training does not enhance cognitive ability: A comprehensive meta-analytic investigation. *Psychological Bulletin*, *144*(2), 111–139.

Saline, S. (1999). The most recent dreams of children ages 8–11. *Dreaming, 9*, 173–181.

Sämann, P., Wehrle, R., Hoehn, D., Spoormaker, V., Peters, H., Tully, C., Czisch, M. (2011). Development of the brain's default mode network from wakefulness to slow wave sleep. *Cerebral Cortex*, *21*, 2082–2093.

Sameroff, A. J., & Haith, M. M. (1996). *The five to seven year shift: The age of reason and responsibility*. University of Chicago Press.

Samson, D. R., Crittenden, A., Mabulla, I., Mabulla, A., & Nunn, C. L. (2017). Hadza sleep biology: Evidence for flexible sleep-wake patterns in hunter-gatherers. *American Journal of Physical Anthropology*, *162*(3), 573–582. https://doi.org/10.1002/ajpa.23160

Sastre, J.-P., Sakai, K., & Jouvet, M. (1981). Are the gigantocellular tegmental field neurons responsible for paraxodical sleep? *Brain Research*, *229*(1), 147–161.

Sato, J. R., Salum, G. A., Gadelha, A., Picon, F. A., Pan, P. M., & al., e. (2014). Age effects on the default mode and control networks in typically developing children. *Journal of Psychiatric Research*, *58*, 89–95.

Savagian, A., & Fernandez-Duque, E. (2017). Do predators and thermoregulation influence choice of sleeping sites and sleeping behavior in Azara's owl monkeys (Aotus azarae azarae) in northern Argentina? *International Journal of Primatology*, *89*, 80–99

Schacter, D. L. (1999). The seven sins of memory: Insights from psychology and cognitiveneuroscience. *American Psychologist*, *54*(3), 182–203. https://doi.org/10.1037/0003-066X.54.3.182

Schacter, D., Addis, D., & Buckner, R. (2008). Episodic simulation of future events: Concepts, data, and applications. *Annals of the New York Academy of Sciences*, *1124*, 39–60. https://doi.org/10.1196/annals.1440.001

Schaefer, A., Kong, R., Eickhoff, S., & Yeo, B. (2018). Local-Global parcellation of the human cerebral cortex from intrinsic functional connectivity MRI. *Cerebral Cortex*, *28*, 3095–3114. https://doi.org/10.1093/cercor/bhx179

Scheeringa, R., Bastiaansen, M., Petersson, K., Oostenveld, R., Norris, D., & Hagoort, P. (2008). Frontal theta EEG activity correlates negatively with the default mode network in resting state. *International Journal of Psychophysiology*, *67*, 242–251.

Schmidt, M. H. (2014). The energy allocation function of sleep: a unifying theory of sleep, torpor, and continuous wakefulness. *Neuroscience Biobehavioral Review*, *47*, 122–153. https://doi.org/10.1016/j.neubiorev.2014.08.001

Schneider, A., & Domhoff, G. W. (1995). *DreamResearch.net: The Quantitative Study of Dreams*. http://dreamresearch.net/

Schneider, A., & Domhoff, G. W. (1999). *The DreamBank*. http://dreambank.net/

Schneider, E. (1953). *Coleridge, opium, and Kubla Khan*. University of Chicago Press.

Schredl, M. (2000). The relationship between dream recall and dream content: Negative evidence for the salience hypothesis. *North American Journal of Psychology*, *2*(2), 243–246.

Schredl, M. (2022). Incorporation of waking experiences into dreams. In M. Kryger, B. J. Roth, C. Goldstein, & W. Dement (Eds.), *Principles and Practices of Sleep Medicine* (Seventh ed., pp. 600–605). Elsevier.

Schredl, M. (2024). *Analyzing a long dream series: What can we learn about how dreaming works?* Routledge.

Schredl, M., & Doll, E. (1998). Emotions in diary dreams. *Consciousness & Cognition*, *7*(4), 634–646.

Schredl, M., & Göritz, A. (2017). Dream recall frequency, attitude toward dreams, and the Big Five personality factors. *Dreaming*, *27*, 49–58.

Schredl, M., & Hofmann, F. (2003). Continuity between waking activities and dream activities. *Consciousness and Cognition*, *12*, 298–308.

Schredl, M., & Schweickert, R. (2022). Social network in the 2015 dreams of a male dreamer. *International Journal of Dream Research*, *15*(1), 118–125.

Schredl, M., Petra, C., Bishop, A., Golitz, E., & Buschtons, D. (2003). Content analysis of German students' dreams: Comparison to American findings. *Dreaming*, *13*, 237–243.

Schredl, M., Remedios, A., Marin-Dragu, S., Sheikh, S., Forbes, A., Iyer, R. S., Orr, M., & Meier, S. (2022). Dream recall frequency, lucid dream frequency, and personality during the Covid-19 pandemic. *Imagination, Cognition and Personality*, *42*(2), 113–133. https://doi.org/10.1177/02762366221104214

Schweickert, R. (2007a). Properties of the organization of memory for people: Evidence from dream reports. *Psychonomic Bulletin & Review*, *14*, 270–276.

Schweickert, R. (2007b). Social networks of characters in dreams. In D. Barrett & P. McNamara (Eds.), *The new science of dreaming: Cultural and theoretical perspectives* (Vol. 3, pp. 277–297). Praeger.

Schweickert, R. (2007c). The structure of semantic and phonological networks and the structure of a social network in dreams. In J. S. Nairne (Ed.), *The foundations of remembering: Essays in honor of Henry L. Roediger, III*. (pp. 281–296). Psychology Press.

Schweickert, R., & Xi, Z. (2010). Metamorphosed characters in dreams: Constraints of conceptual structure and amount of theory of mind. *Cognitive Science*, *34*, 665–684.

Schweickert, R., & Xi, Z. (2011). Theory of Mind and metamorphoses in dreams: *Dr. Jekyll & Mr. Hyde* and *The Metamorphosis*. In P. Leverage, H.

Mancing, R. Schweickert, & J. William (Eds.), *Theory of mind and literature* (pp. 219–228). Purdue University Press.

Schweickert, R., Zhuangzhuang, X., Viau-Quesnel, C., & Zheng, X. (2020). Power law distribution of frequencies of characters in dreams explained by random walk on semantic network. *International Journal of Dream Research*, *13*, 192–201.

Seeley, W. W., Menon, V., Schatzberg, A. F., Keller, J., Glover, G. H., Kenna, H., Reiss, A. L., & Grecius, M. D. (2007). Dissociable intrinsic connectivity networks for salience processing and executive control. *Journal of Neuroscience*, *27*(9), 2349–2356.

Seth, A. K., & Bayne, T. (2022). Theories of consciousness. *Nature Reviews Neuroscience*, *23*, 439–452. https://doi.org/10.1038/s41583-022-00587-4

Shapiro, D., & Notowitz, D. (1988/2016). *Night Wars: The Nightmares of Vietnam Veterans*. www.youtube.com/watch?v=R_aURpo3Als

Sherman, L., Rudie, J., Pfeifer, J., Masten, C., McNealy, K., & Dapretto, M. (2014). Development of the default mode and central executive networks across early adolescence: A longitudinal study. *Developmental Cognitive Neuroscience*, *10*, 148–159.

Shpak, O. V., Lyamin, O. I., Manger, P. R., Siegel, J. M., & Mukhametov, L. (2009). Rest and activity states in the Commerson's dolphin (Cephalorhynchus commersonii). *Zhurnal evoliutsionnoi biokhimii i fiziologii* (English edition), *45*(1), 97–104.

Siclari, F., Baird, B., Perogamvros, L., Bernardi, G., Boly, M., & Tononi, G. (2017). The neural correlates of dreaming. *Nature Neuroscience 20*, 872–878.

Siegel, E., Sands, M. K., Chang, Y., & Barrett, L. F. (2018). Emotion fingerprints or emotion populations? A meta-analytic investigation of autonomic features of emotion categories. *Psychological Bulletin*, *144*, 343–393. https://doi.org/10.1037/bul0000128

Siegel, J. M. (2001). The REM sleep-memory consolidation hypothesis. *Science*, *294*, 1058–1063.

Siegel, J. M. (2021). Memory consolidation is similar in waking and sleep. *Current Sleep Medicine Reports*, *7*, 15–18.

Siegel, J. M. (2022a). Defining sleep. In M. Kryger, B. J. Roth, & W. Dement (Eds.), *Principles and practices of sleep medicine* (7th ed., pp. 52–53). Elsevier.

Siegel, J. M. (2022b). Evolution of mammalian sleep. In M. Kryger, T. Roth, & W. Dement (Eds.), *Principles and practices of sleep medicine* (7th ed., pp. 93–105). Elsevier.

Siegel, J. M. (2022c). Rapid Eye Movement sleep control and function. In M. Kryger, T. Roth, C. Goldstein, & W. Dement (Eds.), *Principles and practices of sleep medicine* (7th ed., pp. 68–86).

Siegel, J. M. (2022d). Sleep function: An evolutionary perspective. *Lancet*, 937–946.

Siegel, J. M., & McGinty, D. (1977). Pontine reticular formation neurons: Relationship of discharge to motor activity. *Science*, *196*, 678–680.

Siegel, J. M., & McGinty, D. (1986). Location of the systems generating REM sleep: Lateral versus medial pons. *Behavioral and Brain Sciences*, *9*, 420–421.

Siegel, J. M., Manger, P., Nienhuis, R., Fahringer, H. M., & Pettigrew, J. D. (1996). The echidna Tachyglossus aculeatus combines REM and NREM aspects in a single sleep state: Implications for the evolution of sleep. *Journal of Neuroscience*, *16*(10), 3500–3506. https://doi.org/10.1523/jneurosci.16-10-03500.1996

Siegel, J. M., Manger, P., Nienhuis, R., Fahringer, H. M., Shalita, T., & Pettigrew, J. D. (1999). Sleep in the platypus. *Neuroscience*, *91*(1), 391–400. https://doi.org/10.1016/s0306-4522(98)00588-0

Siegel, J. M., McGinty, D., & Breedlove, S. M. (1977). Sleep and waking activity of pontine gigantocellular field neurons. *Experimental Neurology*, *56*, 553–573.

Siegel, J. S., Subramanian, S., Perry, D., Kay, B. P., Gordon, E. M., Laumann, T. O., Reneau, T. R., Metcalf, N. V., Chacko, R. V., Gratton, C., Horan, C., Krimmel, S. R., Shimony, J. S., Schweiger, J. A., Wong, D. F., Bender, D. A., Scheidter, K. M., Whiting, F. I., Padawer-Curry, J. A., Shinohara, R. T., Chen, Y., Moser, J., Yacoub, E., Nelson, S. M., Vizioli, L., Fair, D. A., Lenze, E. J., Carhart-Harris, R., Raison, C. L., Raichle, M. E., Snyder, A. Z., Nicol, G. E., & Dosenbach, N. U. F. (2024). Psilocybin desynchronizes the human brain. *Nature*, *632*(8023), 131–138. https://doi.org/10.1038/s41586-024-07624-5

Sikka, P., Feilhauer, D., Valli, K., & Revonsuo, A. (2017). How you measure is what you get: Differences in self- and external ratings of emotional experiences in home dreams. *The American Journal of Psychology 130*, 367–384.

Sikka, P., Revonsuo, A., Sandman, N., Tuominen, J., & Valli, K. (2018). Dream emotions: A comparison of home dream reports with laboratory early and late REM dream reports. *Journal of Sleep Research*, *27*, 206–214. https://doi.org/10.1111/jsr.12555

Sikka, P., Valli, K., Virta, T., & Revonsuo, A. (2014). I know how you felt last night, or do I? Self- and external ratings of emotions in REM sleep dreams. *Consciouness and Cognition*, *25*, 51–66.

Simons, J. S., Ritchey, M., & Fernyhough, C. (2022). Brain mechanisms underlying the subjective experience of remembering. *Annual Review of Psychology*, *73*, 159–186. https://doi.org/10.1146/annurev-psych-030221-025439

Simor, P., Horváth, K., Ujma, P. P., Gombos, F., & Bodizs, R. (2013). Fluctuations between sleep and wakefulness: Wake-like features indicated by increased EEG alpha power during different sleep stages in nightmare disorder. *Biological Psychology*, *94*, 592–600.

Singer, J. L. (1966). *Daydreaming*. Random House.

Singer, J. L. (1975). *The inner world of daydreaming*. Harper and Row.

Singer, J. L., & Singer, D. G. (2013). Historical overview of research on imagination in children. In M. Taylor (Ed.), *The Oxford handbook of the development of imagination* (pp. 11–27). Oxford University Press.

Smith, M., & Hall, C. S. (1964). An investigation of regression in a long dream series. *Journal of Gerontology*, *19*, 66–71.

Snyder, F. (1969). Sleep and REM as biological enigmas. In A. Kales (Ed.), *Sleep: Physiology and psychology* (pp. 266–280). J. B. Lippincott Company.

Snyder, F. (1970). The phenomenology of dreaming. In L. Madow & L. Snow (Eds.), *The psychodynamic implications of the physiological studies on dreams* (pp. 124–151). Charles C. Thomas.

Social-desirability bias. (2025, May 25). In "*Wikipedia*. https://en.wikipedia.org/w/?title=Social-desirability_bias&oldid=1291871635

Solms, M. (1997). *The neuropsychology of dreams: A clinico-anatomical study*. Erlbaum.

Solms, M. (2000). Freudian dream theory today. *Psychologist*, *13*, 618–619.

Solms, M. (2004). Freud returns. *Scientific American*, *290*(5), 83–88.

Solms, M. (2018). The neurobiological underpinnings of psychoanalytic theory and therapy. *Frontiers in Behavioral Neuroscience*, *12*. https://doi.org/10.3389/fnbeh.2018.00294

Solms, M., & Turnbull, O. (2002). *The brain and the inner world*. Other Press.

Sparks, J., & Ledgerwood, A. (2019). Age attenuates the negativity bias in reframing effects. *Personality and Social Psychology Bulletin*, *45*, 1042–1056.

Spreng, R. N., Madore, K., & Schacter, D. (2018). Better imagined: Neural correlates of the episodic simulation boost to prospective memory performance *Neuropsychologia*, *113*, 22–28. https://doi.org/10.1016/j.neuropsychologia.2018.03.025

Sridhar, S., Khamaj, A., & Asthana, M. K. (2023). Cognitive neuroscience perspective on memory: Overview and summary. *Frontiers Human Neuroscience*, *17*, 1–15. https://doi.org/10.3389/fnhum.2023.1217093

St-Cyr-Leroux, B. (2024, September 26). Michelle Carr: Manipulating dreams to improve mental health. In *UdeM Nouvelles*. https://nouvelles.umontreal.ca/en/article/2024/09/26/michelle-carr-manipulating-dreams-to-improve-mental-health/

Stevner, A., Vidaurre, D., Cabral, J., Rapuano, K., Nielsen, S., Tagliazucchi, E., Kringelbach, M. (2019). Discovery of key whole-brain transitions and dynamics during human wakefulness and non-REM sleep *Nature Communications*, *10*(1035), 1–14. https://doi.org/10.1038/s41467-019-08934-3

Stickgold, R. (1998). Sleep: off-line memory reprocessing. *Trends in Cognitive Sciences*, *2*, 484–492. https://doi.org/10.1016/S1364-6613(98)01258-3

Stickgold, R. (2005). Why we dream. In M. Kryger, T. Roth, & W. Dement (Eds.), *Principles and practices of sleep medicine* (4th ed., pp. 579–587). Elsevier.

Stickgold, R., & Wamsley, E. (2017). Why we dream. In M. Kryger, T. Roth, & W. Dement (Eds.), *Principles and practices of sleep medicine* (6th ed., pp. 509–514). Elsevier.

Stickgold, R., James, L., & Hobson, J. A. (2000). Visual discrimination learning requires sleep after training *Natural Neuroscience*, *3*, 1237–1238.

Stickgold, R., Malia, A., Fosse, R., & Hobson, J. A. (2001). Brain-mind states: Longitudinal field study of sleep/wake factors influencing mentation report length. *Sleep*, *24*(2), 171–179.

Stickgold, R., Scott, L., Rittenhouse, C., & Hobson, J. A. (1999). Sleep-induced changes in associative memory. *Journal of Cognitive Neuroscience*, *11*, 182–193.

Stiles, P. G. (1897-1898). A Dream Journal. *DreamBank*. https://dreambank.net/more_info.cgi?further=1&series=physiologist

Storm, B. C. (2011). The Benefit of Forgetting in Thinking and Remembering. *Current Directions in Psychological Science*, *20*(5), 291–295. https://doi.org/10.1177/0963721411418469

Storm, B. C. (2018). Measures of Forgetting. In H. Otani & B. Schwartz (Eds.), *Handbook of research methods in human memory* (pp. 36–49). Routledge. https://doi.org/10.4324/9780429439957

Strange, D., Clifasefi, S., & Garry, M. (2007). False memories. In M. Garry & H. Hayne (Eds.), *Do Justice and Let the Sky Fall: Elizabeth F. Loftus and Her Contributions to Science, Law, and Academic Freedom* (pp. 137–168). Lawrence Erlbaum Associates.

Strauch, I. (2003). Träume im Alter (Dreams in old age). In B. Boothe & B. Ugolini (Eds.), *Lebenshorizont Alter* (pp. 171–187). Vdf, Hochschulverlag AG an der ETH Zürich.

Strauch, I. (2004). Traume im Ubergang von der Kindheit ins Jugendalter: Ergebnisse einer Langzeitstudie (Dreams in the transition from childhood to adolescence: Results from a longitudinal study). Huber.

Strauch, I. (2005). REM dreaming in the transition from late childhood to adolescence: A longitudinal study. *Dreaming*, *15*, 155–169.

Strauch, I. (2014). *The most recent dreams of elderly men and women.* University of Zurich.

Strauch, I., & Lederbogen, S. (1999). The home dreams and waking fantasies of boys and girls ages 9–15. *Dreaming*, *9*, 153–161.

Strauch, I., & Meier, B. (1996). *In search of dreams: Results of experimental dream research.* State University of New York Press.

Stumbrys, T., Erlacher, D., & Schredl, M. (2013). Testing the involvement of the prefrontal cortex in lucid dreaming: A tDCS study. *Consciouness and Cognition*, *22*(4), 1214–1222. https://doi.org/10.1016/j.concog.2013.08.005

Supekar, K., Uddin, L. Q., Prater, K., Amin, H., Greicius, M. D., & Menon, V. (2010). Development of functional and structural connectivity within the default mode network in young children. *Neuroimage*, *52*, 290–301.

Tagliazucchi, E., & Laufs, H. (2014). Decoding wakefulness levels from typical fMRI resting-state data reveals reliable drifts between wakefulness and sleep. *Neuron*, *82*(3), 695–708. https://doi.org/10.1016/j.neuron.2014.03.020

Tagliazucchi, E., von Wegner, F., Morzelewski, A., Brodbeck, V., Jahnke, K., & Laufs, H. (2013). Breakdown of long-range temporal dependence in default mode and attention networks during deep sleep. *Proceedings of the National Academy of Science*, *110*, 15419–15424.

Tamaki, M., Bang, J., Watanabe, T., & Sasaki, Y. (2016). Night watch in one brain hemisphere during sleep associated with the first-night effect in humans. *Current Biology*, *9*, 1190–1194. https://doi.org/10.1016/j.cub.2016.02.063

Tamaki, M., Nittono, H., Hayashi, M., & Hori, T. (2005). Examination of the first-night effect during the sleep-onset period. *Sleep*, *28*, 195–202.

Tan, K. M., Daitch, A., Pinheiro-Chagas, P., Fox, K., J., P., & Lieberman, M. D. (2022). Electrocorticographic evidence of a common neurocognitive sequence for mentalizing about the self and others. *Nature Communications*, *13*, 1–17.

Tanaka, M., Hayashi, M., & Hori, T. (1996). Statistical features of hypnagogic EEG measured by a new scoring system. *Sleep*, *19*(9), 731–738. https://doi.org/10.1093/sleep/19.9.731

Tart, C. (1969). *Altered states of consciousness: A book of readings.* John Wiley & Sons, Inc.

Tartarini, F., & Schiavon, S. (2020). Skin temperature sampling period for longitudinal thermal comfort studies. *Proceedings of the Indoor Air Association.* https://escholarship.org/uc/item/9jn57924

Tarun, A., Wainstein-Andriano, D., Perogamvros, L., Solms, M., Schwartz, S., & Van De Ville, D. (2021). NREM sleep stages specifically alter dynamical integration of large-scale brain network. *iScience*, *24*. https://doi.org/10.1016/j.isci.2020.101923

Taylor, M. (2013). Imagination. In P. Zelazo (Ed.), *The Oxford handbook of developmental psychology (Vol. 1): Body and mind* (pp. 793–831). Oxford University Press.

Tonay, V. (1990/1991). California women and their dreams: A historical and subcultural comparison of dream content. *Imagination, Cognition, and Personality*, *10*, 83–97.

Tonay, V. (1993). Personality correlates of dream recall: Who remembers? *Dreaming*, *3*, 1–8.

Touroutoglou, A., Lindquist, K., Dickerson, B. C., & Barrett, L. F. (2015). Intrinsic connectivity in the human brain does not reveal networks for 'basic' emotions. *Social Cognitive and Affective Neuroscience*, *10*, 1257–1265.

Townley, R. (1998). *Night errands: How poets use their dreams*. University of Pittsbugh Press.

Tucker, M., Humiston, G., T., S., & E., W. (2020). Comparing the effects of sleep and rest on memory consolidation. *Nature and Science of Sleep*, *12*, 79–91. https://doi.org/10.2147/NSS.S223917

Tulving, E. (1974). Cue dependent forgetting. *American Scientist*, *62*, 74–82.

Tulving, E. (2005). Episodic memory and autonoesis. In H. S. Terrace & J. Metcalf (Eds.), *The missing link in cognition: Origins of self-reflective consciousness* (pp. 3–56). Oxford University Press.

Tulving, E., & Thomson, D. M. (1973). Encoding specificity and retrieval processes in episodic memory. *Psychological Review*, *80*(5), 352–373. https://doi.org/10.1037/h0020071

Tuominen, J., Stenberg, T., Revonsuo, A., & Valli, K. (2019). Social contents in dreams: An empirical test of the social simulation theory. *Consciouness and Cognition*, *69*, 133–145. https://doi.org/10.1016/j.concog.2019.01.017

Tuttle, R. (2024). Theories of bipedalism. In *Encyclopedia Britannica*. www.britannica.com/topic/language/Historical-attitudes-toward-language

Tylor, E. B. (1871/1958). *Primitive culture* (Vol. 2). Harper & Row.

Tyson, P., Ogilvie, R., & Hunt, H. T. (1984). Lucid, prelucid, and nonlucid dreams related to the amount of EEG alpha activity during REM sleep. *Psychophysiology*, *21*(4), 442–451.

Uchitel, J., Blanco, B., Vidal-Rosas, E., Collins-Jones, L., & Cooper, R. J. (2022). Reliability and similarity of resting state functional connectivity networks imaged using wearable, high-density diffuse optical tomography in the home setting. *Neuroimage*, *263*, 1–11. https://doi.org/10.1016/j.neuroimage.2022.119663

Uddin, L. Q. (2015). Salience processing and insular cortical function and dysfunction. *Nature Reviews Neuroscience*, *16*, 55–61.

Uddin, L. Q., Supekar, K. S., Ryali, S., & Menon, V. (2011). Dynamic reconfiguration of structural and functional connectivity across core neurocognitive brain networks with development. *Journal of Neuroscience*, *31*(50), 18578–18589. https://doi.org/10.1523/jneurosci.4465-11.2011

Uddin, L. Q., Yeo, B., & Spreng, R. (2019). Towards a universal taxonomy of macro-scale functional human brain networks. *Brain Topography*, *32*, 926–942. https://doi.org/10.1007/s10548-019-00744-6

Uitermarkt, B. D., Bruss, J., Hwang, K., & Boes, A. D. (2020). Rapid eye movement sleep patterns of brain activation and deactivation occur within unique functional networks. *Human Brain Mapping*, *41*, 3984–3992. https://doi.org/10.1002/hbm.25102

Vallat, R., Eichenlaub, J. B., Nicolas, A., & Ruby, P. (2018). Dream recall frequency is associated with medial prefrontal cortex white-matter density *Frontiers in Psychology*, *9*, Article 1856. https://doi.org/10.3389/fpsyg.2018.01856

Vallat, R., Lajnef, T., Eichenlaub, J.-B., Berthomier, C., Jerbi, K., Morlet, D., & Ruby, P. (2017). Increased evoked potentials to arousing auditory stimuli during sleep: Implication for the understanding of dream recall. *Frontiers in Human Neuroscience: Cogntive Neuroscience*, *11* (Article 132), 1–12. https://doi.org/10.3389/fnhum.2017.00132

Vallat, R., Nicolas, A., & Ruby, P. (2020). Brain functional connectivity upon awakening from sleep predicts interindividual differences in dream recall frequency. *Sleep*, *43*(12), 1–11. https://doi.org/10.1093/sleep/zsaa116

Valli, K., & Revonsuo, A. (2009). The threat simulation theory in light of recent empirical evidence: A review. *American Journal of Psychology*, *122*, 17–38.

van Eeden, F. (1913). *Proceedings of the Society for Psychic Research*, *13*, 431–461.

van Rijn, E., Reid, A., Edwards, C., Malinowski, J., Ruby, P., & Blagrove, M. (2018). Daydreams incorporate recent waking life concerns but do not show delayed ('dream-lag') incorporations. *Consciousness and Cognition*, *58*, 51–59.

Vanhaudenhuyse, A., Demertzi, A., Schabus, M., Noirhomme, Q., Bredart, S., Boly, M., & Laureys, S. (2011). Two distinct neuronal networks mediate the awareness of environment and of self. *Journal of Cognitive Neuroscience*, *23*, 570–578.

Vanhaudenhuyse, A., Noirhomme, Q., Tshibanda, L., Bruno, M., Boverou, P., Schnakers, C., Boly, M. (2010). Default network connectivity reflects the level of consciousness in non-communicative brain-damaged patients. *Brain*, *133*, 161–171.

Vargha-Khadem, F., Gadian, D. G., Watkins, K. E., Connelly, A., Paesschen, W. V., & Mishkin, M. (1997). Differential effects of early hippocampal pathology on episodic and semantic memory. *Science*, *277*, 376–380. https://doi.org/10.1126/science.277.5324.376

Vartanian, O. (2012). Dissociable neural systems for analogy and metaphor: Implications for the neuroscience of creativity. *British Journal of Psychology*, *103*, 302–316.

Vaughn, B., & D'Cruz, O. N. (2017). Cardinal manifestations of sleep disorders. In M. Kryger, B. J. Roth, & W. Dement (Eds.), *Principles and Practices of Sleep Medicine* (Vol. 6, pp. 576–586). Elsevier.

Vecchio, F., Miraglia, F., Gorgoni, M., Ferrara, M., & De Gennaro, L. (2017). Cortical connectivity modulation during sleep onset: A study via graph theory on EEG data. *Human Brain Mapping*, *38*, 5456–5464. https://doi.org/10.1002/hbm.23736

Verendeev, A., & Sherwood, C. C. (2017). Human brain evolution. *Current Opinion in Behavioral Sciences*, *16*, 41–45. https://doi.org/10.1016/j.cobeha.2017.02.003

Verghese, A., Garner, K. G., Mattingley, J., & Dux, P. E. (2016). Prefrontal cortex structure predicts training-induced improvements in multitasking performance. *The Journal of Neuroscience*, *36*, 2638–2645.

Vertes, R. (1995). Memory consolidation in REM sleep: Dream on. *Bulletin of the Sleep Research Society*, *1*, 27–32.

Vertes, R., & Eastman, K. (2000). The case against memory consolidation in REM sleep. *Behavioral and Brain Sciences*, *23*, 867–876.

Vertes, R., & Siegel, J. M. (2005). Time for the sleep community to take a critical look at the purported role of sleep in memory processing. *Sleep*, *28*, 1228–1229.

Vidal-Rosas, E. E., von Lühmann, A., Pinti, P., & Cooper, R. J. (2023). Wearable, high-density fNIRS and diffuse optical tomography technologies: A perspective. *Neurophotonics*, *10*(2). https://doi.org/10.1117/1.NPh.10.2.023513

Vogt, B., & Laureys, S. (2005). Posterior cingulate, precuneal and retrosplenial cortices: Cytology and components of the neural network correlates of consciousness. *Progress in Brain Research*, *150*, 205–217.

von der Ohe, C. G., Darian-Smith, C., Garner, C. C., & Heller, H. C. (2006). Ubiquitous and temperature-dependent neural plasticity in hibernators. *Journal of Neuroscience*, *26*, 10590–10598. https://doi.org/10.1523/jneurosci.2874-06.2006

Voss, U., Holzmann, R., Tuin, I., & Hobson, J. A. (2009). Lucid dreaming: A state of consciousness with features of both waking and non-lucid dreaming. *Sleep*, *32*, 1191–1200.

Wagner, U., Gais, S., Haider, H., Verleger, R., & Born, J. (2004). Sleep inspires insight. *Nature*, *427*, 352–355.

Walker, J. M., Garber, A., Berger, R., & Heller, H. C. (1979). Sleep and estivation (shallow torpor): Continuous processes of energy conservation. *Science*, *2014*(4397), 1098–1100. https://doi.org/10.1126/science.221974

Wamsley, E., & Stickgold, R. (2011). Memory, sleep, and dreaming: Experiencing consolidation. *Sleep Medicine Clinics*, *6*, 97–108.

Wamsley, E., & Summer, T. (2020). Spontaneous entry into an "offline" state during wakefulness: A mechanism of memory consolidation? *Journal of Cognitive Neuroscience*, *32*(9), 1714–1734. https://doi.org/10.1162/jocn_a_01587

Wamsley, E., Hirota, Y., Tucker, M., Smith, M., Doan, T., & Antrobus, J. (2007). Circadian and ultradian influences on dreaming: A dual rhythm model. *Brain Research Bulletin*, *71*, 347–354.

Wang, S. Y., Baker, K. C., Culbreth, J. L., Tracy, O., Arora, M., & Wamsley, E. (2021). 'Sleep-dependent' memory consolidation? Brief periods of post-training rest and sleep provide an equivalent benefit for both declarative and procedural memory. *Learning & Memory*, *28*(6), 195–203. https://doi.org/10.1101/lm.053330.120

Warbrick, T. (2022). Simultaneous EEG-MRI: What Have We Learned and What Does the Future Hold? *Sensors*, *6*. https://doi.org/10.3390/s22062262

Waters, F., Dirk Blom, J., Dang-Vu, T., Cheyne, A., Alderson-Day, B., Woodruff, P., & Collerton, D. (2016). What Is the Link Between Hallucinations, Dreams, and Hypnagogic-Hypnopompic Experiences? *Schizophrenia Bulletin*, *42*, 1098–1109. https://doi.org/10.1093/schbul/sbw076

Watson, R., & Rechtschaffen, A. (1969). Auditory awakening thresholds and dream recall in NREM sleep. *Perceptual and Motor Skills*, *29*, 635–644.

Watts, D., & Strogatz, S. (1998). Collective dynamics of small world networks. *Nature*, *393*, 440–442.

Webb, E., Campbell, D., Schwartz, R., Sechrest, L., & Grove, J. (1966/1981/2000). *Nonreactive measures in the social sciences*. Sage.

Webb, M. A., & Tangney, J. P. (2022). Too good to be true: Bots and bad data from Mechanical Turk. *Perspectives on Psychological Science*, 1–4.

Wehr, T. A. (1992). A brain-warming function for REM sleep. *Neuroscience Biobehavioral Review*, *16*(3), 379–397.

Weisberg, R. (1986). *Creativity: Genius and other myths*. W. H. Freeman.

Weizmann, I. (2017). Resolution revolution: Modern microscopy's impact on science. *Weizmann Magazine*, *11*. www.weizmann.ac.il/WeizmannCompass/sections/features/resolution-revolution

Wheeler, R., & Gabbert, F. (2017). Using self-generated cues to facilitate recall: A narrative review. *Frontiers in Psychology*, *27*(8), 1830. https://doi.org/10.3389/fpsyg.2017.01830

White, S. H. (1965). Evidence for a hierarchical arrangement of learning processes. *Advances in child development and behavior*, 2, 187–220.

Whitman, R. M., Pierce, C. M., Maas, J. W., & Baldridge, B. J. (1962). The dreams of the experimental subject. *Journal of Nervous & Mental Disease*, *134*(5), 431–439.

Wick, A., Combertaldi, S., & Rasch, B. (2020). The first-night effect of sleep occurs over nonconsecutive nights in unfamiliar and familiar environments. *Sleep*, *47*(10), 1–13. https://doi.org/10.1093/sleep/zsae179

Wilson, M., & McNaughton, B. (1994). Reactivation of hippocampal ensemble memories during sleep. *Science*, *265*, 676–679.

Windt, J. (2015). *Dreaming: A conceptual framework for philosophy of mind and empirical research*. MIT Press.

Wirebring, L., Stillesjö, S., Eriksson, J., Juslin, P., & Nyberg, L. (2018). A similarity-based process for human judgment in the parietal cortex. *Frontiers in Human Neuroscience*, *13*. https://doi.org/10.3389/fnhum.2018.00481

Wollman, M., & Antrobus, J. (1987). Cortical arousal and mentation in sleeping and waking subjects. *Brain and Cognition*, *6*, 334–340.

Woolley, J. D., & Boerger, E. (2002). Development of beliefs about the origins and controllability of dreams *Developmental Psychology*, *38*, 24–41.

Woolley, J. D., & Wellman, H. M. (1992). Children's conceptions of dreams. *Cognitive Development*, *7*(3), 365–380.

Worsley, A. (1988). Personal experiences in lucid dreaming. In J. Gackenbach & S. LaBerge (Eds.), *Conscious mind, sleeping brain: Perspectives on lucid dreaming* (pp. 321–341). Plenum.

Wrangham, R. (2019). *The goodness paradox: The strange relationship between virtue and violence in human evolution*. Vintage Books.

Yale Medicine. (2024). *Parasomnias*. Yale Medical School. www.yalemedicine.org/conditions/parasomnias

Yan, X., Kong, R., Xue, A., Yang, Q., Orban, C., An, L., Holmes, A. J., Qian, X., Chen, J., Zuo, X., Zhou, J. H., Fortier, M. V, Tan, A. P., Gluckman, P., Chong, Y. S., Meaney, M. J., Bzdok, D., Eickhoff, S. B., & Yeo, B. T. T. (2023). Homotopic local-global parcellation of the human cerebral cortex from resting-state functional connectivity *Neuroimage*, *273*, Article 120010. https://doi.org/10.1016/j.neuroimage.2023.120010

Yellott, J. I. (2007). A chronological history of vision research: 1600–1960. In *Course Material on Vision Research*. https://homepages.hass.rpi.edu/ruiz/IDIspring07/stereo_history/text/visionsc.html

Yeo, B., Krienen, F., Sepulcre, J., Sabuncu, M., Lashkari, D., Hollinshead, M., Buckner, R. (2011). The organization of the human cerebral cortex estimated by intrinsic functional connectivity *Journal of Neurophysiology*, *106*, 1125–1165.

Yetish, G., Kaplan, H., Gurven, M., Wood, B., Pontzer, H., Manger, P., Siegel, J. M. (2015). Natural sleep and its seasonal variations in three pre-industrial societies *Current Biology*, *25*, 2862–2868. https://doi.org/10.1016/j.cub.2015.09.046

Yoo, J., Min, S., Lee, S.-K., & Han, S. (2021). Neural correlates of episodic memory modulated by temporally delayed rewards. *PLoS One*, *16*(4), Article e0249290. https://doi.org/10.1371/journal.pone.0249290

Yuan, H., Li, X., & Wei, B. (2024). Modeling default mode network patterns via a universal spatio-temporal brain attention skip network. *Neuroimage*, *287*, 1–10. https://doi.org/10.1016/j.neuroimage.2024.120522

Zadra, A., Desjardins, S., & Marcotte, É. (2006). Evolutionary function of dreams: A test of the threat simulation theory in recurrent dreams. *Consciousness and Cognition*, *15*(2), 450–463. https://doi.org/10.1016/j.concog.2005.02.002

Zadra, A., Nielsen, T., & Donderi, D. (1998). Prevalence of auditory, olfactory and gustatory experiences in home dreams. *Perceptual & Motor Skills*, *87*(3), 819–826. https://doi.org/10.2466/pms.1998.87.3.

Zepelin, H., Siegel, J. M., & Tobler, I. (2005). Mammalian sleep. In M. Kryger, B. J. Roth, & W. Dement (Eds.), *Principles and practice of sleep medicine* (4th ed., pp. 91–100). Elsevier.

Zhang, R., & Volkow, N. (2019). Brain default-mode network dysfunction in addiction. *NeuroImage*, *200*, 313–331 https://doi.org/10.1016/j.neuroimage.2019.06.036

Zimmerman, W. B. (1970). Sleep mentation and auditory awakening thresholds. *Psychophysiology*, *6*, 540–549.

Zmigrod, L., Garrison, J. R., Carr, J., & Simons, J. S. (2016). The neural mechanisms of hallucinations: A quantitative meta-analysis of neuroimaging studies. *Neuroscience Biobehavioral Review*, *69*, 113–123.

INDEX